AF316579

Fractures
of the
Calcaneus

Video Contents

Fractures of the Calcaneus

Second Edition

Editor

Mandeep S Dhillon
MBBS MS (Ortho) FAMS FRCS (Eng)
Professor and Chairperson
Department of Orthopedic Surgery
Head, Department of Physical Medicine and Rehabilitation
In-charge, Sports Injury Clinic
Postgraduate Institute of Medical Education and Research
Chandigarh, India
President, Indian Biologics Orthopaedic Society

Foreword

Mark Myerson

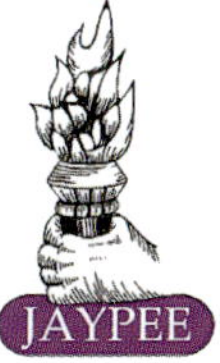

JAYPEE BROTHERS MEDICAL PUBLISHERS
The Health Sciences Publisher
New Delhi | London

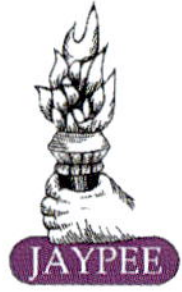

Jaypee Brothers Medical Publishers (P) Ltd

Headquarters

Jaypee Brothers Medical Publishers (P) Ltd
EMCA House, 23/23-B
Ansari Road, Daryaganj
New Delhi 110 002, India
Landline: +91-11-23272143, +91-11-23272703
+91-11-23282021, +91-11-23245672
Email: jaypee@jaypeebrothers.com

Corporate Office

Jaypee Brothers Medical Publishers (P) Ltd
4838/24, Ansari Road, Daryaganj
New Delhi 110 002, India
Phone: +91-11-43574357
Fax: +91-11-43574314
Email: jaypee@jaypeebrothers.com

Overseas Office

JP Medical Ltd.
83, Victoria Street, London
SW1H 0HW (UK)
Phone: +44 20 3170 8910
Fax: +44 (0)20 3008 6180
Email: info@jpmedpub.com

Website: www.jaypeebrothers.com
Website: www.jaypeedigital.com

© 2024, Jaypee Brothers Medical Publishers

Inquiries for bulk sales may be solicited at: jaypee@jaypeebrothers.com

Fractures of the Calcaneus

First Edition: 2013
Second Edition: **2024**

ISBN: 978-93-5465-665-1

Printed at: Samrat Offset Pvt. Ltd.

Contributors

Aman Hooda
MBBS MS DNB MNAMS Dip SICOT
Assistant Professor
Department of Emergency Medicine
Division of Orthopedics
Dr BR Ambedkar State Institute
of Medical Sciences
Mohali, Punjab, India

Andrew Sands
MD FAAOS FAOA Dip ABOS
Chief
Foot and Ankle Surgery
Downtown Orthopedic Associates
Clinical Associate Professor
Department of Orthopedic Surgery
Weill Cornell Medical College
New York, NY, USA

Ankit Khurana
MBBS MS DNB FRCS (Tr & Ortho)
Assistant Professor
Department of Orthopedics
Dr BSA Medical College
and Hospital
New Delhi, India

Balvinder Rana
MS (Ortho)
Senior Consultant
Max Hospital
New Delhi, India

Bibek Adhya BPT MSPT
Senior Physiotherapist
Department of Physical Medicine and
Rehabilitation
Postgraduate Institute of Medical
Education and Research
Chandigarh, India

Cristian Ortiz MD
Consultant
Department of Foot and Ankle Surgery
IFFAS President 2020–2023
Clínica Universidad de los Andes
Avenida Plaza 2.501
Las Condes, Santiago

Devendra K Chouhan MBBS MS
Professor
Department of Orthopedics
Postgraduate Institute of Medical
Education and Research
Chandigarh, India

Donald McBride FRCS (Ortho)
Consultant
Trauma and Orthopedic Surgeon
University Hospital of North Staffordshire
Stoke on Trent
Staffordshire, UK

Felipe López-Oliva Muñoz MD PhD
Chief of Section
Department of Orthopedic Surgery
Jiménez Díaz Foundation Hospital
Madrid, Spain

Francisco Forriol Campos MD PhD
Professor
Department of Orthopedic Surgery
San Pablo CEU University
Madrid, Spain

Harman Chaudhry MD
Research Fellow
Division of Orthopedic Surgery
McMaster University
Hamilton, Canada

Herman Singh Johal MD FRCS
Associate Professor
Department of Surgery
McMaster University
Hamilton, Ontario, Canada

Himmat S Dhillon BPT MPT
Consultant Physiotherapist
Director
Sports Health Physio & Sports Injury Clinic
Melbourne, Australia

HK Verma MS MCh MSc (Ortho, Eng)
Director
Biomedical Technology Wing
Sree Chitra Tirunal Institute for Medical
Sciences and Technology
Thiruvananthapuram, Kerala

Joris Hermus MD
Orthopedic and Trauma Surgeon
Maastricht University Medical Center
Maastricht, Netherlands

Karthick Rangasamy MS DNB MNAMS
Assistant Professor
Department of Orthopedic Surgery
Postgraduate Institute of Medical
Education and Research
Chandigarh, India

KV Menon MS (Ortho)
Professor
Department of Orthopedics
Bharati Vidyapeeth Medical College
Pune, Maharashtra, India

Mandeep S Dhillon
MBBS MS (Ortho) FAMS FRCS (Eng)
Professor and Chairperson
Department of Orthopedic Surgery
Head, Department of Physical Medicine
and Rehabilitation
In-charge, Sports Injury Clinic
Postgraduate Institute of Medical
Education and Research
Chandigarh, India
President
Indian Biologics Orthopaedic Society

Marianne Comeau-Gauthier
Department of Orthopedic Surgery
McMaster University
Hamilton, Canada

Michael Swords DO
Chair
Department of Orthopedic Surgery
Director of Orthopedic Trauma
Sparrow Hospital
Michigan Orthopedic Center
Lansing MI, USA

Mohit Bhandari MD PhD FRCSC
Professor and Academic Chairperson
Division of Orthopedic Surgery
McMaster University
Hamilton, Canada

Nicola Maffulli
MD MS PhD FRCP FRCS (Ortho) FFSEM
Professor
Department of Trauma and
Orthopedic Surgery
Consultant Trauma and
Orthopedic Surgeon
Department of Medicine, Surgery
and Dentistry
University of Salerno, Italy
School of Pharmacy and Bioengineering
Keele University School of Medicine
Thornburrow Drive, Stoke on Trent
England
Queen Mary University of London
Barts and the London School of Medicine
and Dentistry, Centre for Sports and
Exercise Medicine, Mile End Hospital, 275
Bancroft Road, London E1 4DG, England

Nicole Fraticelli DO
Department of Orthopedic Surgery
Sparrow Medical Group
Orthopedic Trauma
Sparrow Hospital
Lansing, MI, USA

Nikolaos Gougoulias MD PhD
Consultant Orthopedic Surgeon
Department of Orthopedics
General Hospital of Katerini
Litochoro Pierias, Greece

Nirmal Raj Gopinathan MS MAMS
Professor
Department of Orthopedic Surgery
Postgraduate Institute of Medical
Education and Research
Chandigarh, India

Prasoon Kumar MBBS MS Dip SICOT
Assistant Professor
Department of Orthopedics
Postgraduate Institute of Medical
Education and Research
Chandigarh, India

Rahul Banerjee MD FACS
Orthopedic Trauma Surgeon
Parkland Memorial Hospital
Assistant Professor Residency Program
Director
Department of Orthopedic Surgery
University of Texas Southwestern Medical
Center
Dallas, TX, USA

Rajesh Kumar Rajnish
MBBS MS (Ortho)
Assistant Professor
Department of Orthopedics
All India Institute of Medical Sciences
Jodhpur, Rajasthan, India

Rajiv Shah MS (Ortho)
Director and Chief
Foot and Ankle Orthopedics
Department of Orthopedics
Sunshine Global Hospitals
Vadodara, Gujarat, India

Raman Mundi MD FRCSC
Assistant Professor
Department of Orthopedic Surgery
University of Toronto
Toronto, ON, Canada

Richard E Buckley MD FRCS
Professor
Department of Surgery
University of Calgary
Calgary, AB, Canada

Sampat D Patil MS (Ortho)
Director
Department of Orthopedics
Sahyadri Superspecialty Hospital
Pune, Maharashtra, India

Sandeep Patel
MS (Ortho) FRCS (Ortho and Trauma)
Eng DNB (Ortho) MAMS
Assistant Professor
Department of Orthopedics
Postgraduate Institute of Medical
Education and Research
Chandigarh, India

Sarvdeep Dhatt MBBS MS MNAMS
Professor
Department of Orthopedics
Postgraduate Institute of Medical
Education and Research
Chandigarh, India

Shivam Shah MS (Ortho)
Consultant Orthopedic Surgeon
Department of Orthopedics
Sunshine Global Hospital
Vadodara, Gujarat, India

Sidak Dhillon MD (Sports Medicine)
Team Physician
Department of Talent Performance—
Sports
Round Glass FC

Siddhartha Sharma
MS (Ortho) DNB (Ortho) FRCS (Trauma & Ortho)
Post Doc Fellow
Associate Professor
Department of Orthopedic Surgery
Postgraduate Institute of Medical
Education and Research
Chandigarh, India

SS Suresh MS (Ortho) MCh (Ortho) FACS
Head, Department of Orthopedics
Ibri Regional Referral Hospital
Ibri, Sultanate of Oman

Stefan Rammelt MD PhD
Professor
Head of the Foot and Ankle Center
University Center of Orthopedic, Trauma
and Plastic Surgery
University Hospital Carl Gustav Carus at
TU Dresden
Dresden, Germany

Stephen W Pournaras III MD
Resident
Department of Orthopedic Surgery
One Brooklyn Health
New York, NY, USA

Tim Schepers MD PhD
Associate Professor
Department of Trauma Unit
Department of Surgery
Amsterdam UMC
Amsterdam, The Netherlands

Tun Hing Lui
MBBS (HK) FRCSEd FHKCOS FHKAM (Ortho)
Consultant
Department of Orthopedics and
Traumatology
North District Hospital
Hong Kong, China
Honorary Professor
Department of Orthopedics
The Second Affiliated Hospital
Shenzhen University
Shenzhen, China

Vikas Bachhal MBBS MS
Associate Professor
Department of Orthopedic Surgery
Postgraduate Institute of Medical
Education and Research
Chandigarh, India

Vishal Kumar MBBS MS (Ortho) DNB
Additional Professor
Department of Orthopedics
Postgraduate Institute of Medical
Education and Research
Chandigarh, India

Foreword

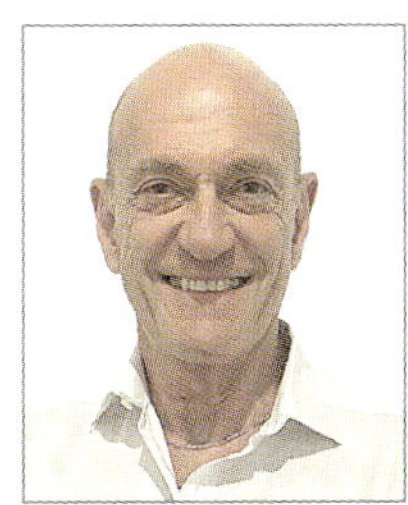

This book is an extraordinary compilation of techniques and insights into managing fractures of the calcaneus and a true compendium for any surgeon with an interest in managing these challenging deformities. Kudos to Dr Mandeep S Dhillon for an outstanding addition to the literature. The illustrations are artfully and accurately presented in a consistent manner throughout the book, and these are extraordinarily useful to understand the three-dimensional correction of deformity. There is an extensive and thorough presentation of the advantages of operative and nonoperative treatment alternatives, the various approaches to acute correction, indications and techniques for primary arthrodesis, and treatment of complications of these fractures.

The chapter by Bhandari et al. on "Evidence-based Orthopedics: What is Optimal for Calcaneus Fracture Today" is extraordinarily well written and for any reader interested in understanding the outcomes of treatment this chapter is a real classic. Perhaps it will be surprising to the readers that "all systematic reviews and meta-analyses reviews have come to essentially the same conclusion", that there are not enough high-quality studies to make a definitive decision on the difference between operative and non-operative treatment. One of the points highlighted by these authors is that outcomes of treatment, even today, are determined by the institutional volume and surgeon experience. Although many of the more extensive studies have been performed at institutions with vast surgical experience with calcaneus fractures, this should still place the burden of decision making on each individual surgeon according to his or her experience.

Continuing on the thinking about the outcomes of these fractures, there are so many variables to consider, and one that I find particularly interesting is the range of motion of the hindfoot following fracture treatment (whether operative or nonoperative).

While the indications for a primary arthrodesis have historically been listed as Sanders type IV or on occasion type III fractures, the indications should be expanded.

The outcomes of treatment of calcaneus fractures are variables, including the obvious parameters such as rates of complications, revision surgery, subsequent need for arthrodesis, as well as multiple patient outcome measures. The range of motion of the subtalar joint and return to work are variables which I have found to be extremely important in decision making. Many calcaneus fractures occur in young workers, who, by the very nature of the injury have difficulty returning to their occupation, and oftentimes lack incentive to return to work. This is then compounded substantially by treatments that are not perceived by the patient as being successful. When one considers that the primary goal of fracture surgery is the restoration of anatomy and not necessarily recovery of a normal subtalar range of motion, it surprises me that primary subtalar arthrodesis is not a more popular procedure. To think about this slightly differently, the range of motion of the subtalar joint following adequate open reduction internal fixation is not always optimal, and indeed with what appears to be a good reduction, subtalar motion may be *absent*. With this in mind, therefore, why not perform more primary arthrodesis procedures? Performing a primary arthrodesis of the subtalar joint has generated less interest and enthusiasm than expected, yet this is an extraordinarily important procedure that must be part of the surgeon's armamentarium. The chapter on this topic is addressed by Muñoz et al. and I would encourage surgeons to consider this as an excellent treatment alternative in selected cases. The goal of primary arthrodesis is no different than that of open reduction and internal fixation, since the anatomic reduction of the hindfoot is essential, and this should not be performed as an "open internal arthrodesis" (OIA). Primary arthrodesis cannot be successfully accomplished unless the anatomy is simultaneously restored.

The chapter on managing malunion of the calcaneus by Sands et al. is particularly well written and illustrated with interesting clinical examples. The decision making for an in situ versus a structural bone block arthrodesis of the subtalar joint is always challenging. An approach to correction of malunion must take into consideration not only the architecture, but also biomechanics and clinical function of the hindfoot and ankle. The restoration of anatomy should optimize push off strength, as well as maintain or improve the range of motion of the ankle joint. Any procedure which restores the talar declination angle is, therefore, a necessary adjunct to reconstruction of malunion however, the same technique for restoring height to the

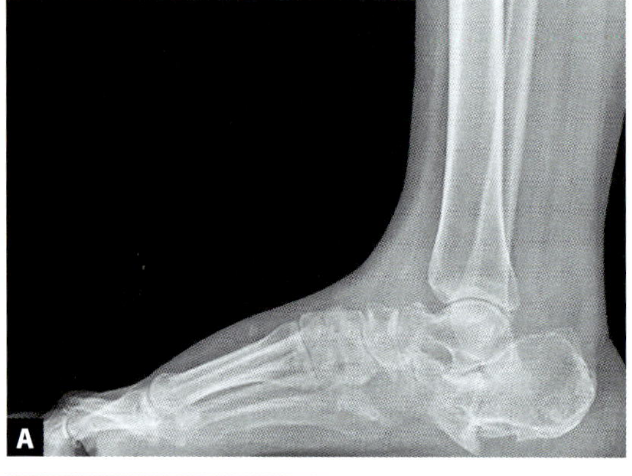

hindfoot with a subtalar arthrodesis cannot always be used. When the tuberosity is tilted cephalad and associated with additional collapse, it is not easy to restore the architecture of the hindfoot as well as the talar declination with a standard bone block arthrodesis. Below is a technique **(Figs. A to G)** which I have found to be very useful for these malunions, where, in addition to profound joint depression, there is a sagittal plane angular malunion of the tuberosity (A).

Unlike a vertical osteotomy which neither restore the alignment nor architecture of the hindfoot, one approaches the calcaneus as for a bone block arthrodesis with a vertical posterolateral incision and a generous ostectomy of the lateral wall performed (B).

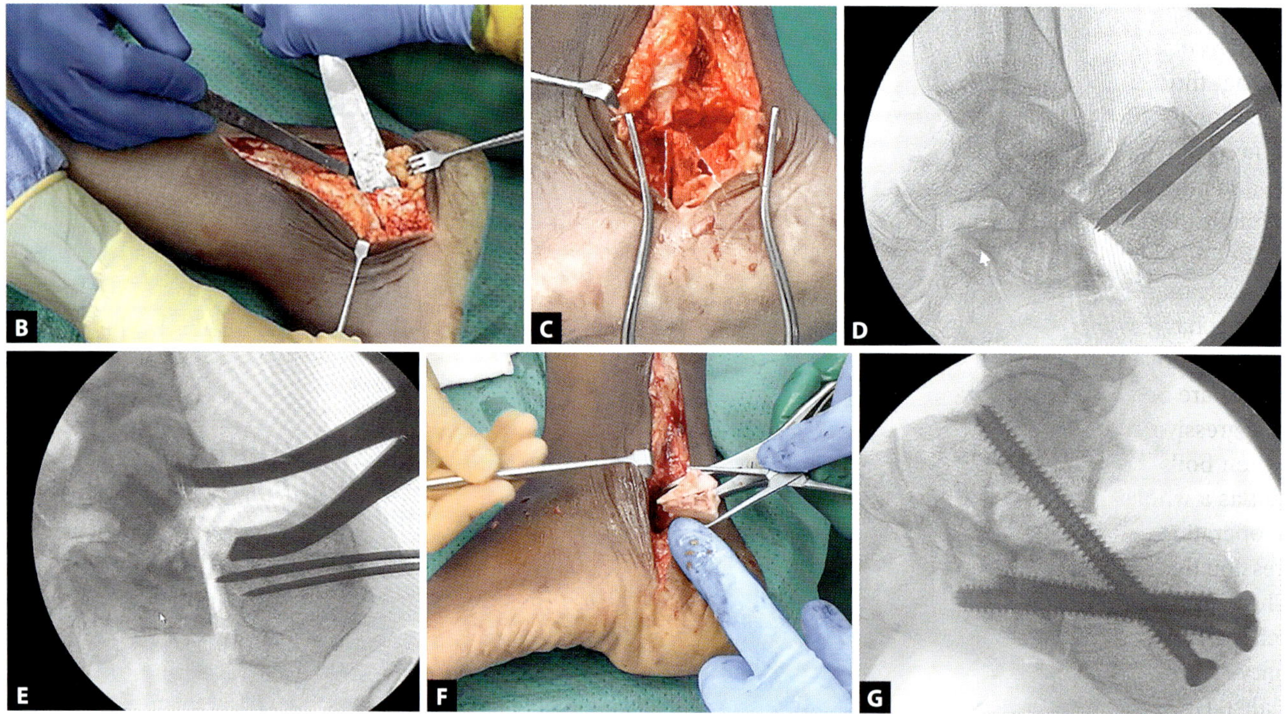

A triangular osteotomy with the base plantar is now made at the apex of the malunion (C).

Following the osteotomy, the triangular bone wedge is removed for use as a structural block graft (D). The tuberosity is then shifted inferiorly, and the osteotomy closed, restoring the pitch angle and height of the heel (E).

This is then pinned temporarily; the bone graft is inserted into the subtalar joint (F) to restore the height of the hindfoot as well as the declination angle of the talus and definitive fixation performed (G).

This is a veritable treatise on the management of all aspects of calcaneus trauma and subsequent salvage. It contains a wealth of historic information and includes current technical guides and tips which are invaluable in treating the complex variety and scope of these injuries. My congratulations to Dr Mandeep S Dhillon and all the contributors.

Mark Myerson MD
President and Founder
Steps2Walk
Greenwood Village, CO, USA
Professor
Department of Orthopedic Surgery
University of Colorado, Denver, USA
Past President
American Orthopaedic Foot and Ankle Society

Preface to the Second Edition

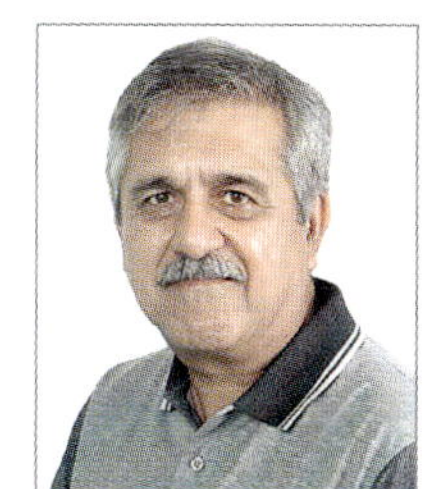

12 years on, life has changed; when I wrote the preface to the 1st edition, many moons ago, I started that preface as *"In the 21st century, trauma surgery has reached a stage where specialists focused on specific areas are becoming necessary to manage many complex fractures. The spine is one such area, as is the pelvis. The foot and ankle have received little or no attention, and many times the injuries to this important weight-bearing structure are managed "conservatively", often due to lack of confidence or ability to reconstruct complex fractures in this area."*

At that time, the focus had changed from mostly conservative management to aggressive surgical interventions, and the mainstay of such management was the popular extensile approach. Much water has flowed under the bridge in the last 12 years, and in 2023, the extensile approach is now reserved for a specific group of cases, and minimally invasive interventions have come to the forefront. So, we have changed this book accordingly, keeping much of the old, with additions and revisions, and adding a lot based on what we now know with our evolving understanding and better techniques.

The calcaneus still remains the most fractured bone in the foot, in addition to being the largest, and has a major role in the biomechanics of the whole foot. With specialization in focused areas of the body becoming the flavor of the day, Asia has seen a whole new generation interested in solving problems of the foot and ankle. The controversy as to whether the outcomes are better with or without surgery, rears up every few years; this may be due to the fact that foot specialists are more aggressive in surgical interventions, while general orthopedic and trauma surgeons may tend to be more conservative. This then boils down to understanding not only the fracture anatomy and its classification, but also understanding the patient as a whole. I personally feel that the data that creates this controversy may be skewed somewhat by the fact that some operations on fractured calcaneus are done by inexperienced surgeons, leading to more complications and, hence, the impression that surgery may not be so beneficial.

The structure of this book was thus designed for surgeons at all levels of training and experience. The original edition had chapters on radiology, patient selection, surgical exposures, rehabilitation, and outcomes. I had included chapters on primary arthrodesis, minimally invasive surgery, malunion corrections and role of arthroscopy which were meant for the specialist. However, the huge success of the first edition, as evidenced by the fact that it was sold out, made me envisage a wider audience with the addition of more chapters in the subsequent edition. Percutaneous reduction and fixation have been rewritten, peripheral fractures have been given the specific focus (Sustentaculum tali, anterior end of the calcaneus and tuberosity avulsions are individual chapters), two unique chapters on calcaneus fractures in children and stress fractures have been added. For the specialist, we have new chapters on interlocking nailing for calcaneus fractures and arthroscopic management of complications. These 27 chapters make the current edition of the book perhaps the most comprehensive treatise on this common fracture published in the world.

For this, I have to thank the plethora of authors who are world leaders in this field, who have contributed with the chapters and the best available data, with the singular aim of helping the reader manage any type of calcaneal fracture that they encounter, at any stage of their career. As I said in the previous preface, it is my hope that this aim is achieved, as one of my passions is educating the young minds of today, especially in areas of interest that are dear to me.

Mandeep S Dhillon

Preface to the First Edition

In the 21st century, trauma surgery has reached a stage where specialists focused on specific areas are becoming necessary to manage many complex fractures. The spine is one such area, as is the pelvis. The foot and ankle have received little or no attention, and many times the injuries to this important weight-bearing structure are managed "conservatively", often due to lack of confidence or ability to reconstruct complex fractures in this area.

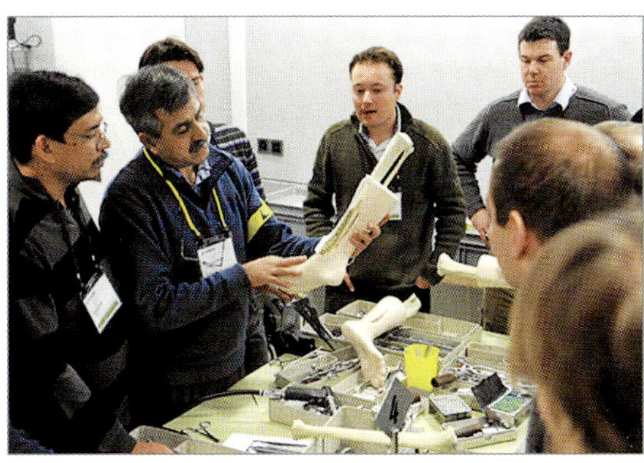

In modern orthopedics, the recognition that inadequate treatment of foot injuries can have lifelong disastrous complications are coming to the forefront. Surgeons realize that complex midfoot injuries need to be accurately reconstructed, calcaneus fractures benefit from well-applied surgical interventions, and the talus needs an accurate reduction and stabilization.

The calcaneus, or "os calcis" is the most commonly fractured bone in the foot, in addition to being the largest, and has a major role in the biomechanics of the whole foot. Nevertheless, controversy still exists as to whether the outcomes are better with or without surgery. I personally feel that this data may be skewed somewhat by the fact that some operations on fractured calcaneus may have been done by inexperienced surgeons, leading to more complications and, hence, the impression that surgery may not be so beneficial in these cases.

The purpose of this book is to dispel this myth. There is enough evidence in the literature that if surgery is done in well-selected patients, in a proper way, using appropriate implants, the outcomes could be significantly improved. The structure of this book is thus designed for surgeons of all levels of training and experience. There are chapters, which talk about radiology, patient selection, surgical exposures, and rehabilitation, which would help the trauma surgeon doing all kinds of fracture surgeries. Chapters on primary arthrodesis, minimally invasive surgery, malunion corrections and role of arthroscopy are meant for the specialist foot surgeons. And, of course, there are specific chapters, which discuss how outcomes are measured, and how patients are rehabilitated. Perhaps, one of the most important chapters reviews the evidence-based medicine for calcaneal fracture management.

In a nutshell, I have tried to compile the best available data, contributed by the best minds currently working in their respective fields, with the singular aim of helping the reader manage any type of calcaneal fracture that they encounter, at any stage of their career. I hope that this aim is achieved, as one of my passions is educating the young minds of today, especially in areas of interest that are dear to me.

Mandeep S Dhillon

Acknowledgments

My educative process has been so complex that a standard dedication may not suffice for this book on a complex fracture. Let's start by naming my first orthopedic teacher, Professor RL Mittal of Patiala, who inculcated a specific interest in me about problems of the foot; this was taken forward by my subsequent chief Professor ON Nagi of Chandigarh, who encouraged me to focus on this often-neglected area of orthopedics. Dr Sureshwar Pandey, the pioneer who started the Indian Foot Society was another guiding light, and along the way, many associates, friends, and colleagues have influenced me. The list is too long to name, and some of these may have been my students as we published and did a lot of research with their help and support.

On the personal front, the usual suspects come to the forefront. My wife of many years, Rima, who does not mind the many hours on the computer and at work; my mother (of longer years!), Dr Ganda Singh, who gave me the gift to clearly express myself in my formative years. Unfortunately, my parents are no longer in this world, but they would be looking down from heaven with indulgent smiles, as I publish the second edition of the book. And, of course, my two sons, Himmat Dhillon and Dr Sidak Dhillon, who have stoically borne my absences from their lives while I struggled with my academic aspirations as I wrote the first book. Perhaps, they are better off for it; they are now both medical specialists in their own right, and in the current edition they have contributed a chapter each. I also have new additions to the family since I published the 1st edition; Aarzoo Dhillon, my daughter-in-law and the ever-smiling Veer Dhillon, my grandson, who is playing in my lap while I write the acknowledgments in Melbourne. It is their love and support that keeps me motivated.

I have to acknowledge the many patients, who form the basis of much of the knowledge that I have gained to reach this level of understanding. And, of course, all the authors who have contributed to this work, from India and abroad, without whom the value of this book would be much diminished.

Collectively, I thank you all.

Contents

Historical Aspects of Calcaneus Injury

Mandeep S Dhillon, Vikas Bachhal

"Those who cannot remember the past are condemned to repeat it".
–George Santayana, The Life of Reason, 1905

◼ INTRODUCTION

History of fracture treatment dates back to the Neolithic period. Clark, in his review of the history of fractures, documented many injuries which have been recorded over the ages.[1] He stated that due to the mechanics of fracture being the same in the first and the twentieth century, basic treatments and principles of immobilization have changed very little, with splints and bandaging being the mainstay of fracture management over the last two millennia.

Throughout history, man has broken his limbs; the humble "bonesetter" was accorded recognition by man over the ages, and this is documented in most of our civilization's history. These were usually self-trained persons or people who had apprenticed to other bonesetters. The modern profession of treating bone fractures was given the name "*Orthopedics*" by Andre; Jones expanded the specialty to include fractures and the treatment of adults.[2] Countless other medical men and surgeons developed manipulative and surgical procedures to increase the knowledge base in this field over the last 150 years, to achieve what we now know as modern-day fracture care. However, even today, one of the most controversial bones to break is the calcaneus;[3] in the whole of the last century, there have been diametrically opposed opinions with regard to the optimal management of this particular group of fractures.

The calcaneus is a unique bone with a unique mechanism of fracture; even though isolated calcaneal fractures are not life-threatening, the associated disability is often significant and cases have been often crippled due to badly deformed heels. Even in the famous *Edwin Smith Surgical Papyrus*, sketchy references to fractures of the clavicle, the humerus, and the cervical spine are noted, but none to the calcaneus.[4] From archeological excavations found in the Nubian Desert, several specimens of forearm fractures were found, which are now in the museum of the Royal College of Surgeons in London.[1] This fracture was common, perhaps due to the fact that the forearm was often used to protect a person from blows. Calcaneal fractures were less commonly seen, as falls from great heights were few, and often people did not survive these falls. Road accidents in the previous eras were usually low-velocity injuries, in contrast to the modern era, and so heel fractures and injuries have been less commonly documented over the passage of time.

Hippocrates has spoken of many treatments for fractures;[5] he described a method for reducing fractures of the spine. "*The patient was bound to a ladder, which was then raised perpendicularly with ropes and pulleys and let down suddenly, so that the jolting might reduce the deformity*". He has also described the appearance of a heel of a patient who had fallen from a height; however, he did not probably recognize a "calcaneal fracture", making this case perhaps the first documented missed calcaneal fractures in history.[1]

It is pertinent to note that Theodoricus, in 1546, and others following him, denied that the calcaneus was ever fractured: "*Calcaneus non fragitur, quia os durum est et protectum ligamentis*". "*Nullo pacto calcis accidit fractura*".[6] Malgaigne distinguished two separate mechanisms for calcaneus fracture by avulsion due to muscular action and by crushing force **(Figs. 1A and B)**.[7] Abel, in 1878, reported three cases of fracture of the sustentaculum tali and was surprised at the lack of literature on the subject at that time, further emphasizing the fact that not much was known about this injury at that time.[6]

Joseph-François Malgaigne was a French surgeon and medical historian who is well known for his work on fractures. In his most famous work, Traité des Fractures et des Luxations, which appeared in 1847, he described two types of fractures of calcaneus—one due to muscular action (avulsion) and second due to crushing—forming the first rudimentary classification system for these fractures (**Figs. 1 and 2**).

Understanding the pathomechanics and optimal treatment for calcaneal fractures during the 20th century has been as controversial as was the realization of existence of these fractures in the century before that (1800s). Possibly, the first documented description of the treatment of calcaneal fracture was in 1720 by Petit and DeSault.[8] They advocated rest and limb elevation which remained the principal treatment till the end of the 19th century. Paszkowski was the first to recommend immobilization in a

cast as a treatment for calcaneal fractures in 1880.[8] Although, with better understanding of these fractures, more focused treatment methods have evolved, cast immobilization still remained a viable method of treatment till recently. This was emphasized by proponents of this method principally because of the inability to obtain uniformly acceptable results and relatively poor outcomes using other methods.

The advent of roentgenograms, in 1895, kindled the desire of restoring the distorted anatomy of this bone. This resulted in development of methods of closed reduction, and several methods were described in the first half of the last century. Cotton and Wilson[9] first described such a method in 1908 and were the first to recognize the importance of reducing the lateral wall of the calcaneus, which we now know is vital for restoring the width of the heel. They understood the injury enough to propose disimpaction of the fracture (they were unclear about the tuberosity disimpaction) with traction applied on a metal rod behind the Achilles tendon, followed by sharp blows to the point of the heel (**Fig. 3**).

Frederic J. Cotton (**Fig. 4**) *was a founding member of the American College of Surgeons and served as a member of the first Board of Regents of the College and a founding member of the Committee on Fractures. Being an accomplished artist, he provided several illustrations in his book on Dislocations and Fractures, first published in 1910, and was the first to suggest the importance of reducing lateral wall in calcaneus fractures in order to reduce the width of heel.*

With regards to calcaneus fracture, Cotton commented in 1916: "a man who breaks his heel bone is done …".[9,10]

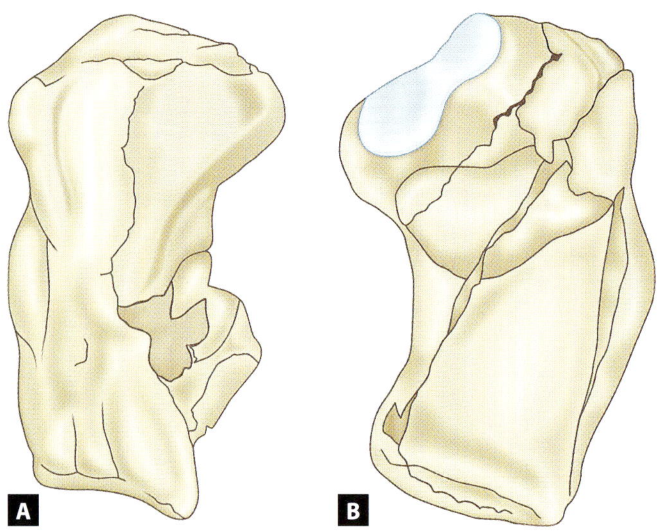

Figs. 1A and B: First anatomical description of calcaneus fracture given by Malgaigne JF in 1847.
Source: Adapted from Malgaigne (1847).[7]

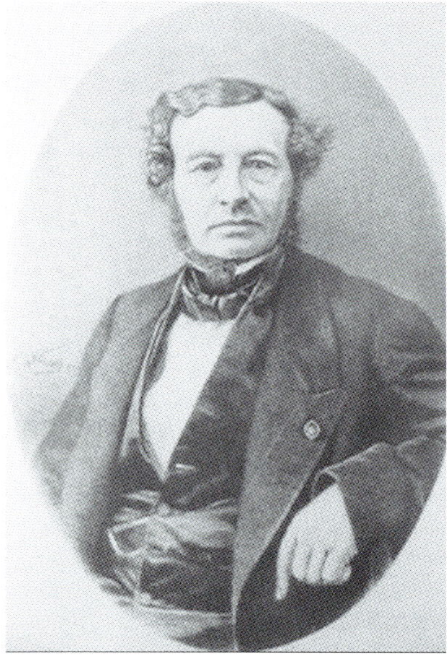

Fig. 2: Joseph-François Malgaigne (1806–1865).

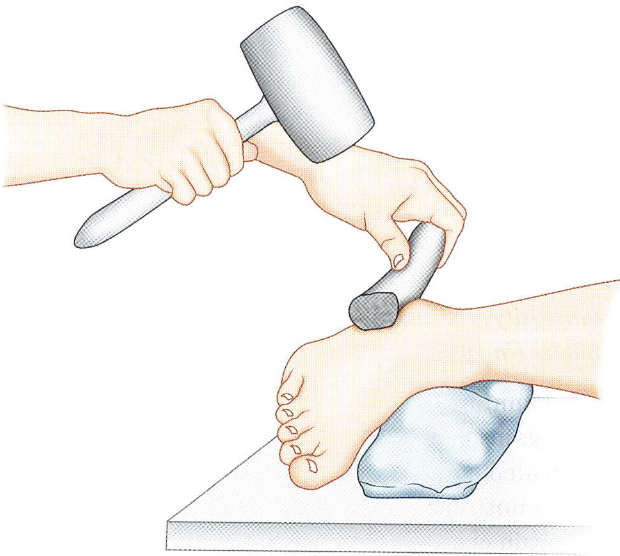

Fig. 3: Artist's rendition of an attempt to reduce the blown-out lateral wall of the calcaneus after a fracture.
Source: Adapted from Cotton FJ. Dislocations and Joint-fractures. Philadelphia: WB Saunders; 1910.

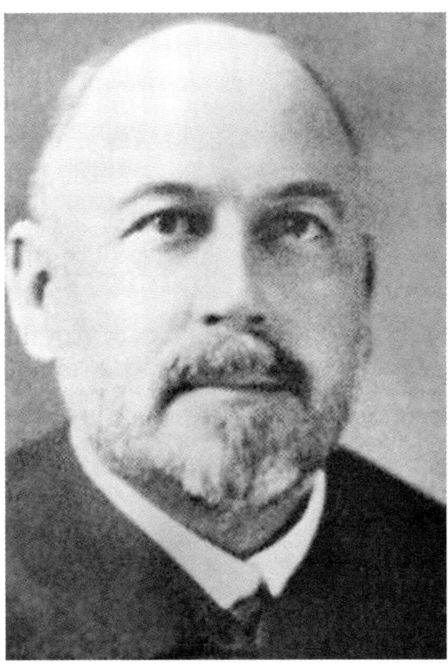

Fig. 4: Frederic Jay Cotton (1869–1938).

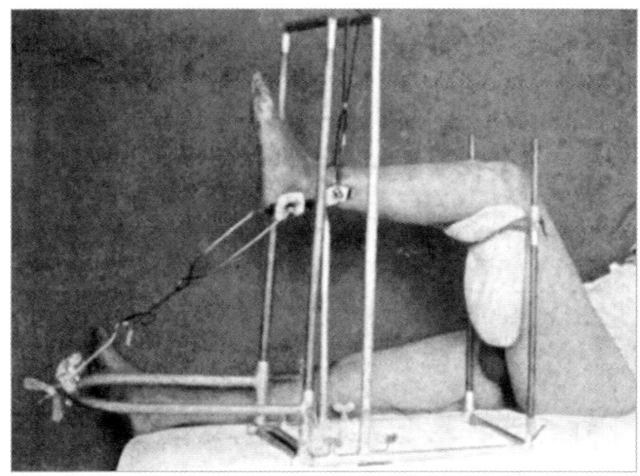

Fig. 5: Screw traction apparatus for reduction of fractures of calcaneus as described by Böhler.
Source: Adapted from Böhler (1931).[11]

In 1931, Böhler described his modification of closed reduction[11] where traction was provided by a pin in the calcaneal tuberosity, along with a pin in the tibia for countertraction (perhaps the forerunner of the modern distractor?) **(Fig. 5)**; lateral compression was provided by a specially designed clamp applied over the skin for this purpose **(Fig. 6)**. He also emphasized the importance of restoring the tuberosity joint angle (Böhler's angle).

Professor Lorenz Böhler **(Fig. 7)** *was an Austrian surgeon who pioneered the fracture treatment during the first half of the 20th century. He established and served as Director of Allgemeine Unfallversicherungsanstalt (AUVA) Hospital in Vienna, Brigittenau, which was later named after him: Lorenz-Böhler-Unfallkrankenhaus. His organizational skills combined with meticulous records helped him in publishing his most notable work in the form of his book: Treatment of Fractures. which made him the foremost authority on the subject during his time. He described his classification and method of reducing and treating calcaneus fractures and emphasized on restoring the tuberosity angle (later named after him as Böhler's angle) Böhler (in 1931) also developed a classification system.*

Hermann, in 1937,[12] further modified this method by using tongs instead of a pin for traction while countertraction was provided by the surgeon's weight applied to a crutch placed against the plantar surface of the foot. Arnesen, in 1966,[13] again changed the method by adding a pin through the metatarsal bases, along with a calcaneal pin to provide longitudinal traction. This was the time when surgeons were beginning to understand the fracture mechanics and were using aids to disimpact and maybe reduce the fracture.

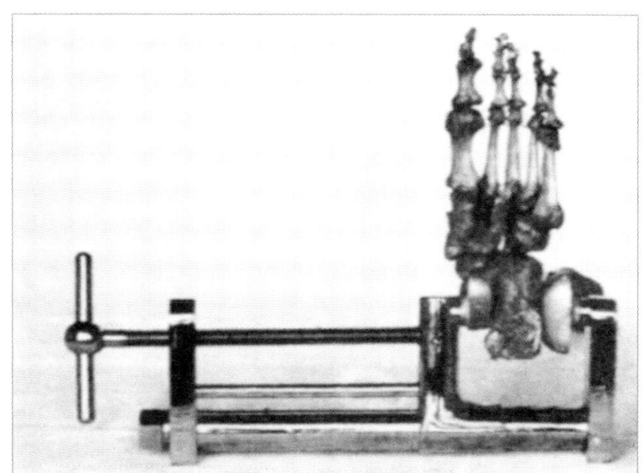

Fig. 6: Böhler's os calcis clamp in the screw vise.
Source: Adapted from Böhler (1931).[11]

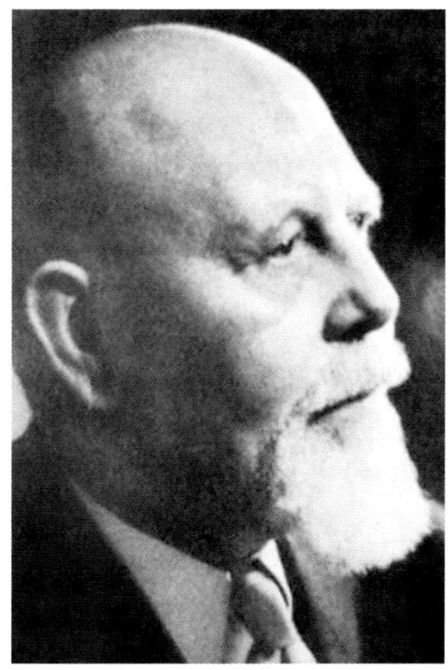

Fig. 7: Lorenz Böhler (1885–1973).

Essex-Lopresti, in his classic publication,[14] provided a somewhat better understanding of the unique pathoanatomy of calcaneal fractures; he divided these fractures into two basic types, the tongue type and the joint depression type, and this concept is used in understanding the fracture even today. He further reported that good results were obtainable with closed reduction of tongue-type fracture while advocating open reduction for joint depression. His method of closed reduction involved driving a Steinmann pin along the length of calcaneus while reducing the fracture by levering the posterior fragment with a Steinmann pin. His method in principle has stood the test of time and is still being used with favorable results for tongue-type fractures.

Peter Essex-Lopresti **(Fig. 8)** *trained at the London Hospital, qualifying in 1937. He joined the Royal Army Medical Corps, serving as a surgical specialist in an airborne division during World War II. He published a report on the injuries sustained during over 20,000 parachute jumps made by the Sixth British Airborne Division and is remembered for describing the Essex-Lopresti fracture and for his work on classification and treatment of fractures of the calcaneus. He distinguished intra-articular fractures of the calcaneus from extra-articular ones, and they correctly associated the intra-articular variety with a poorer long-term prognosis.*[14,15]

Alongside the popular attempts at refining methods of closed reduction, operative techniques were also being increasingly used by some physicians in the early 20th century. Operative procedures used during this period were either open reduction or primary arthrodesis. First, such recorded instance dates back to 1902 where Morestin

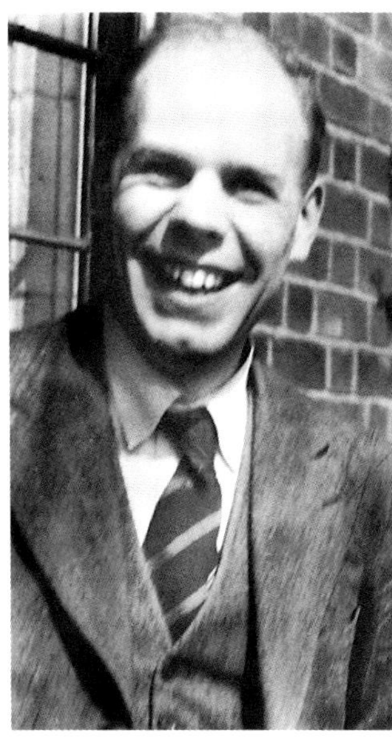

Fig. 8: Peter Gordon Lawrence Essex-Lopresti (1916–1951).

recommended the direct lateral approach to elevate the depressed fragment of the posterior fragment.[8] This was followed by recommendation of primary arthrodesis by Van Stockum in 1912.[8] Both these operative methods were evolving simultaneously, and various authors reported early good results with either method, without any definitive randomized comparative study. Although primary arthrodesis gained some support (mostly during the 1950s and 1960s) with several reports of favorable outcomes, continued development of better surgical techniques and superior devices for internal fixation led to open reduction with internal fixation becoming the preferred treatment for significantly displaced fractures of the calcaneus. Presently, subtalar arthrodesis is primarily reserved as a salvage procedure for disabling pain after initial treatment with other methods, with the recommended time for this procedure being at least 2 years after failed primary treatment.

Palmer, in 1948,[16] disappointed with results of primary subtalar arthrodesis as a treatment option, reported on results of his open reduction technique which formed the principal basis of modern open reduction techniques. During the early days, there were several proponents of medial, lateral, or combined approaches to the fractures and all three approaches were used without clear evidence of superiority of one over another. McReynolds[8] was one such staunch supporter of the medial approach and emphasized the importance of medial displacement and medial rotation of the superomedial fragment. This concept was challenged by Stephenson in 1983,[17] who used computed tomography (CT) scans to ascertain that the superomedial fragment essentially remained in its position, while the rest of the posterior facet was displaced inferiorly and rotated. The use of CT has perhaps had the most dramatic effect on the understanding and management of the calcaneus fractures and has become an indispensable tool in the diagnosis and treatment planning of these fractures. Based on coronal CT images, Sanders[18] developed a classification system which forms the pillar for fracture understanding and treatment planning in the modern era.

With growing popularity of open reduction, the need for better fixation devices was an obvious consequence. In the initial phases, multiple wires or stout Steinmann pins were employed to hold the displaced tuberosity; the three-dimensional reconstruction was a concept that was understood only in the last half of the 20th century. Subsequent developments led to the use of screws to hold the displaced facet after elevation, semitubular or reconstruction plates to span the fracture, and ultimately the development of specialized plates manufactured solely for use in calcaneal fracture. The 1990s saw the development of the low profile, multilimbed titanium plates, which could hold various parts of the fracture, allowed fixed angle locked or compression screws, and have a low enough profile to avoid impingement on the lateral soft tissues. Although these newer plates have been very successful in the past few decades, all open procedures have associated wound healing problems which prompted surgeons of the 21st century to explore the possibility of using minimally invasive or less invasive techniques for selected fracture patterns. Such efforts have yielded generally positive results in recent past, extending our understanding of these fractures and supporting the idea of accurate reduction of intra-articular posterior facet injuries along with maintaining the shape of tuberosity in terms of its height, width, and length, and its alignment in coronal plane.[19,20]

Rehabilitation after the calcaneus fracture has had fewer controversies than other aspects of treatment of these fractures.[21-23] A new approach of early mobilization began with the report by Day in 1950[21] and many subsequent authors including Essex-Lopresti strongly supported the concept. Lindsay and Dewar in 1958[22] and later Lance et al. in 1963[23] reported favorable results after early mobilization of calcaneal fractures, even when treated conservatively. This approach was widely used during 1960s when many believed that attempts at reduction (closed or open) did not offer any clear advantage, while inviting potential complications which would seem unnecessary in the scenario. Although this approach of early mobilization without any attempt at reduction has since been challenged, early mobilization after calcaneal fractures has remained the cornerstone of current treatment strategies.

Understanding and management of calcaneus fractures can be broadly divided into three time periods paralleling with advances in imaging and understanding of biology of fracture healing and biomechanics. Before 1900, these were largely unknown and poorly understood injuries. The first half of the last century saw rising numbers perhaps reflecting a higher number of falls with vertical growth of human dwellings. Physicians of this era experimented with closed reductions with limited but significant success; however, the latter half of the century saw exponential growth in numbers reflecting life in the fast lane and ensuing collisions. With increasing severity of injuries during high-energy trauma, closed treatment of past seemed obviously inadequate, prompting surgeons to adopt aggressive strategies involving open surgical procedures. This had improved the outcomes significantly; however, a surgeon's endeavor for improving results has ushered the era of minimally or less invasive approaches in recent decades which has shown promising results.

One fact in our evolution of knowledge about calcaneal fractures is pertinent. Perhaps more has been written in the past quarter century about this fracture, which was unknown in the Middle Ages, than all the combined published literature prior to that.[3,24] Our knowledge and understanding of these fractures have changed immensely in the past few decades, but such is the nature and complexity of this fracture that all is not yet known about it. Our continued endeavor will perhaps keep shedding light on all facets of this fracture which shall aid our treatment strategies in future. Future generations may still say that the surgeons of 2020 had limited knowledge about this fracture. But such is the nature of history.

■ REFERENCES

1. Clark WA. History of fracture treatment up to the sixteenth century. J Bone Joint Surg (Am). 1937;19:47-63.
2. Mostofi SB. Who's Who in Orthopaedics. London: Springer-Verlag London; 2005.
3. Dhillon MS, Bali K, Prabhakar S. Controversies in calcaneus fracture management: a systematic review of the literature. Musculoskelet Surg. 2011;95(3):171-81.
4. Breasted JH. The Edwin Smith Surgical Papyrus. Hieroglyphic Transliteration, Translation, and Commentary, vol. 1. Chicago, IL: The University of Chicago Press; 1930. pp. 350-7.
5. The Genuine Works of Hippocrates: Translated from the Greek with a Preliminary Discourse and Annotations, vol. 2. New York: William Wood and Company; 1891. pp. 23-156.
6. Ely LW. Old fracture of the tarsus: with a report of seventeen cases. Ann Surg. 1907;45(1):69-89.
7. Malgaigne JF. Traité des Fractures et des Luxations; 1847.
8. McReynold IS. Trauma to the Os calcis and heel cord. In: Jahss MH (ed) Disorders of the foot. WB Saunders, Philadelphia. 1982. pp. 1497-1542.
9. Cotton FJ, Wilson LT. Fractures of the os calcis. Boston Med Surg J. 1908;159(18):559-65.
10. Cotton FJ, Henderson FF. Results of fractures of the os calcis. Am J Orthop Surg. 1916;14:290-8.
11. Böhler L. Diagnosis, pathology, and treatment of fractures of the os calcis. J Bone Joint Surg. 1931;13:75-89.
12. Hermann OJ. Conservative therapy for fracture of the os calcis. J Bone Joint Surg. 1937;19:709-18.
13. Arnesen A. Treatment of fracture of the os calcis with traction and manipulation. Acta Chir Scand. 1966;132:566-73.
14. Essex-Lopresti P. The mechanism, reduction technique, and results in fractures of the os calcis. Br J Surg. 1952;39(157):395-419.
15. Essex-Lopresti P. The hazards of parachuting. Br J Surg. 1946;34(133):1-13.
16. Palmer I. The mechanism and treatment of fractures of the calcaneus; open reduction with the use of cancellous grafts. J Bone Joint Surg Am. 1948;30A:2-8.
17. Stephenson JR. Displaced fractures of the os calcis involving the subtalar joint: the key role of the superomedial fragment. Foot Ankle. 1983;4:91-101.
18. Sanders R, Fortin P, DiPasquale T, Walling A. Operative treatment in 120 displaced intraarticular calcaneal fractures. Results using a prognostic computed tomography scan classification. Clin Orthop Relat Res. 1993;(290):87-95.

19. Feng Y, Shui X, Wang J, Cai L, Yu Y, Ying X, et al. Comparison of percutaneous cannulated screw fixation and calcium sulfate cement grafting versus minimally invasive sinus tarsi approach and plate fixation for displaced intra-articular calcaneal fractures: a prospective randomized controlled trial. BMC Musculoskelet Disord. 2016;17:288.

20. Xia S, Wang X, Lu Y, Wang H, Wu Z, Wang Z. A minimally invasive sinus tarsi approach with percutaneous plate and screw fixation for intra-articular calcaneal fractures. Int J Surg. 2013;11(10):1087-91.

21. Day FG. Treatment of fractures of os calcis. Can Med Assoc J. 1950;63:373-6.

22. Lindsay WR, Dewar FP. Fractures of the os calcis. Am J Surg. 1958;95:555-76.

23. Lance EM, Carey Jr EJ, Wade PA. Fractures of the os calcis. Treatment by early mobilization. Clin Orthop Relat Res. 1963;30:76-90.

24. Wells C. Fractures of the heel bones in early and prehistoric times. Practitioner. 1976;217(1298):294-8.

General Considerations in Calcaneal Fracture Treatment

Mandeep S Dhillon, Sampat D Patil

"The best way to become acquainted with a subject is to write a book about it".
–Benjamin Disraeli (1804–1881)

"I have but one lamp by which my feet are guided, and that is the lamp of experience".
–Patrick Henry

FIRST AID

Like any lower limb injury, first aid for a calcaneus fracture involves the RICE regimen (rest, icing, compression and elevation). A simple plaster of Paris (POP) slab with a crepe bandage, or a plastic-molded back splint, elevated over two to three pillows helps in decreasing the pain and swelling. Nonsteroidal anti-inflammatory drugs (NSAIDs) and intermittent icing also help in reducing the swelling, and toe mobilization is encouraged. The patient should be kept nonweightbearing (NWB).

RADIOLOGY

Simple X-rays are often enough to determine the fracture type; history and clinical examination would give evidence of bilaterality, and contralateral X-rays may be needed. Special X-rays and how to take them are described in another Chapter.

Computed tomography (CT) scans are the key in cases where surgical intervention is planned (Chapter 4).

DECISION FOR TREATMENT

Nonoperative or operative management depends on many factors, including age, type of fractures, associated injuries, facilities available, comorbidity, etc. Nonoperative protocols are described in Chapter 6, and POP is often not given in cooperative patients as splintage elevation and avoiding weight bearing can work. POP may be needed in certain scenarios such as ours, as patients are noncooperative.

Surgery is often indicated and should be planned keeping in mind all factors including available resources.

TIMING OF SURGERY

For surgery planned with a conventional extensile approach, immobilization and elevation are continued till wrinkling of the skin is evident over the heel (positive wrinkle sign), usually by 7–10 days (see Chapters 7 and 9). If a limited open or minimally invasive approach is planned, then earlier fixation is easier as it allows fragment manipulation. The same can be combined with another procedure such as fixation of a spine injury if required. Often, the decision to operate is mandated by an open fracture, where the timing and protocols are different (see Chapter 16) and often staged surgery is needed.

TOURNIQUET

A pneumatic tourniquet is invariably used as it helps decrease bleeding and shortens surgery time. Many experienced surgeons may forego tourniquet inflation (after application) and inflate the cuff as and when required. A tourniquet is not required if using a percutaneous approach or external fixation only.

The tourniquet is typically placed on the thigh as high as possible. A large tourniquet is applied over a layer of cotton with care to avoid wrinkles in the cotton and injury to the external genitalia in males.

The ideal cuff pressure should be kept 100 mm Hg over the mean arterial pressure. The maximum time duration for tourniquet inflation should not typically exceed 120 minutes, when it should be deflated and reinflated if needed after 20 minutes.

ANTIBIOTICS

The incidence of surgical site infections in calcaneus surgery (up to 25%) is higher than for other orthopedic procedures, due to poor vascularity in the skin of this area and limited muscle cover. Most surgeries are done under antibiotic cover, starting with a dose of intravenous (IV) antibiotics administered to all patients with closed fractures preoperatively before tourniquet inflation (1,500 mg cefuroxime or 1,000 mg cefazolin). At our center, we give two or three doses postoperatively. Patients with open fractures with contamination or farm injuries receive extended IV antibiotics for 3–5 days (cefuroxime with amikacin and metronidazole on hospital admission), till definitive intraoperative culture reports become available.

ANESTHESIA

Options for anesthesia are multiple; we prefer regional/spinal anesthesia in most unilateral cases. General anesthesia (GA) is preferred in case of spine injuries (prone position) or polytrauma (multiple interventions) or those on anticoagulants; even in bilateral cases, which can be done in the same sitting, GA may be better as patients do not tolerate a prone position for prolonged periods.

PATIENT AND C-ARM POSITIONING

For most calcaneus surgeries, after tourniquet application, the patient is placed in the lateral decubitus position **(Figs. 1 and 2)**.

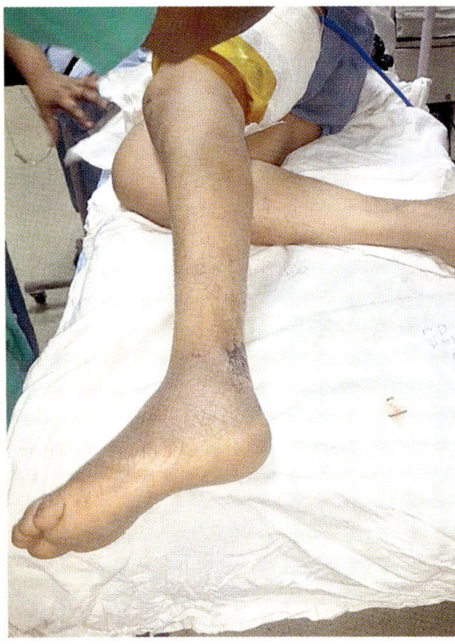

Fig. 1: Patient position with tourniquet in place. Never start the calcaneus case unless you see a good axial view, and never leave the operating theater (OT) unless you see a good Broden's view. Sometimes, the metal edge of the operation table will overlap the C-arm view intraoperatively.

The bony prominences (elbow, pelvis, knee, ankle) are adequately cushioned. Care is taken to especially pad the peroneal nerve of the lower leg, as it winds around the fibular head (may lead to iatrogenic foot drop). The underlying lower limb is folded away from the operative field for better radiology. The foot to be operated is brought as distal as possible with the operating surgeon at the foot end of the table. A sterile rolled sheet or bump is used under the foot while operating. This facilitates C-arm positioning from the side.

Patients undergoing concomitant spine injuries can be placed in the prone position **(Fig. 3)**.

However, it is difficult to do the conventional extensile approach in prone position. Percutaneous or limited open approaches may be more suitable if surgery has to be performed in the prone position.

SKIN PREPARATION[1,2]

The surgical site is first disinfected with povidone-iodine, followed by alcohol-based/chlorhexidine solution and then draped free. Sequential application has been shown to decrease the presence of viable cutaneous bacteria than either agent used alone. The toes are draped out of the surgical field using adhesive sterile surgical drapes. We do not, as a routine, use adhesive drapes to cover the entire surgical field as no definitive evidence of reduction of infection is available in the literature; however, we do cover the toes to take them out of the sterile field of surgery.

ESSENTIAL INSTRUMENTS

Standard instruments **(Fig. 4)** include small Langenbeck retractor, no. 10 and no. 15 scalpel blades, grasping forceps (toothed and plain), small osteotomes, periosteum elevators, multiple straight and curved artery forceps, and multiple Kirschner wires 1.5–2.0 mm (sharp at one end only to avoid injury).

Specialized instruments such as Hintermann retractor, distractors, or external fixation devices **(Fig. 5)** may be required depending upon the specifics of the case. Powered instruments are very helpful.

IMPLANTS

Implants specific to the procedure should be procured, and multiple options should be available in the operating theater (OT). If minimally invasive surgery (MIS) is planned (see Chapter 8), then all types and sizes of screws and wires should be available, along with external fixation devices to supplement fixation in complex cases. For an extensile approach (see Chapter 9), calcaneal plates and partially and fully threaded small and large fragment cancellous screws

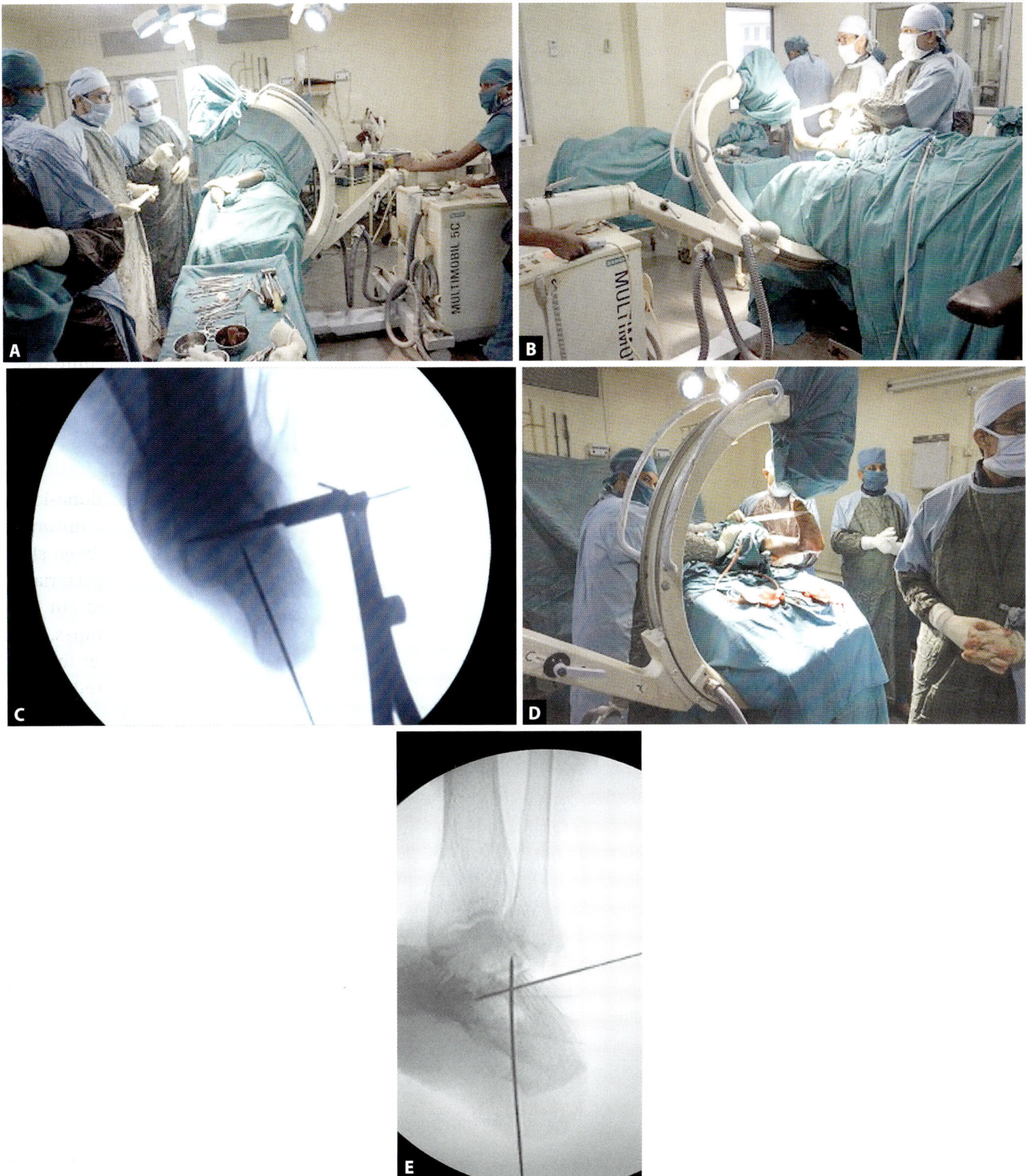

Figs. 2A to E: (A) Position of C-arm for lateral and axial views; (B) Position of C-arm for lateral and axial views and use of sterile bandage to hold foot in dorsiflexion; (C) Axial view of calcaneus; (D) Position of C-arm for Broden's view; (E) Broden's view of the calcaneus.

should be available. Specialized approaches such as the subtalar approach may require specialized plates tailored to the approach.

WOUND CLOSURE AND DRESSING

Wound closure is performed with subcutaneous Vicryl sutures combined with Allgöwer-Donati Ethilon sutures

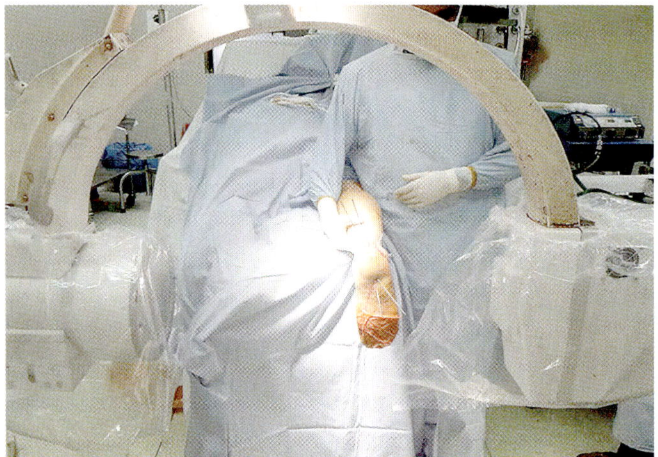

Fig. 3: Patient positioned prone, with C-arm positioned for a lateral view.

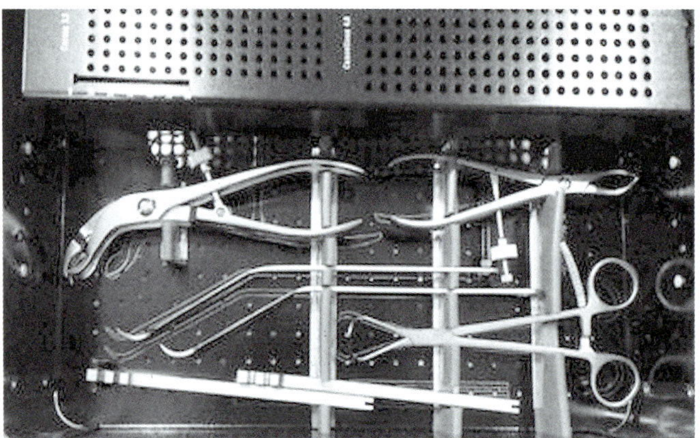

Fig. 4: Instruments needed for reduction of the calcaneus.

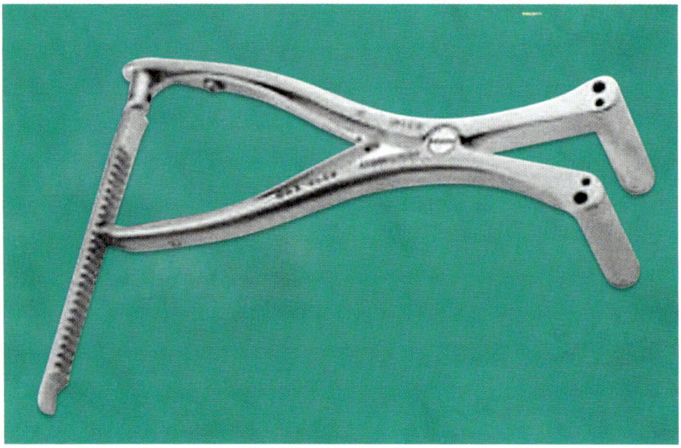

Fig. 5: Hintermann retractor.

(*Ethicon, Division of Johnson & Johnson, Somerville, NJ*), with placement of a closed suction drain (10 Fr). This drain is removed postoperatively when drainage is <30 mL after 24 hours; many surgeons deflate the tourniquet prior to

wound closure and do a meticulous hemostasis. A drain may not be required in this scenario. After the extensile approach, sutures are tied sequentially from the periphery to the apex, in order to minimize the chances of flap necrosis. All patients are hospitalized after primary surgery and are discharged when pain is under control and the suture line is dry; we often delay stitch removal. All patients remain NWB for a period of 10–12 weeks postoperatively and mobilize with crutches.

IMMOBILIZATION, REHABILITATION, AND WEIGHT-BEARING PRECAUTIONS

Postoperative immobilization must balance the requirements necessary to prevent loss of fixation, encourage soft-tissue healing, and minimize immobilization of joints. Range-of-motion (ROM) exercises should be started as soon as possible, as early motion, even if NWB, allows for better healing of articular cartilage, ligament, and soft-tissue injuries and helps prevent muscle atrophy of the surgical limb.

Loss of motion can result from prolonged immobilization. Long-term disability can occur from immobilization in the incorrect position, particularly equinus. With few exceptions (e.g., tuberosity avulsion fractures, Chapter 13), the foot should be kept immobilized in a plantigrade neutral position using a removable split or POP slab, which is removed multiple times daily for exercises.

PHYSICAL THERAPY

A good collaboration with physiotherapists is essential as therapy progresses in stages (see Chapter 26). ROM exercises are essential for regaining function, but equinus contractures also must not be allowed to develop. Crutch training to avoid weight on operated foot is important, as unregulated weight bearing can lead to implant failure. As the fracture heals, the foot is placed under increasing load and stress.

ANTICOAGULATION

The overall incidence of clinically significant extremity deep vein thrombosis (DVT) following calcaneal fractures surgery is low.[3] The clinical benefit of formal anticoagulation after foot and ankle surgery remains unclear.

SPECIAL PRECAUTIONS FOR OPEN FRACTURES

Details of management of open fractures have been dealt within Chapter 16. The principles remain the same as for any other fracture and involve thorough debridement of all necrotic and devitalized tissue, copious lavage with normal saline, and minimal internal and external fixation until soft-tissue consolidation. Early soft-tissue coverage may require the assistance of plastic surgeons with skin grafting or soft-tissue flaps and is essential to help preserve bone and minimize the risk of infection.[4-6]

■ REFERENCES

1. Patrick S, McDowell A, Lee A, Frau A, Martin U, Gardner E, et al. Antisepsis of the skin before spinal surgery with povidone iodine-alcohol followed by chlorhexidine gluconate-alcohol versus povidone iodine-alcohol applied twice for the prevention of contamination of the wound by bacteria: a randomised controlled trial. Bone Joint J. 2017;99-B(10):1354-65.
2. Moores N, Rosenblatt S, Prabhu A, Rosen M. Do iodine-impregnated adhesive surgical drapes reduce surgical site infections during open ventral hernia repair? A comparative analysis. Am Surg. 2017;83:617-22.
3. SooHoo NF, Eagan M, Krenek L, Zingmod DS. Incidence and risk factors for thromboembolism following surgical treatment of ankle fractures. #235. Presented at the American Academy of Orthopaedic Surgeons 76th Annual Meeting, Las Vegas, February 25–28, 2009.
4. Dhillon MS, Bali K, Prabhakar S. Controversies in calcaneus fracture management: a systematic review of the literature. Musculoskelet Surg. 2011;95(3):171-81.
5. Dhillon MS, Prabhakar S. Treatment of displaced intra-articular calcaneus fractures: a current concepts review. SICOT J. 2017;3:59.
6. Rammelt S, Swords M, Dhillon MS, Sands AK. Manual of Fracture Management: Foot & Ankle Surgery. New York: Thieme Medical Publishers; 2019.

3 Clinical Anatomy and Injury Mechanics

KV Menon, SS Suresh

"People see only what they are prepared to see".

–Emerson RW

INTRODUCTION

Appreciation of the structural and functional anatomy of the hindfoot is critical to the understanding of injuries of the heel bone. The skeleton of the human foot depicts the evolution of the organism to erect bipedal ambulation. It has been structurally and functionally adapted to the specific gait pattern comprising the foot flat stance to the push-off phases of normal adult walking. Unlike many animals (the digitigrade and unguligrade mammals as opposed to the plantigrade ones) where the calcaneus has no role in weight bearing, the human foot is placed horizontally during locomotion and the calcaneus bears a major part of the body weight **(Fig. 1)**. But similar to the animal hindfoot, the calcaneus is the attachment of the major propulsive force of the leg—the gastro-soleus musculotendinous unit. The posterior extent of the calcaneus from the coronal midline of the tibia is the lever arm of the tendoachilles and is obviously longer for fast-running primates. During the heel strike phase of normal gait and during the same phase in running, the entire body weight plus its multiples due to the ground reaction force is transmitted through the calcaneus alone. Restoration of the structure and function of the heel bone and its surrounding soft tissues assumes greater significance in this context.

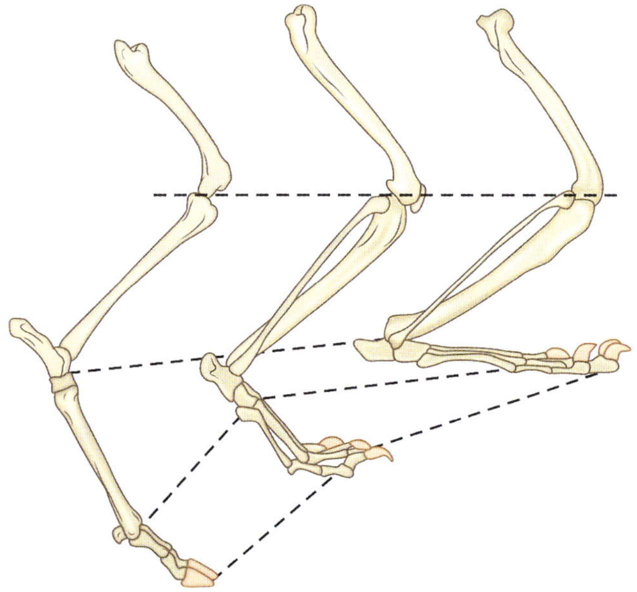

TOPOGRAPHICAL ANATOMY

The os calcis is described as an irregular bone, predominantly cancellous in structure and enveloped in a shell of thin cortical bone.[1-3] It represents the largest of the seven tarsal bones in man. It can be imagined as a rectangular solid placed horizontally in the anteroposterior (AP) axis and possessing six surfaces **(Fig. 2)**. The anterior surface

Fig. 1: The plantigrade foot is the only one where the calcaneus contacts the ground during weight bearing in mammals (BIO 342; Comparative vertebrate anatomy lecture notes 5—Skeletal system IV appendicular skeleton).

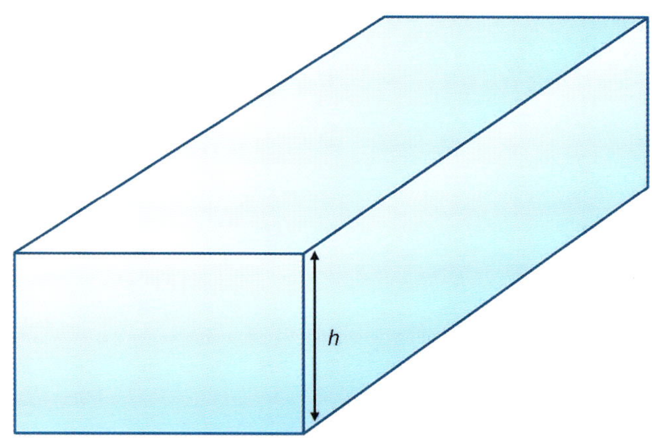

Fig. 2: The six surfaces represent the surfaces of the os calcis. (*h:* height)

articulates with the cuboid and the superior articulates with the talus. The inferior surface bears most of the distal muscle attachments. The posterior surface receives the insertion of the achilles tendon. The medial side is related to the major neurovascular bundle and the tendons of the foot and the lateral surface of the minor neurovascular bundle and the tendons of the ankle and the hindfoot.[5]

The most striking feature of the os calcis is its tuberosities. On the anterosuperior aspect of its medial surface is the large, sustentaculum tali **(Fig. 3)**. This horizontal bony prominence is structurally the strongest part of the bone and is therefore the key to reduction and stabilization in fractures of this bone. Attached to it are the strong plantar calcaneonavicular ligament and the anterior fibers of the deltoid ligament. The tibialis posterior tendon gives off fibers to insert here and the flexor hallucis longus and the flexor digitorum longus pass under it **(Fig. 4)**. Also related to the

under surface and the medial surface of the calcaneus are the posterior tibial vessels and nerves.[5] The superior surface of the sustentaculum tali bears the middle talocalcaneal joint. On the middle part of the lateral surface is the peroneal tubercle which is quite small in comparison and along with the peroneal trochlea attached to it transmits the peroneus brevis and longus tendons **(Fig. 5)**. Also attached to the lateral surface is the calcaneofibular ligament of the ankle joint. The posterior half is called the tuber calcaneus and the middle third of its posterior surface gives attachment to the tendoachilles and the plantaris muscles. The upper part is covered by the achilles bursa and the superior surface of the tuberosity by a large fat pad. On the plantar surface at its posterior end lies the calcaneal tubercle whose medial process bears the origin of the abductor hallucis and the flexor digitorum brevis, its lateral process to the abductor digiti quinti, and the central part to the plantar aponeurosis and the quadratus plantae muscle.

The os calcis articulates with two bones—the talus and the cuboid. The talocalcaneal articulation consists of three discrete joints—the anterior middle and posterior ones **(Fig. 6)**. The anterior one located over the anterior end of the superior surface and the middle one on the dorsum of the sustentaculum are smaller joints, located in the horizontal axis and play a lesser role in weight bearing. The posterior subtalar joint which is the primary weight bearer is located in the middle of the superior surface of the calcaneum and is oriented facing anteriorly and superiorly by about 45°. It is supported by strong compression trabeculae under the surface called the thalamic portion of the bone. The posterior subtalar joint is a saddle-shaped joint and supports the eversion and inversion of the hindfoot.[1,3,7] Between the

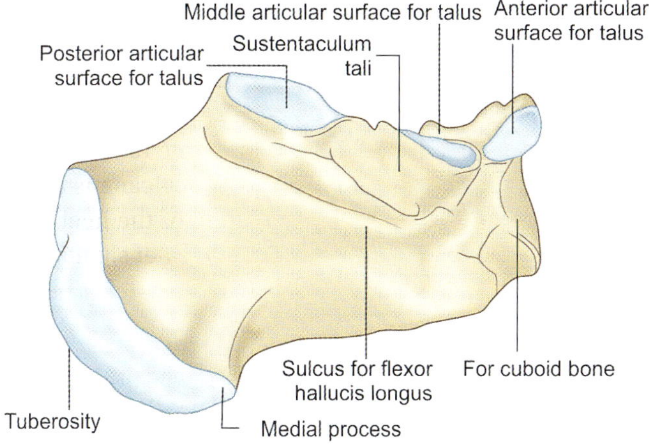

Fig. 3: Medial view of the calcaneus.

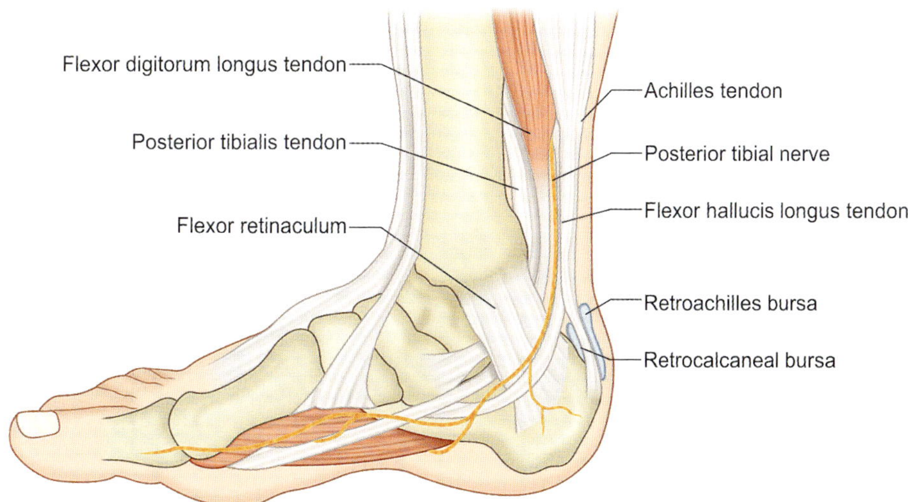

Fig. 4: Soft tissues in relation to the medial surface of the hindfoot.

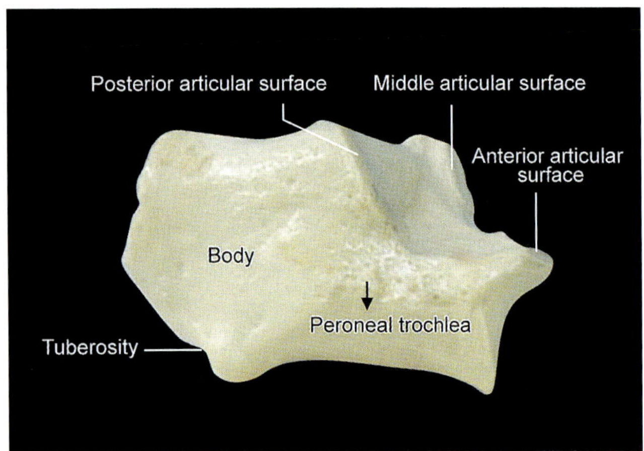

Fig. 5: Lateral view of the calcaneus.

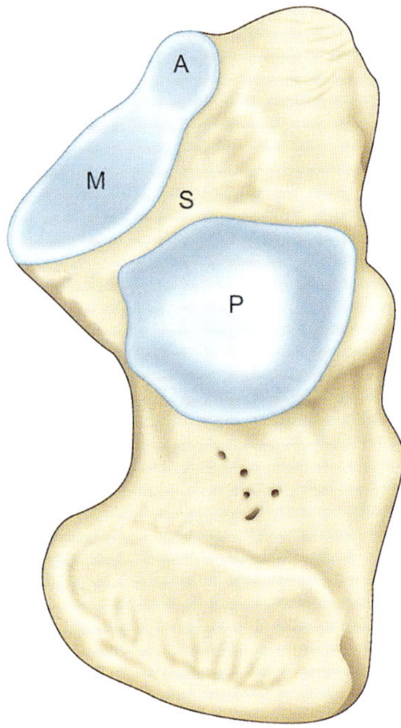

Fig. 6: The superior surface shows the three subtalar articular facets and the large tuberosity. (A: anterior facet; M: Middle facet; P: posterior facet; S: sinus tarsi)

posterior and middle facets lies the calcaneal sulcus which together with the similar groove on the talus forms the sinus tarsi. The sinus tarsi lodges the artery of the sinus tarsi and the interosseous talocalcaneal ligament. Anterior to the anterior facet, the bifurcate Y ligament is attached and lateral to it is the origin of the extensor digitorum brevis.

■ FUNCTIONAL ANATOMY

The axis of the calcaneus in the standing position is oriented in the posteroanterior direction and slightly laterally (15–35° between the talometatarsal line and the calcaneal axis) directed. In the sagittal plane, it can be seen inclined to the floor by approximately 25° which is called the

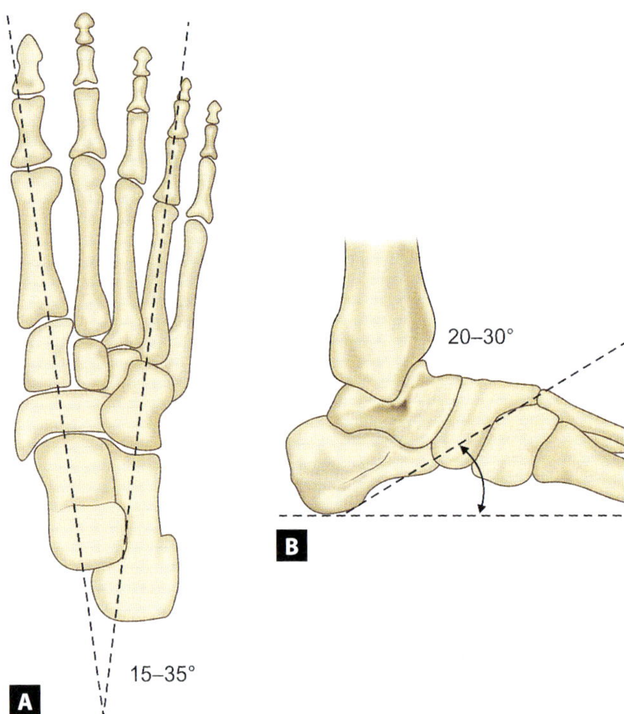

Figs. 7A and B: The orientation of the calcaneus in the axial and sagittal planes.

pitch **(Figs. 7A and B)**. This angle is crucial to maintain the longitudinal arch of the foot, and restoration is sought during reconstruction after fractures. Similarly, the inclination of the posterior subtalar joint to the horizontal or the long axis of the calcaneum forms the basis of Gissane's angle and Bohler's angle, both of which are considered critical and need to be restored **(Fig. 8)**. In normal instance, the calcaneus is tilted by 5–10° in the coronal plane giving it a slight valgus placement **(Fig. 9)**.[2,7,13]

It is also important to appreciate that the talus is placed in the middle and anterior third of the calcaneus leaving a large part of the posterior third free to provide the lever arm for the achilles tendon. Restoration of this length after fractures of the calcaneum is predictably crucial for effort-free propulsion during locomotion.

The trabecular pattern in the foot as a whole and especially the os calcis reflects the design requirements of erect locomotion and weight bearing and they develop according to Wolff's law **(Fig. 10)**. The principal compressive trabeculae run from the posterior subtalar joint to the point of the heel and is the primary load-bearing column. The secondary compression group runs from the posterior subtalar joint to the posterior surface and possibly represents the load borne during heel strike phase of gait. The major tensile load is borne by the principal tensile trabeculae starting at the insertion of the achilles tendon and spanning down in the same axis into the bone. The secondary tensile trabeculae

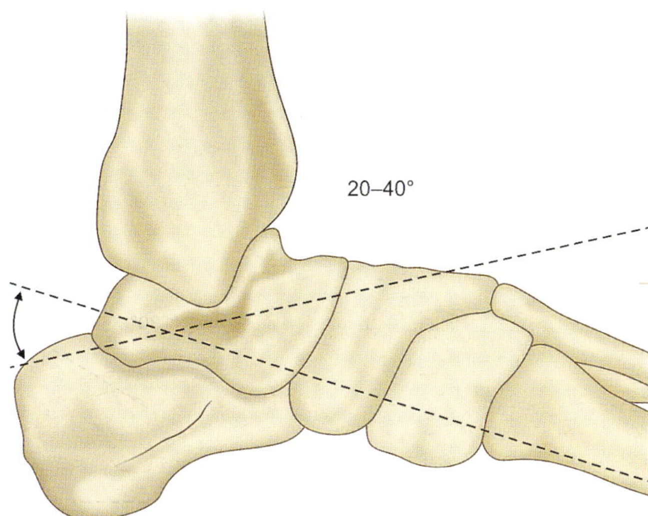

Fig. 8: The Bohler's angle represents the sagittal plane relation between the talus and the calcaneus and also the integrity of the posterior subtalar joint.

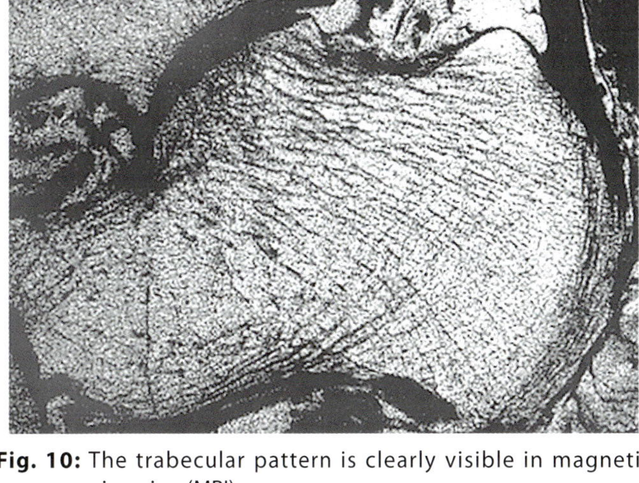

Fig. 10: The trabecular pattern is clearly visible in magnetic resonance imaging (MRI).
Source: Link TM, Lotter A, Beyer F, Christiansen S, Newitt D, Lu Y, et al. Changes in calcaneal trabecular bone structure after heart transplantation: an MR imaging study. Radiology. 2000;217:855-62.

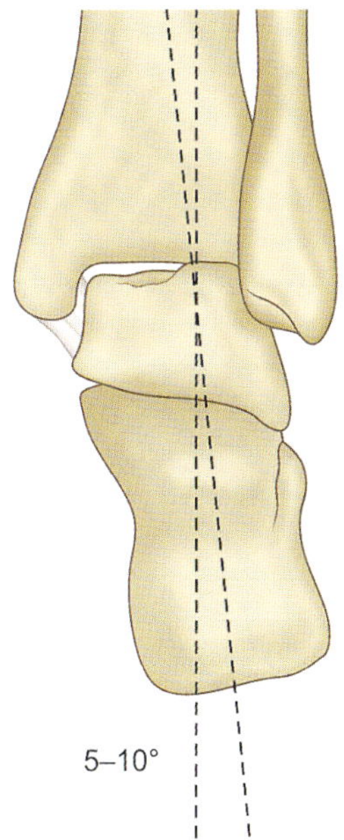

Fig. 9: The coronal plane alignment of the normal os calcis.

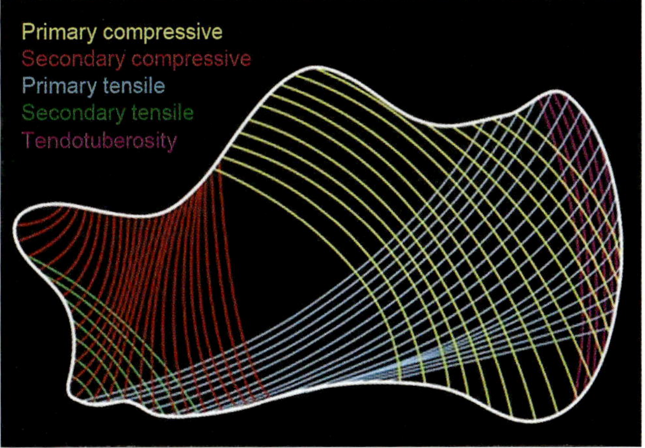

Fig. 11: The compression trabeculae under the posterior subtalar joint, the tension trabeculae, and the neutral triangle are represented (Roentgen Ray Reader: Calcaneal trabecular bone architecture).
Courtesy: Behrang Amini.

support the arch of the foot and are thought to represent the tensile forces required to maintain the longitudinal arch of the foot or in other words counter the pull of the plantar fascia. There is an area under the thalamic segment of the bone with relatively sparse trabeculae called the neutral triangle referring perhaps to the mutual cancellation of compression and tension forces **(Fig. 11)**. This area has been considered traditionally as having little significance in the pathological anatomy of fractures, but we feel that when the posterior subtalar joint is depressed, crushing the thalamic compression trabeculae, the vacuous neutral triangle might fail to support the articular surface even after it has been elevated to its original state. This, the authors feel, is an argument in favor of grafting the region in depressed fractures affecting this area.

Several studies have looked at the trabecular pattern and analyzed the stress transfer mechanisms in the os calcis.[7,11,15,17] The authors propose a new hypothesis based on the "da Vinci's bridge" concept **(Figs. 12A and B)**. This hypothesis presupposes an asymmetrical bridge comprising two longitudinal arches—the medial longitudinal arch of the foot and the lateral longitudinal arch. Needless to say, these are of different heights, lengths, and radii of curvature. The two transverse arches are along the balls of the feet

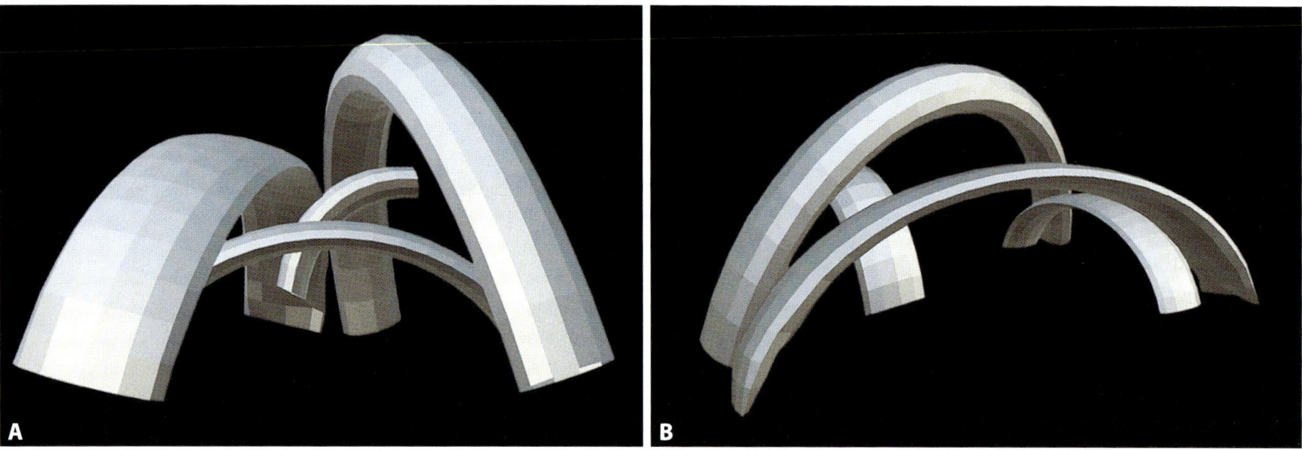

Figs. 12A and B: Schematic representation of the da Vinci's bridge concept applied to the foot. Note the medial and lateral longitudinal and the proximal and distal transverse arches.

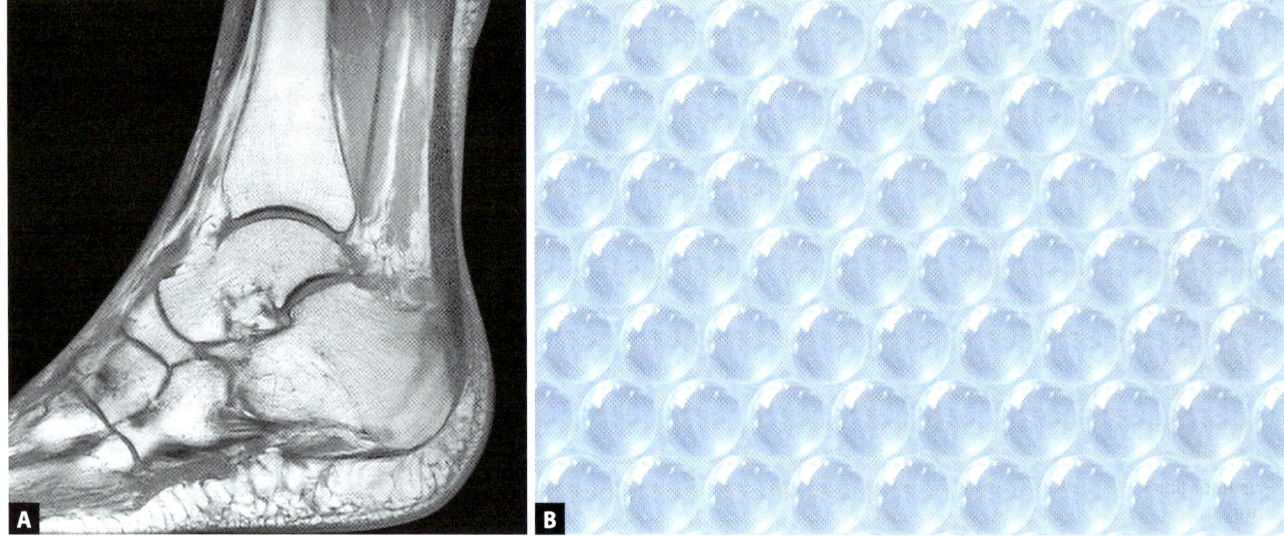

Figs. 13A and B: The calcaneal fat pad acts as a functional "bubble pack" to protect the bone during weight bearing.

and the midfoot region, the latter being a "quarter circle" arc as depicted in the illustration. The tensile trabeculae of the entire foot lie along these arches reflecting their inherent role in maintaining load-bearing function of the longitudinal arches. Should the integrity of these trabeculae be disrupted (as in foot fractures), the load-bearing function is also disrupted and will be reorganized after healing, depending on the posthealing anatomy. Hence, restoration of the trabecular anatomy along with the arches is of prime importance in all foot injuries; the authors hypothesize that in calcaneal fractures the posterior part of the arches, measured primarily as the pitch of the calcaneus, needs restoration to achieve this function.

Of particular importance is the calcaneal fat pad. The heel pad is a structure that functions exactly like the "bubble pack". The periosteum sends vertical septe into the deep fascia of the foot dividing the soft tissue layer into multiple pockets, each filled with compressed fat **(Figs. 13A and B)**. This heel pad has been shown to have a significant function in compressive load bearing and also takes the shear stresses on the heel during walking on uneven grounds and running. Injury to the fat pad is inevitable in most fractures of the calcaneum, and this can result in painful weight bearing for several months. Similarly, surgical access should protect the fat pad as much as possible.

■ VASCULAR ANATOMY

The vascular anastomoses around the ankle and heel are crucial for several reasons. Avascular necrosis of the calcaneus is rare compared to that of the talus due to its profuse muscular, tendinous, and ligamentous attachments; however, skin flap viability over the fractured bone is often tenuous when treated operatively and sometimes nonoperatively as well. Dissection of the tissues in this region mandates one layer,[4] reflection of flaps including skin, fascia, subcutaneous tissues, and periosteum as a whole to prevent necrosis of these flaps.

The posterior tibial artery, the main supplier to the foot and ankle, divides into medial and lateral plantar vessels and also gives off the direct calcaneal branches. The anterior tibial artery gives off the medial and lateral malleolar branches and the lateral tarsal artery which in turn supplies the sinus tarsi region. The artery of the tarsal sinus anastomoses with these latter branches. This artery arises from the peroneal perforating artery which also supplies the calcaneum directly by several small branches **(Figs. 14A and B)**.[4,14] The surgical implications of this extensive arterial network are that avascular necrosis of the calcaneal bone is relatively rare.[22] The placement of surgical incisions to

preserve the vascularity of the bone appears to be less critical than it is to preserve the blood supply of the overlying skin and soft tissues—the latter frequently undergoing ischemic necrosis after surgical procedures on the calcaneus. Purely from the anatomical viewpoint, the posterior plantar approach appears to be the least damaging to the overlying soft tissue vasculature—whether the surgical access to the pathology is adequate, is another matter.

ANATOMY AND PATHOMECHANICS OF OS CALCIS FRACTURE

The vast majority of calcaneal fractures are due to direct vertical compression injury, and this is what will be dealt with here.[18-20] There is a smaller group of extra-articular avulsion fractures and open fractures due to high-velocity injuries which are outside the ambit of this treatise.[21]

Direct compression forces transmitted through the talus to the calcaneus are manifest as a sequence of structural changes.[6] The talar tuberosity impales the superior surface of the os calcis and acts as a wedge driven into the bone splitting the bone at its structurally weakest point **(Fig. 15)**. This results in a primary fracture line running between the anterior and middle facets in the anterolateral to posteromedial direction. The direction of this primary fracture line has been of some debate and has been described differently by different authors;[7-10,12,16] nevertheless, it is agreed that it lies anterior to the posterior subtalar joint and is primarily in the coronal plane **(Figs. 16A to D)**. Simultaneously, the posterior articular facet is impacted down into the void created by the neutral triangle **(Fig. 17)**. The pull of the tendoachilles elevates the point of the heel thus distorting the pitch and the Bohler's angles; often this pull gives rise to a secondary fracture line avulsing the tuberosity of the os calcis horizontally—described as the tongue fracture **(Fig. 18)**. The horizontal fracture line may actually run just behind the posterior facet joint. As the

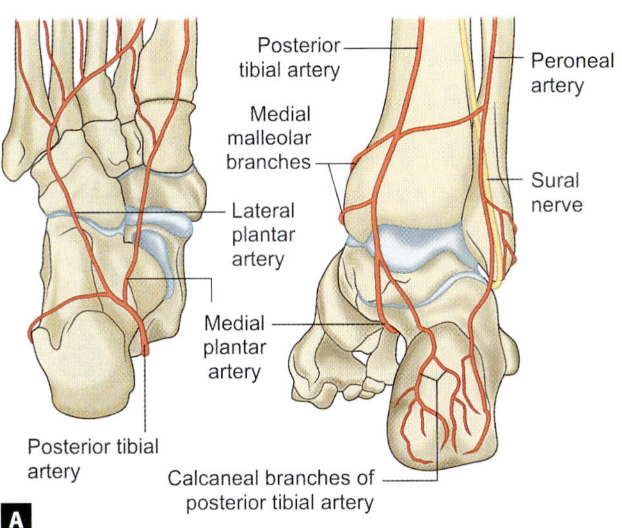

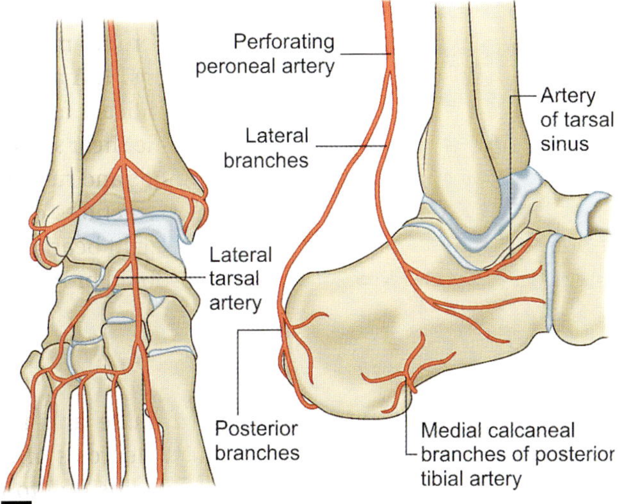

Figs. 14A and B: Arterial anastomosis around the ankle.

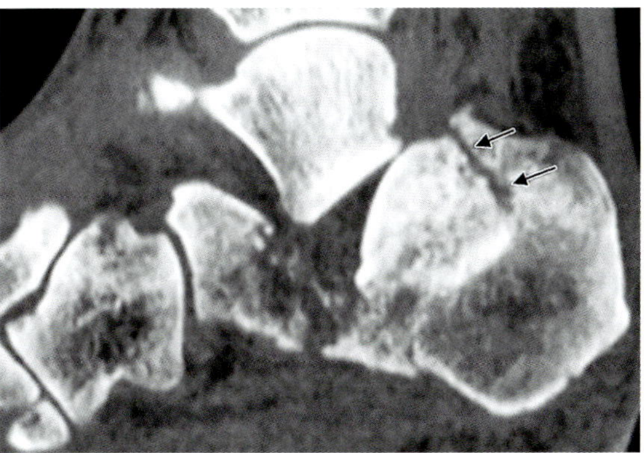

Fig. 15: Lateral process of Talus wedging into body of the calcaneus is clearly seen.

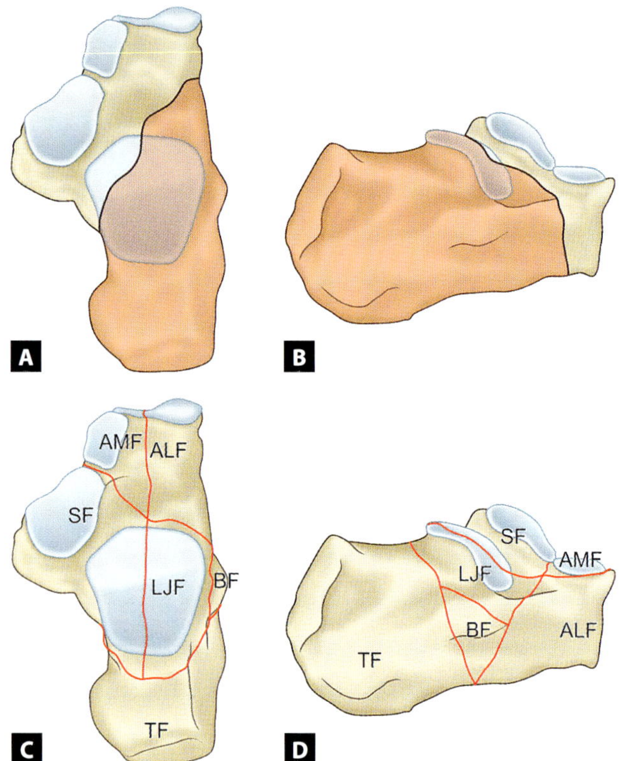

Figs. 16A to D: The two depictions of the primary fracture line are shown in red. (ALF: anterolateral fragment; AMF: anteromedial fragment; BF: blowout fragment; LJF: lateral joint fragment; SF: sustentacular fragment; TF: tuberosity fragment)

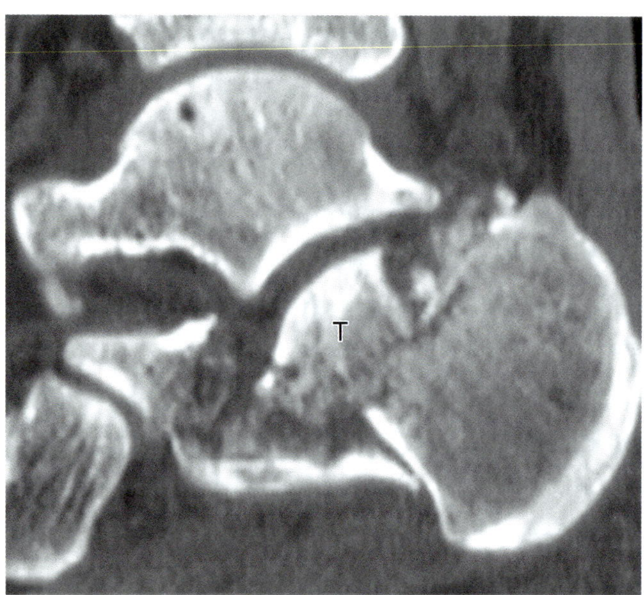

Fig. 17: The posterior subtalar joint is impacted into the neutral triangle.

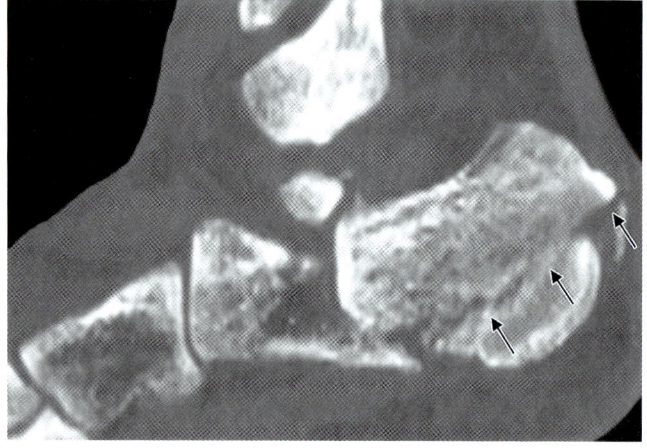

Fig. 18: The tongue-shaped fragment is elevated due to the tendoachilles pull.

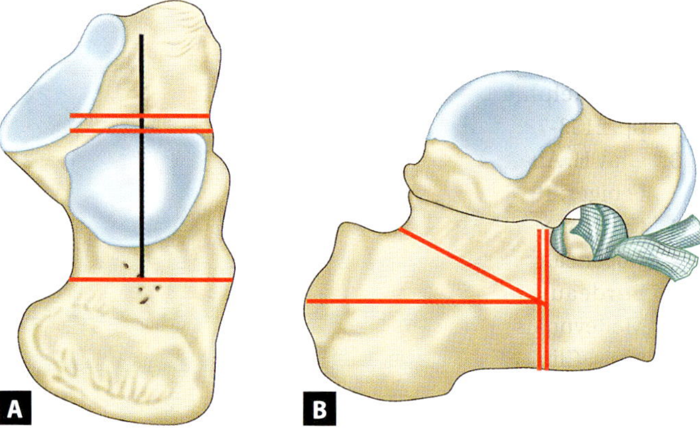

Figs. 19A and B: Secondary fracture lines.

energy dissipation continues, several distinct secondary fracture patterns ensue. The most common variety runs through the posterior subtalar joint in the AP direction splitting the sustentacular fragment medially from the body fragment laterally **(Figs. 19A and B)**. This fracture has been described by several authors as due to a shear component of the force.[11,13,15,16] The exact location and the degree of comminution of these fragments form the basis of Sanders classification. Centrifugal explosive forces may also result in lateral wall bursts in the calcaneus **(Fig. 20)**.

The sustentacular bone is by far the strongest part of the os calcis. Also, its ligamentous attachments ensure that this is most often the least displaced fragment from its normal anatomical locus. Therefore, a reduction is generally attempted against the normally located sustentaculum; also stabilization is attempted against the strong bone therein.

The weakest part of the bone is the neutral triangle. In the intact specimen, this area needs no support; however, when the arch is broken, the authors believe that it does need support till it can be reformed. The thalamic segment bearing the posterior subtalar joint is elevated and held to the sustentaculum fragment and the resulting void is filled with bone graft or even better synthetic ceramic substitutes to maintain that reduction **(Figs. 21A to C)**.

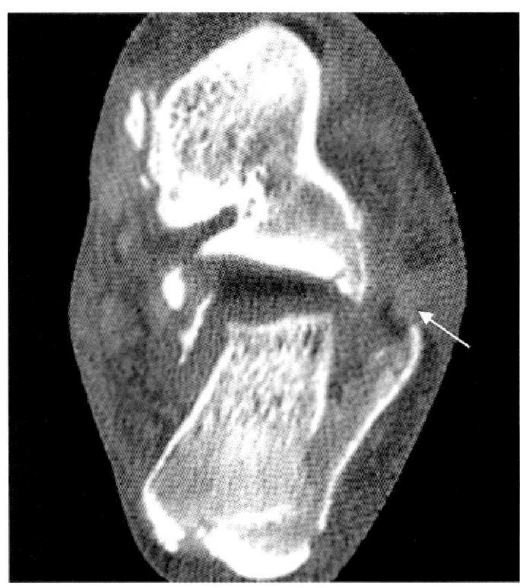

Fig. 20: Lateral wall explosion is often part of the fracture complex.

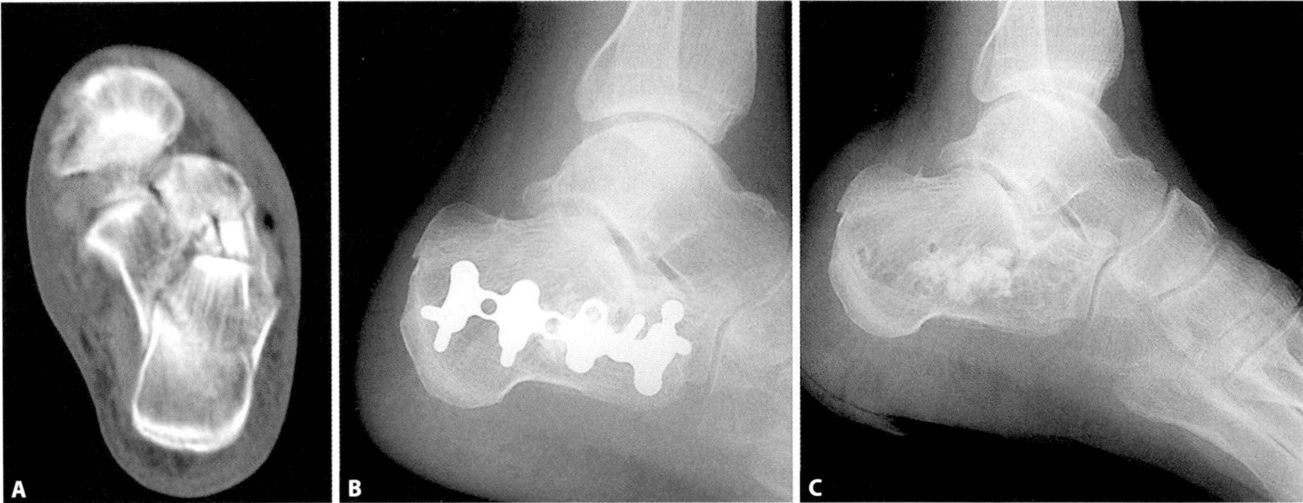

Figs. 21A to C: Calcaneum fracture treated with surgical reconstruction and ceramic augmentation at implant removal after 1 year.

■ REFERENCES

1. Harty M. Anatomic considerations in injuries of the calcaneus. Orthop Clin North Am. 1973;4:179-83.
2. Fitzgibbons T, McMullen ST, Mormino MA. Fractures and dislocations of the calcaneus. In: Bucholz RW, Heckman JD (Eds). Rockwood and Green's Fractures in Adults. Philadelphia, PA: Lippincott Williams & Wilkins; 2001. pp. 2133-79.
3. Gray H. Anatomy of the Human Body. Philadelphia, PA: Lea & Febiger; 1918.
4. Carr JB. Mechanism and pathoanatomy of the intraarticular calcaneal fracture. Clin Orthop Relat Res. 1993;290:36-40.
5. Burdeaux BD. Reduction of calcaneal fractures by the McReynolds medial approach technique and its experimental basis. Clin Orthop Relat Res. 1983;177:87-103.
6. Buckwalter KA, Rydberg J, Kopecky KK, Crow K, Yang EL. Musculoskeletal imaging with multi-slice CT. AJR Am J Roentgenol. 2001;176:979-86.
7. Linsenmaier U, Brunner U, Schöning A, Rieger J, Krötz M, Mutschler W, et al. Classification of calcaneal fractures by spiral computed tomography: implications for surgical treatment. Eur Radiol. 2003;13:2315-22.
8. Carr JB, Hamilton JJ, Bear LS. Experimental intra-articular calcaneal fractures: anatomic basis for a new classification. Foot Ankle. 1989;10:81-7.
9. Eastwood DM, Phipp L. Intra-articular fractures of the calcaneum: why such controversy? Injury. 1997;28:247-59.
10. Essex-Lopresti P. The mechanism, reduction technique, and results in fractures of the os calcis. Br J Surg. 1952;39: 395-419.
11. Myerson M, Manoli A. Compartment syndromes of the foot after calcaneal fractures. Clin Orthop Relat Res. 1993;290:142-50.
12. Paley D, Hall H. Calcaneal fracture controversies: can we put Humpty Dumpty together again? Orthop Clin North Am. 1989;20:665-77.
13. Sanders R, Fortin P, DiPasquale T, Walling A. Operative treatment in 120 displaced intraarticular calcaneal fractures:

results using a prognostic computed tomography scan classification. Clin Orthop Relat Res. 1993;290:87-95.

14. Crosby LA, Fitzgibbons T. Computerized tomography scanning of acute intra-articular fractures of the calcaneus: a new classification system. J Bone Joint Surg Am. 1990;72:852-9.

15. Sanders R, Gregory P. Operative treatment of intra-articular fractures of the calcaneus. Orthop Clin North Am. 1995;26:203-14.

16. Sanders R. Intra-articular fractures of the calcaneus: present state of the art. J Orthop Trauma. 1992;6:252-65.

17. Zwipp H, Tscherne H, Thermann H, Weber T. Osteosynthesis of displaced intraarticular fractures of the calcaneus: results in 123 cases. Clin Orthop Relat Res. 1993;(290):76-86.

18. Furey A, Stone C, Squire D, Harnett J. Os calcis fractures: analysis of interobserver variability in using Sanders classification. J Foot Ankle Surg. 2003;42:21-3.

19. Trnka HJ, Zettl R, Ritschl P. Fracture of the anterior superior process of the calcaneus: an often misdiagnosed fracture. Arch Orthop Trauma Surg. 1998;117:300-2.

20. Kathol MH, el-Khoury GY, Moore TE, Marsh JL. Calcaneal insufficiency avulsion fractures in patients with diabetes mellitus. Radiology. 1991;180:725-9.

21. Squires B, Allen PE, Livingstone J, Atkins RM. Fractures of the tuberosity of the calcaneus. J Bone Joint Surg Br. 2001;83:55-61.

22. Bui-Mansfield LT, Clayton TL. Isolated bone infarct of the calcaneus after fracture. J Comput Assist Tomogr. 2010;34(6):958-60.

Imaging Techniques and Image Interpretation

Rajiv Shah, Sarvdeep Dhatt

"Treat the patient, not the X-ray".

–James M Hunter

"Diagnosis is not the end, but the beginning of practice".

–Martin H Fischer

■ INTRODUCTION

The calcaneus is a bone with a typical shape which is unlike any other in the body; added to that are the multiple articulating surfaces which make interpretation of imaging fairly difficult. For precise interpretation of radiological imaging, a thorough knowledge of the anatomy of bone as well as radiological angles formed with the surrounding bones is essential. It is only after precise analysis of radiology that the surgeon can understand the fracture type, pattern, and displacements, which are essential to formulate the management plan. Multiple factors influence this, principal among which are the number of joints displaced by the fracture; degree of articular step as well as the size of joint displacement; and the overall deformation of the shape of the calcaneus by trauma.[1-3] The decision to be taken is whether to go ahead with conservative management options or to intervene surgically. Even during surgery, the exact determinants of displacements by radiology allow the surgeon to execute a step-by-step restoration of the anatomy. The imaging modalities commonly used are plain radiographs and computed tomography (CT) scanning, with a very limited role of more advanced procedures such as magnetic resonance imaging (MRI).

It is imperative to understand the normal trabecular architecture of the calcaneus as it is important for detecting subtle fractures on radiographs. Calcaneus has tensile and compressive trabeculae.[4]

■ COMPRESSIVE TRABECULAE

- *Thalamus:* It is a Greek word for room or chamber. These are the primary compressive trabeculae and extend from the articular surface of the subtalar joint to the cortex of the posterior tuberosity in a concave anteroinferior curve.
- *Anterior apophyseal:* These are the secondary compressive trabeculae. Curved trabeculations fan out from the region of the sinus tarsi anteroinferiorly to the anterior tuberosity.

■ TENSILE TRABECULAE

- *Inferior plantar:* These are the primary tensile trabeculae. Curved trabeculations extend from the inferior cortex to the cortex of the posterior tuberosity.
- *Anterior plantar:* These are the secondary tensile trabeculae. Trabeculations extend from the anterior part of the inferior cortex anterosuperiorly to the anterior tuberosity.
- *Posterior Achillean:* Also known as the tendo-tuberosity group, these tensile trabeculae run parallel to the posterior tuberosity.

Subtle disruptions in these trabecular patterns can alert you to the possibility of a fracture. Keats has also described a prominent trabeculation along the inferior aspect of the calcaneus on the lateral view that can simulate a stress fracture.

Ward's triangle is a lucent triangular window bounded superiorly by the primary and secondary compressive trabeculae and inferiorly by the tensile trabeculae. It may sometimes be mistaken for a lesion and is referred to as the pseudocyst or pseudolesion of the calcaneus.[5,6]

■ RADIOLOGICAL GOALS

Radiological goals in calcaneus fracture assessment are well defined; the first step is to decide whether the fracture is intra-articular or extra-articular as the management options are different for both types. In intra-articular fractures, the next question is evaluating the number of joints involved, the degree of joint depression, and the degree of displacement of the articular surfaces. It is also essential to determine the deformation of the overall shape of the bone and to assess the status of the medial and lateral walls of calcaneus as all these influence the surgical plan. Exact determination of fragment position, angulation, and displacement allows reduction planning; the degree of communition is also important for assessment, together with information about the quality of the bone itself.

■ PLAIN RADIOGRAPHY

Plain X-rays are the most common primarily done investigation; many a time, it is sufficient by itself in giving satisfactory information. Plain X-ray film findings are so important that the findings of more advanced modalities such as CT are compared and correlated with the plain films. Some radiological views are mandatory and include the routine foot and ankle series, especially lateral view of hindfoot and anteroposterior (AP) and oblique views of the foot. A very important view is the Harris or axial view[7-9] and the standard ankle radiograph series. With the help of these views almost all fractures, subluxations, and/or dislocations can be diagnosed. Mortise view[7-9] may also be employed.

Specialized views are Broden's view[7-9] that visualizes the posterior articular facet of the subtalar joint, along with the subtalar view. Broden's view may be done in an acute setting and is always done intraoperatively. Rarely comparative views can be obtained; this is more required for comparative axial images.

Radiology should not be limited to the foot alone; calcaneus fractures arising out of high-velocity trauma or falls are often associated with concomitant injuries and imaging of spine, pelvis, ipsilateral lower limb as well as contralateral foot (in cases of clinical evidence) is also required.[9] In fact, lumbar spine radiographs should be obtained routinely. If radiographs reveal an intra-articular component, then CT scanning is indicated.[10] In the published literature, multiple other views for fracture calcaneus are described but these views are hard to read and are not consistently reproducible so as to be used routinely.[10,11]

Lateral View of Hindfoot

The hindfoot lateral view **(Fig. 1)** forms the most important diagnostic tool in the initial assessment of calcaneus fractures **(Figs. 2A to D)**. This view must include the lower end of tibia and fibula, along with the entire calcaneus and midfoot. This view shows the posterior facet and the relationship of calcaneus with the talus above. The lateral

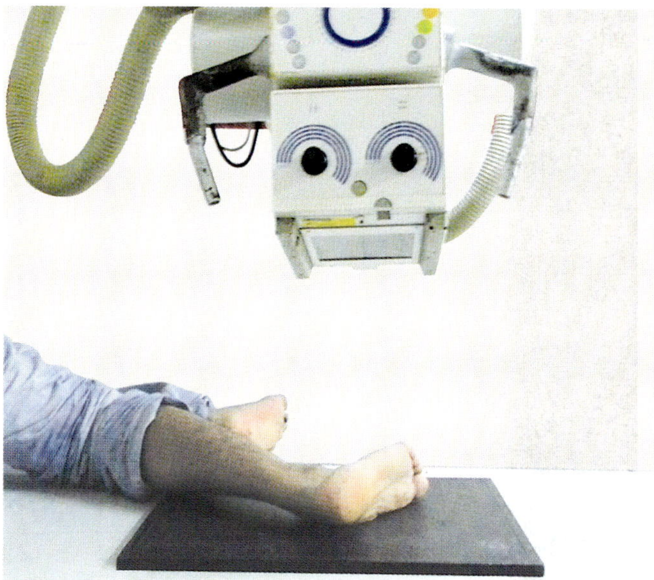

Fig. 1: Positioning of foot and X-ray beam for lateral view of the hindfoot.

process of talus is seen as a downward projection, and this V-shaped process marks the anterior border of the posterior facet.[7-9]

In the lateral view, two angles can easily be evaluated. The angle of Gissane **(Fig. 3A)** is the angle formed between the anterior aspect of the lateral calcaneal border and the lateral border of the posterior facet of calcaneus. Böhler's angle **(Fig. 3B)** is formed at the intersection of two lines; one line is drawn from the apex of posterior tuberosity to the apex of posterior facet, and the second line from the apex of anterior process to the apex of posterior articular facet. This angle usually measures between 20 and 40°.[7-9]

In a fractured calcaneus bone, the lateral view reveals loss of the posterior facet's height. The facet is impacted into the body of the calcaneus (which is shattered like an egg) and is also rotated anteriorly, thus reducing Böhler's angle. Gissane's angle will be increased in all cases where the posterior facet is separated from sustentaculum tali and is depressed.[10]

There can be presence of a radiological sign called "double density" sign.[7-9] In this sign, there is overlap of bony density at the level of the subtalar joint. This reflects partial facet separation and is suggestive of depression of the lateral part of the posterior articular facet only **(Fig. 4)**. In such a case, facet is also depressed but both Gissane's angle and Böhler's angle appear normal.[12]

The type of fracture, whether it is a tongue type or a joint depression type, can easily be noted with the help of lateral film. It is important to realize that in addition to facet displacement, the lateral view also gives an estimate

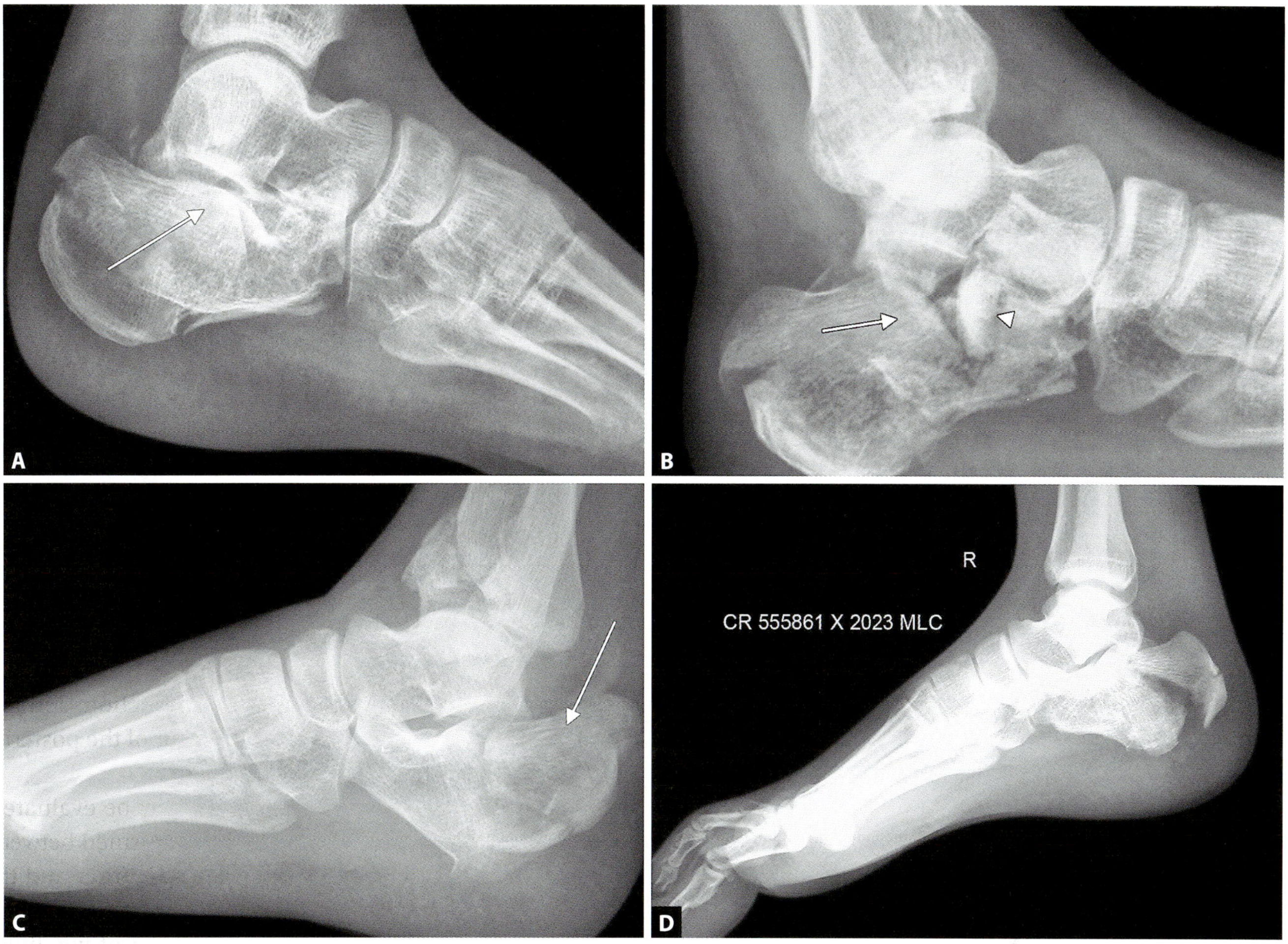

Figs. 2A to D: *Lateral X-rays:* (A) Tongue-type fracture with depressed, attached posterior facet (white arrow); (B) Tongue-type fracture (white arrow) with separated posterior facet in rotated and depressed position (arrowhead); (C) Tongue-type fracture with comminution of the tuberosity (arrow); (D) Avulsed tuberosity fragment.

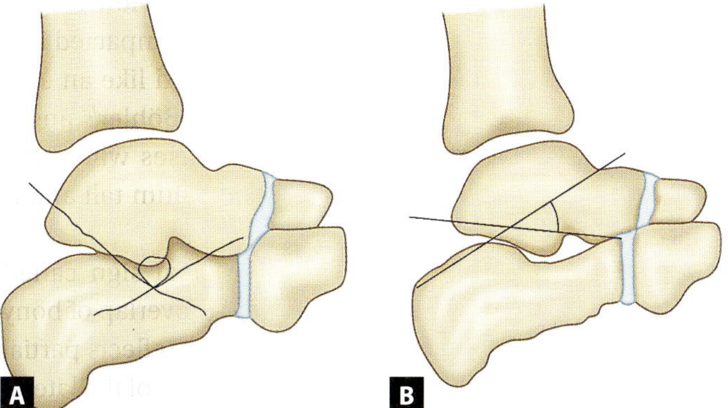

Figs. 3A and B: (A) Critical angle of Gissane; (B) Böhler's angle.

calcaneocuboid joint or not as this may have both therapeutic and prognostic implications.[13]

The most difficult extra-articular fracture to diagnose is a fracture of the anterior process of calcaneus.[5] This fracture is best evaluated in lateral and oblique views. This fracture can be easily overlooked because of overlap and demands a high degree of suspicion. If not diagnosed in time, it can lead to nonunion.[6]

Anteroposterior and Oblique Views of Foot

Anteroposterior and oblique views of foot are important to note or detect anterior extension of fracture line and involvement of calcaneocuboid joint. The AP view **(Fig. 5)** shows calcaneocuboid, calcaneotalar, and calcaneonavicular articulations. The medial oblique view is done with the medial foot surface touching the X-ray cassette and the foot is angled 30–45° inward. This view delineates the third to fifth foot ray and the calcaneocuboid and calcaneonavicular

of the length and height of the calcaneus. In this view, the displaced bony fragments may act like protruded bone, and the protrusions to be noted are plantar and posteriorly located bony prominences. This view also shows whether any fracture line is extending into the anteriorly located

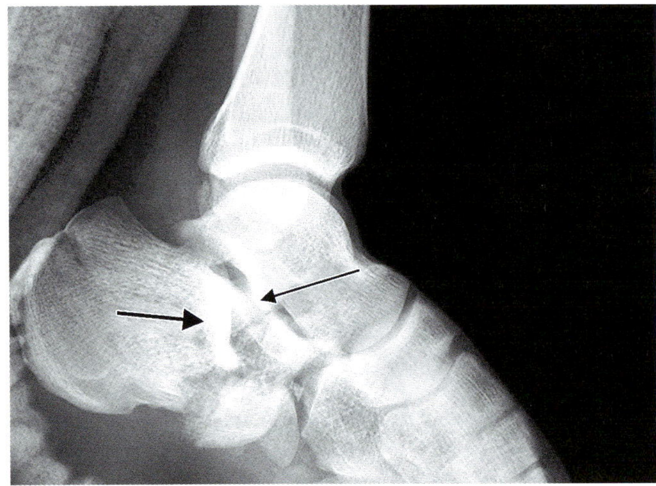

Fig. 4: Lateral X-ray of hindfoot showing a double-density sign of the depressed part of posterior facet (arrows).

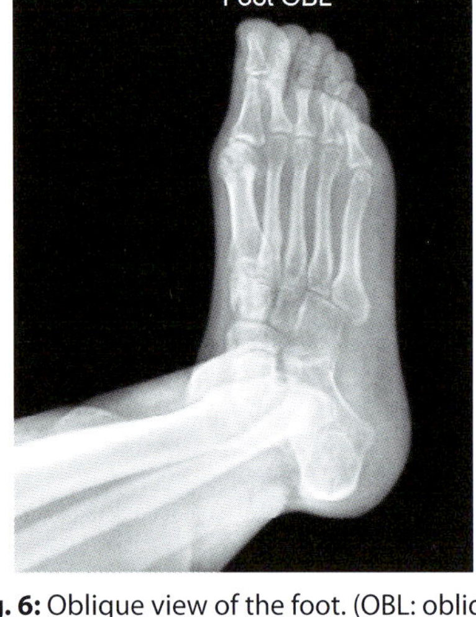

Fig. 6: Oblique view of the foot. (OBL: oblique)

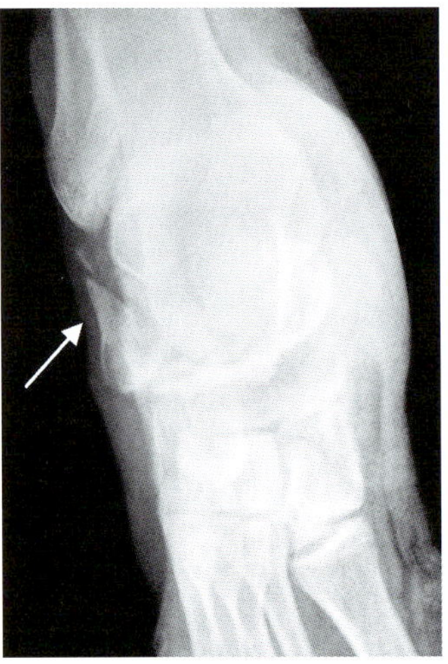

Fig. 5: Anteroposterior view of the foot showing fracture of the anterior end of calcaneus and involvement of the calcaneocuboid joint. The arrow is pointing to displaced fracture fragment from anterior process of calcaneus.

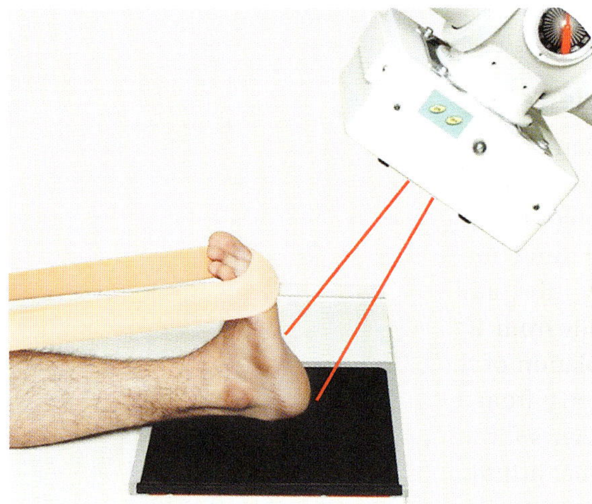

Fig. 7: Harris axial view—positioning of the foot and the X-ray beam.

articulations **(Fig. 6)**. Anterior process fractures can be detected from these X-ray views very clearly.[7-9]

Harris Axial View[7-9]

Harris axial view is perhaps one of the most important radiograph in assessing calcaneal fractures and was an invaluable aid prior to the easy availability of CT scans. The patient is sitting or lying and foot is held at 90° of dorsiflexion; the X-ray beam is then angled cranially to 40° and is focused at the base of metatarsals **(Fig. 7)**. The medial and lateral calcaneal walls, subtalar joints, and calcaneal alignment can be well seen in this view **(Figs. 8A to C)**. This view also demonstrates the position of sustentaculum tali. Sustentacular fractures can be detected very easily through this examination. The amount of heel broadening and heel shortening can also be assessed through Harris view. The lateral or medial bony protrusions can also be noted easily in these views. An underemphasized fact is the angulation of the posterior calcaneal body fragment, which is mainly into varus.[14] The biggest disadvantage in the acute setting is obtaining this view as patient positioning can be difficult because of pain.

Comparative X-Rays

Comparative Harris views are the best for assessing the integrity of fracture. This view shows precise comparison for assessing height, breadth, medial, and lateral blow out of the affected/fractured bone.[8]

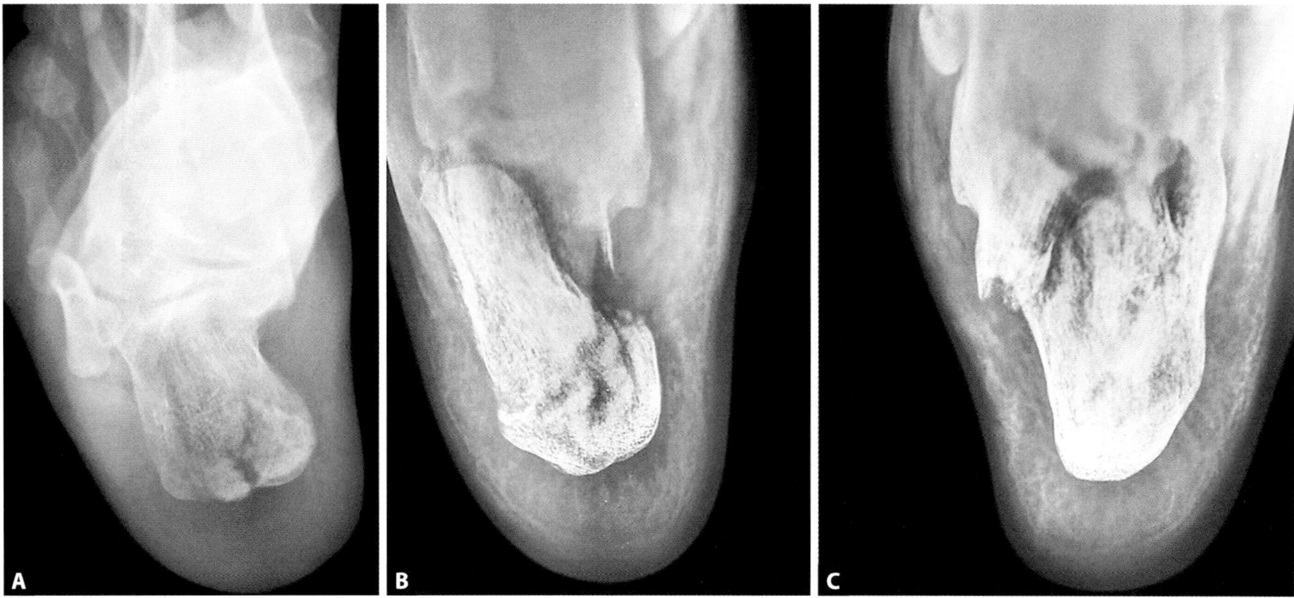

Figs. 8A to C: Harris axial view—X-ray. (A) Heel varus; (B and C) X-rays showing bilateral calcaneus fracture with different patterns of injury.

Broden's View[7-9]

Broden's view is a special view, which delineates the posterior facet very clearly. The foot is rotated to 30–40° of internal rotation and the X-ray beam is centered on the lateral malleolus, is fired with a cranially angled X-ray tube, and the position of the X-ray tube is shifted serially from 40°, 30°, 20°, and 10° **(Figs. 9 and 10)**. As the angulation of the tube changes, the entire posterior facet is shown from anterior to posterior. This view is one of the key views for intraoperative evaluation. In the absence of subtalar arthroscopic examination, subtalar joint reduction assessment intraoperatively is best done through these views. The most important fact with this view is its uniformity and easy reproducibility.

Mortise View

Mortise view is used to delineate the posterior facet and the entire talus **(Fig. 11)**. This is easily done even in an acute setting without causing much pain to the injured foot and demonstrates the posterior facet nicely.

▌ IMAGING OF UNCOMMON EXTRA-ARTICULAR FRACTURES

Fracture of the anterior process of calcaneus is visualized only on oblique view of the foot and is a very commonly missed injury. Tuberosity fractures are also seen more commonly on the lateral view of ankle. Complex fracture dislocations are best demonstrated in routine foot and ankle series views. Avulsion fractures of the posterior angle of calcaneus can also be diagnosed by these X-rays.[6]

Tomograms

Tomograms are rarely required these days as they have been replaced by CT scans.[9] They do not provide any additional information and in fact may fail to show the real extent of articular incongruity and expose the patient to increased dosage of radiation.

Computed Tomography Scan

Availability of CT scan and three-dimensional (3D) reconstructions has revolutionized our understanding of calcaneus fractures. In fact, the CT scan has even allowed outcome assessment and analysis of treatment as this can easily be done postoperatively. Adequate details of all calcaneal articulations are seen with CT scans, and these provide clear information about the various fracture lines, joint surface integrity, and intra-articular fragments. These are essential for all intra-articular fractures.[10-12]

Thinner slices up to 2–3 mm are ideal. CT scans are obtained in the axial, 30° semicoronal, and sagittal planes. For oblique coronal images, the gantry needs to be tilted to 90°, and excellent information with regards to posterior facet and sustentaculum tali can then be obtained. Axial cuts show extension of fracture lines; sagittal cuts show displacement of tuberosity, posterior facet, and anterolateral fragments. These cuts demarcate tongue-type fractures from joint depression-type injuries; 30° semicoronal views show displacements of articular fragments of the posterior facet and sustentacular fragments if any. This view also shows lateral wall widening, shortening of bone, and displacement of body. Thus, with the help of these images, one can classify

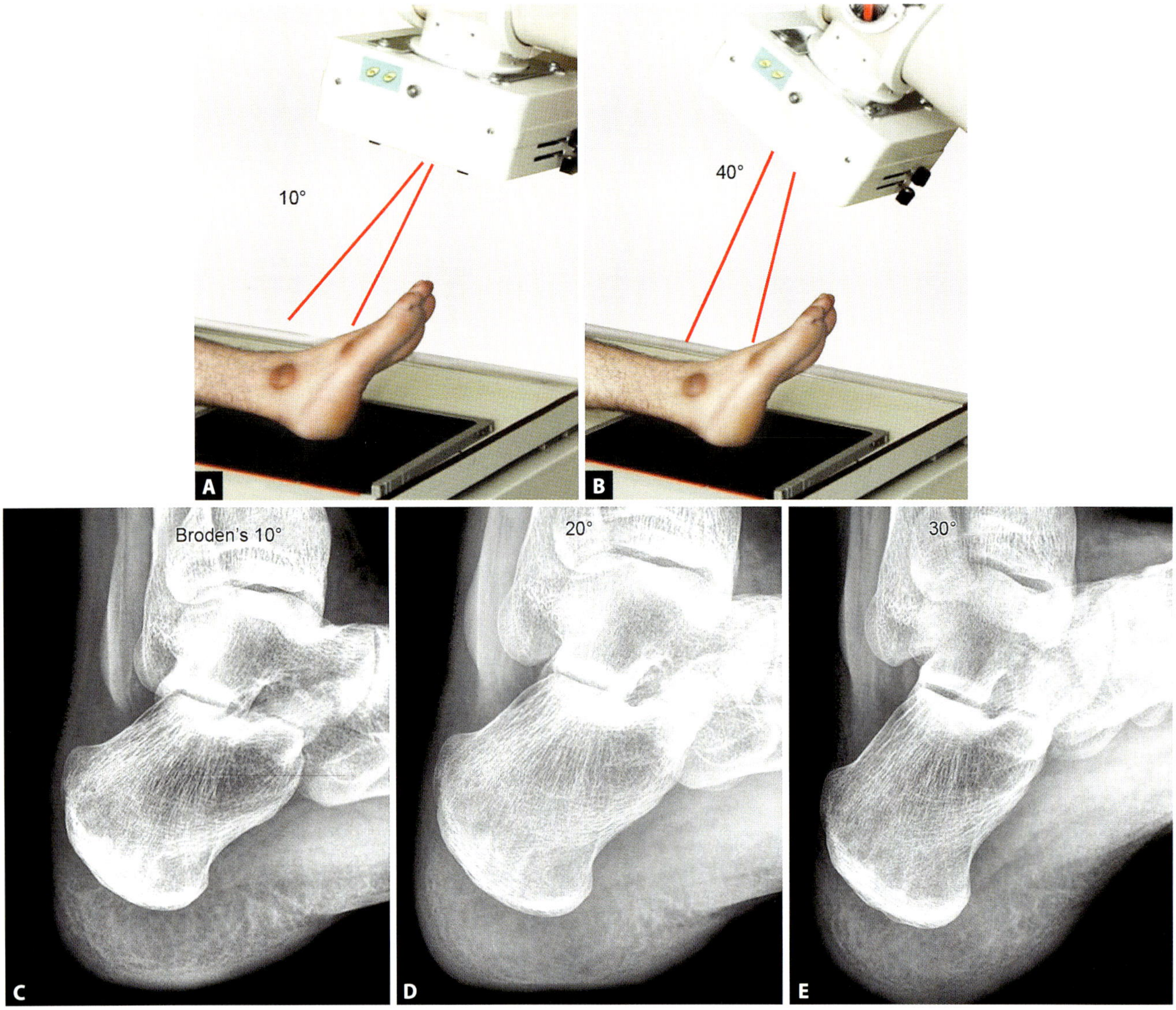

Figs. 9A to E: Broden's view. (A and B) Foot and X-ray beam positioning; (C to E) three images.

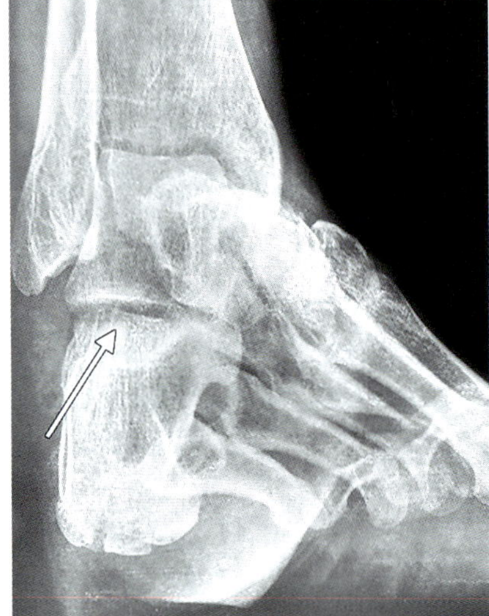

Fig. 10: Broden's view. The arrow is pointing to displcaed articular facet of calcaneus.

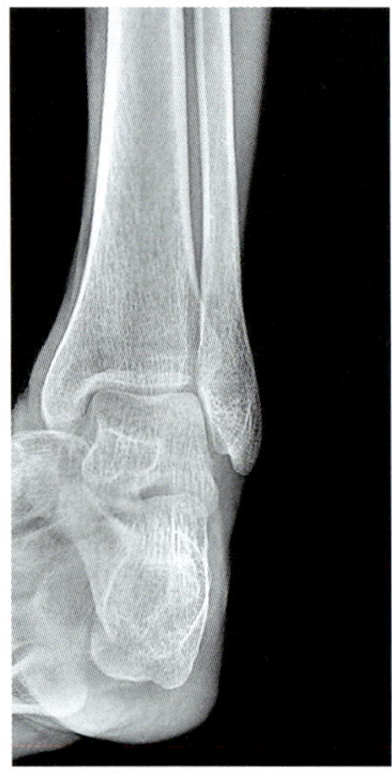

Fig. 11: Mortise view.

the fracture and also devise a plan of management with operative steps **(Figs. 12 and 13)**.

Three-dimensional reconstructions can give a better idea about fracture fragments and their positioning to make operative planning easy.[10-12]

■ RADIOLOGY INTERPRETATION

From various available imaging modalities, the following radiological parameters are analyzed.

Angles

The tuber angle of Böhler is formed between a line drawn from the highest point of the anterior process of the calcaneus to the highest point of posterior facet and a line drawn tangential to the superior edge of the tuberosity of calcaneus. This angle is normally between 20 and 40°. Any reduction in this angle suggests collapse of the posterior weight-bearing articular facet of calcaneus.

The crucial angle of Gissane is formed by two strong cortical struts extending laterally; one along the lateral margin of the posterior facet and the other extending anterior to the beak of the calcaneus. This obtuse angle is seen directly beneath the lateral process of the talus.

The triangle formed anteriorly between traction trabeculae from the inferior cortex of calcaneus and compression trabeculae from posterior and anterior articular facets is known as the neutral triangle and is an indication of the degree of osteoporosis.

Fracture Lines

Fracture lines are important to note while looking at radiological images. The fracture lines could be primary and secondary, and the development of these lines depends on the amount and direction of deforming force applied to the bone.[5,13] The extension of these lines depends on the position of the foot at the time of trauma. The primary fracture line runs laterally from the lateral process of talus to extend medially and sometimes may run anteriorly to exit from the anterior process or through the calcaneocuboid joint. A secondary fracture line may continue posteriorly into the posterior facet, producing a joint depression type of fracture. If the initial force was directed axially, a tongue-type fracture will be produced. Many a time, two primary

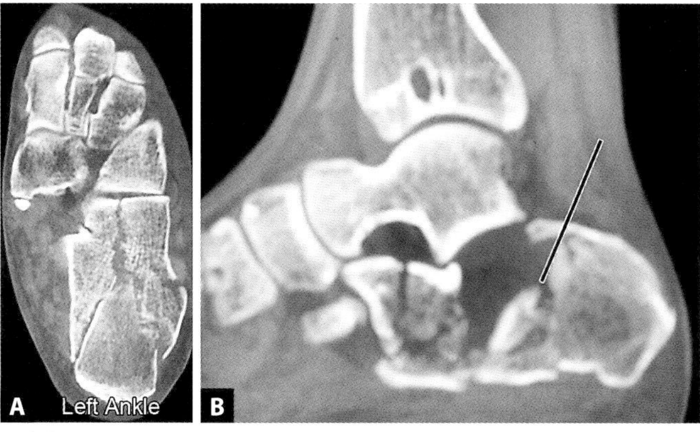

Figs. 12A and B: (A) Computed tomography (CT) scan coronal section showing fracture line at subtalar joint and burst lateral wall; (B) CT scan showing depressed and rotated facet fragment and burst lateral wall.

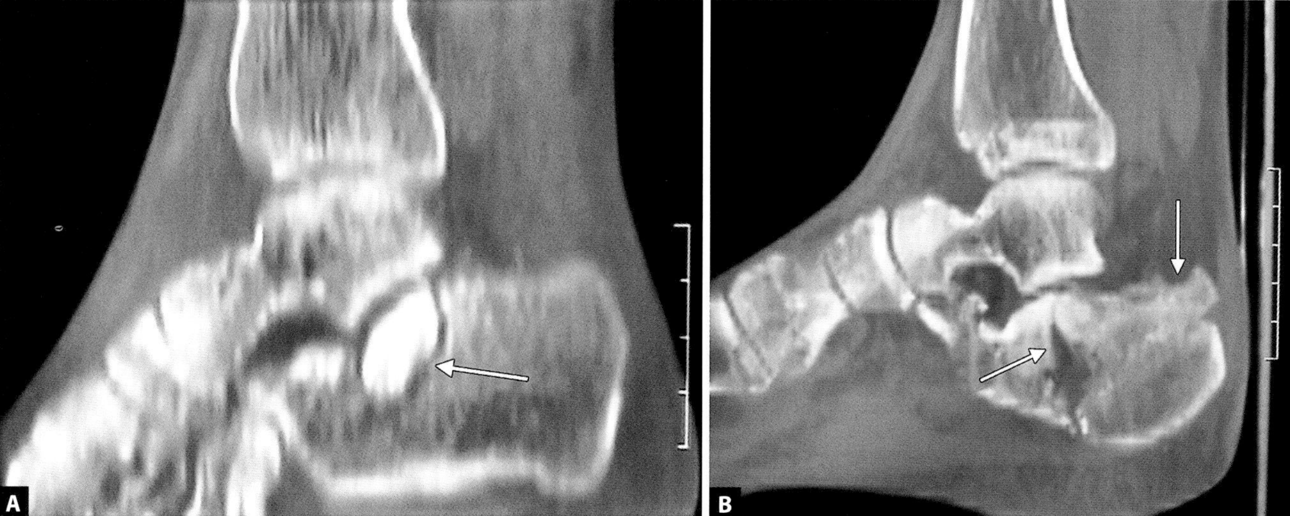

Figs. 13A and B: (A) Computed tomography (CT) scan sagittal section showing depressed rotated posterior facet segment; (B) CT scan sagittal section showing avulsed tuberosity/tongue-type fracture and fracture lines through the subtalar joint.

fracture lines may be noted, making this a combination of fracture patterns, with both tongue type and joint depression type being seen in one bone. CT scan is the best guide for assessing all these fracture lines.

Joints

Two joints are looked at with focus on two major articular surfaces of the calcaneus; these are anteriorly located calcaneocuboid joint and posteriorly located talocalcaneal or subtalar joint. The surfaces are evaluated for comminution and depression. Various CT scan views demonstrate joint integrity much better than plain films.

Shape and Size

Another important parameter to be assessed is the shape and size of calcaneus. The height and width are looked at to assess whether the bone is broadened in transverse plane and is shortened vertically or not.

Heel Position

Noting the position of heel, whether in varus (medially angulated) or in valgus (laterally angulated), helps in deciding the intraoperative corrective maneuvers.

Bony Walls

The medial and lateral walls of calcaneus are assessed for comminution, displacement, and blowout. Lateral wall displacement may damage the surrounding structures such as peroneal tendons and the calcaneofibular ligament. Medial wall displacement may damage structures such as posterior tibial nerve and the tendon of flexor hallucis longus.

Sustentaculum Tali

The position and comminution of sustentaculum tali are important to assess as this is the strongest part of calcaneus and forms the base on to which the reduction of the lateral part of the depressed posterior facet is based during surgical fixation.

Fragments

Fragment-specific diagnosis is important as and it comprises of noting the number of fragments, their displacement direction, angulations, and position. This helps in operative management. Fragments could be located plantarward, posteriorly and medially. Taking note of this is essential for accurate intraoperative correction and helps to prevent malunion.

Bone Quality and Degree of Comminution

A general note of osteoporosis and osteopenia is made on the initial radiographs. This has a huge bearing on fixation techniques. The amount of comminution decides the treatment option and CT scan is the best guide for the same. Those highly comminuted osteoporotic fractures may need supervised neglect or primary arthrodesis.

Classification

The basic radiological fracture classification is either extra-articular or intra-articular type. It may as well be subclassified as tongue-type, joint depression type, or a mixed fracture. A CT scan-based classification described by Zwipp et al.[15] can also be used to better understand the injury pattern. An articular fracture-based classification described by Sanders et al.[10,11] may also be used on coronal plane CT images **(Fig. 14)**.

This classification is based on coronal CT scan cuts. The section showing the widest undersurface of the posterior facet of the talus was arbitrarily used. The talus was divided into three equal columns by two lines. These lines and a third line, located just medial to the medial edge of the posterior facet, divide the posterior facet into three potential pieces: A medial, a central, and a lateral fragment. These fragments and the sustentaculum comprised a total of four potential articular pieces.

All nondisplaced articular fractures, irrespective of the number of fracture lines, are considered as type I fractures.

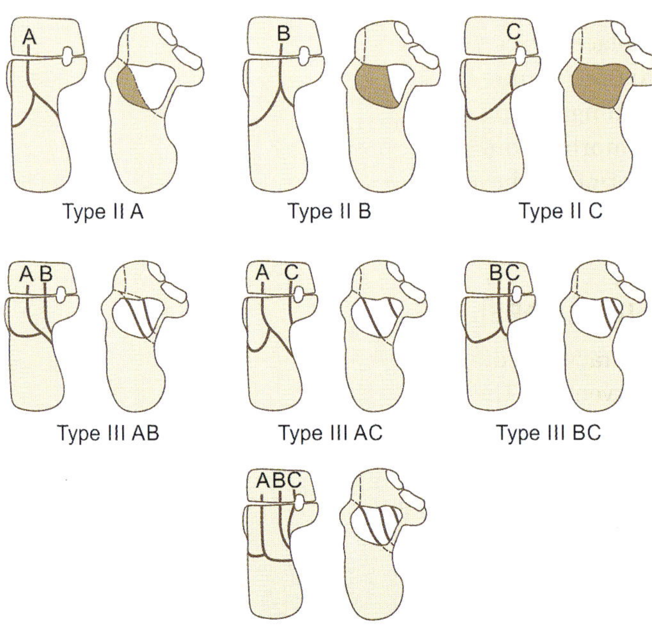

Fig. 14: Classification of intra-articular calcaneal fractures according to Sanders et al.[10,11]

Type II fractures are defined as two-part fractures of the posterior facet. Further, it is subdivided into three subtypes, IIA, IIB, and IIC, based on the location of the primary fracture line.

Type III fractures consisted of three-part fractures characterized by a centrally depressed fragment, similar to a split depressed fracture of the tibial plateau or a die-punch fracture of the distal part of the radius; subtypes included IIIAB, IIIAC, and IIIBC.

Type IV fractures, or four-part articular fractures, were highly comminuted and often had more than four articular fragments.

It is by radiological evaluation of above-listed points that the fracture is easily classified.

RADIOLOGY INTERPRETATION AND ITS ROLE IN MANAGEMENT

The next step is to choose the right method of treatment (closed manipulation and plaster immobilization, minimally invasive fixation, or open reduction and internal fixation), and this too is decided by radiological parameters, in addition to clinical assessment and other patient-related factors. Factors such as age, general condition of patient, associated premorbid conditions, soft tissue and neurovascular status, and associated injuries also dictate the treatment line over and above radiological parameters, and they must be considered together with imaging assessment.

By and large, a majority of extra-articular fractures can be treated conservatively, provided the displacement is not significant. On the other hand, a majority of intra-articular displaced fractures will need open reduction and internal fixation. Minimally invasive methods may be reserved for tongue-type fractures and fractures with associated premorbid conditions. A surgical plan for correction of deformities, the sequential reduction steps, and the fixation techniques can also be formulated based on the radiological information.

INTRAOPERATIVE RADIOLOGY

Accuracy of reduction should be monitored during surgical intervention. The surgeon must be aware of the techniques of various intraoperative radiological imaging. The reduction may be either closed, minimally invasive, or open; precise imaging is deemed for the best outcome. With a patient positioned in a lateral decubitus position, the following four necessary images are needed during surgical intervention.

Lateral View

The patient is positioned in a lateral decubitus position with the affected limb over the top. The image intensifier is positioned diagonally. AP imaging yields a lateral view of the heel **(Fig. 15)**.

Axial View

In the same position of the patient, the image intensifier is rotated laterally. The assistant pulls the toes into dorsiflexion with a bandage sling to yield precise axial imaging **(Video 1)**.

Broden's View

The patient's affected limb is moved into 45° of external rotation with a cranial tilting of the image intensifier to 10°, 20°, 30°, and 40°, where the beam is centered over the tip of

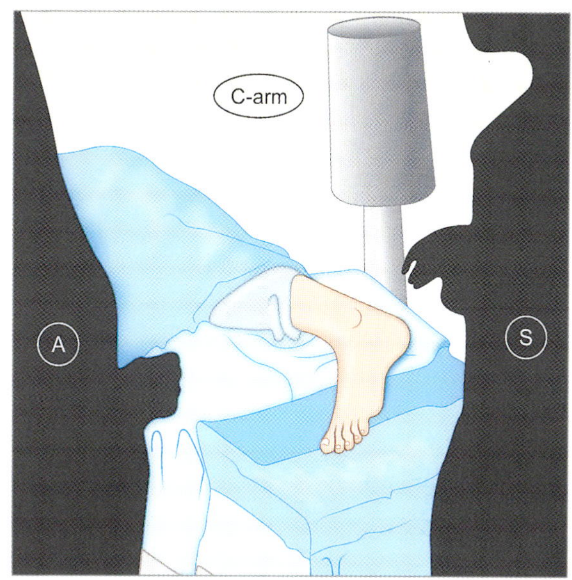

Fig. 15: Intraoperative, anteroposterior positioning of image intensifier (C-arm) to procure a lateral view of the calcaneus. (A: assistant; S: surgeon)

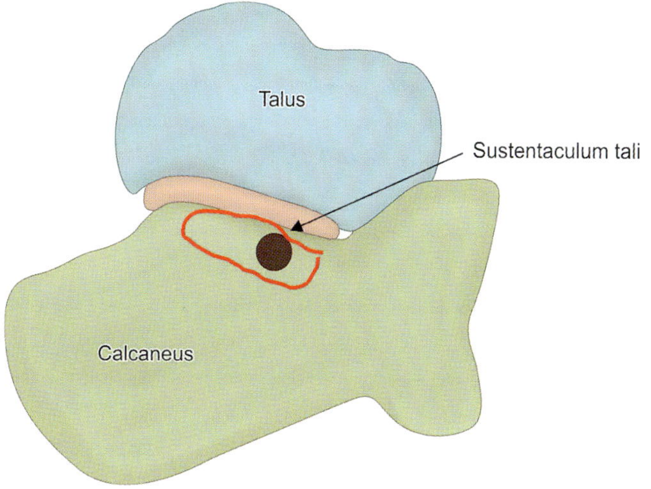

Fig. 16: Diagrammatic picture of the sustentacular view.

the lateral malleolus. Precise sequential delineation of the entire posterior subtalar joint is obtained **(Videos 2A and B)**.

Sustentacular View

During surgery, the surgeon needs to have a precise trajectory of sustentaculum tali. A sustentacular view yields this trajectory **(Fig. 16)**. The view is procured by turning the image intensifier to 30° externally **(Video 3)**.

■ REFERENCES

1. Essex-Lopresti P. The mechanism, reduction technique, and results in fractures of the os calcis. Br J Surg. 1952;39:395-419.
2. Lindsay WR, Dewar FP. Fractures of the os calcis. Am J Surg. 1958;95:555-76.
3. Palmer I. The mechanism and treatment of fractures of the calcaneus: open reduction with the use of cancellous grafts. J Bone Joint Surg Am. 1948;30A:2-8.
4. Guyer BH, Levinsohn EM, Fredrickson BE, Bailey GL, Formikell M. Computed tomography of calcaneal fractures: anatomy, pathology, dosimetry, and clinical relevance. Am J Roentgenol. 1985;145:911-9.
5. Heger L, Wulff K, Seddiqi MS. Computed tomography of calcaneal fractures. Am J Roentgenol. 1985;145:131-7.
6. Utukuri MM, Knowles D, Smith KL, Barrie JL, Gavan D. The value of the axial view in assessing calcaneal fractures. Injury. 2000;31(5):325-6.
7. Isherwood I. A radiological approach to the subtalar joint. J Bone Joint Surg Br. 1961;43:566-74.
8. Bontrager KL. Textbook of Radiographic Positioning and Related Anatomy, 5th edition. St Louis, MO: Mosby; 2001.
9. Brian PL, Mahraj RPM. Imaging of the calcaneus. Foot Ankle Clin. 2005;10:443-61.
10. Sanders R. Displaced intra-articular fractures of the calcaneus. J Bone Joint Surg Am. 2000;82:225-50.
11. Sanders R, Fortin P, DiPasquale T, Walling A. Operative treatment in 120 displaced intraarticular calcaneal fractures. Results using a prognostic computed tomography scan classification. Clin Orthop Relat Res. 1993;(290):87-95.
12. Swanson SA, Clare MP, Sanders RW. Management of intra-articular fractures of the calcaneus. Foot Ankle Clin. 2008;13:659-78.
13. Barei DP, Bellabarba C, Sangeorzan BJ, Benirschke SK. Fractures of the calcaneus. Orthop Clin North Am. 2002;33:236-85.
14. Juliano P, Nguyen HV. Fractures of the calcaneus. Orthop Clin North Am. 2001;32:35-51.
15. Zwipp H, Tscherne H, Thermann H, Weber T. Osteosynthesis of displaced intraarticular fractures of the calcaneus: results in 123 cases. Clin Orthop Relat Res. 1993;(290):76-86.

5

Fracture Classification

Richard E Buckley, Sandeep Patel

"A classification is useful only if it considers the severity of the bone lesion and serves as a basis for treatment and evaluation of the results".

–Professor Maurice Müller

■ INTRODUCTION

Fractures of the calcaneus are relatively rare injuries. They represent only 1.2% of all fractures in adult population.[1] The calcaneus is the most frequently fractured tarsal bone[2] and through the years has received considerable attention from orthopedic surgeons. This is due to the fact that this fracture represents a life-changing injury that mainly affects young active people.[3] The burden to society is significant, with the socioeconomic impact being substantial in terms of days away from work and recreation.[4] Additionally, the management when indirect costs are included appears to be high regardless of operative or nonoperative treatment.[4]

Classification systems in orthopedic trauma surgery serve as tools for identifying fracture patterns, establishing treatment guidelines, and determining the prognosis of an injury. Furthermore, they facilitate data collection and presentation, thus allowing accurate communication among orthopedic surgeons in everyday clinical practice and research.[5] Historically, the first attempts to describe and classify calcaneus fractures were made by Malgaigne in 1843[6] and Hoffa in 1888.[7] Böhler[8] and Palmer[9] followed with their classifications in 1931 and 1948, respectively. Despite the low incidence of calcaneus fractures in the general population, >40 classifications have been described and presented in the orthopedic literature.[10] Most of these classification schemes are not currently in use and are considered to be of historical value. Nevertheless, it should not be forgotten that the historic value of these classifications is priceless. The numerous classification systems can be categorized as being developed before the computed tomography (CT) scans were popular and those after CT scans were commonplace. Nineteen conventional radiographic classifications have been used at least once since 1980, and another 15 are CT

based and are considered contemporary.[10] On the contrary, there are 30 systems left unused or only mentioned in the literature after 1980.[10] In addition to clinically developed classifications, there are two systems that were developed based upon cadaveric models.[11,12] The involvement of the posterior facet determines whether the fracture is extra- or intra-articular. Extra-articular fractures include the tuberosity fracture, the sustentaculum fracture, the anterior process fracture, and the anterior avulsion fracture.[13]

The success of each classification system is measured by defining its reliability and validity. The reliability refers to interobserver reliability and reflects the precision, i.e., the agreement between different observers. The validity measures the accuracy of a classification system and is reflected in intraobserver reliability. This means that a good classification system for calcaneus fractures would be one in which multiple surgeons could classify a fracture as a "type A" (interobserver reliability), and the intraoperative findings would confirm that the type of fracture is indeed a "type A" (validity or intraobserver reliability).[5]

■ EXTRA-ARTICULAR FRACTURES

The extra-articular fractures represent up to 60% of calcaneal fractures in children, and their incidence has been reported to be 25–40% of adult calcaneal fractures.[3,13-16] According to the mechanism of injury, they can generally be classified as compression or avulsion fractures. Another classification scheme categorizes them according to their location in calcaneus. See **Flowchart 1** for the classification of extra-articular fractures.

Fitzgibbons et al. have classified extra-articular fractures into anterior process, middle calcaneal (body, sustentaculum, peroneal tubercle, and lateral tubercle),

Flowchart 1: Classification of extra-articular fractures.

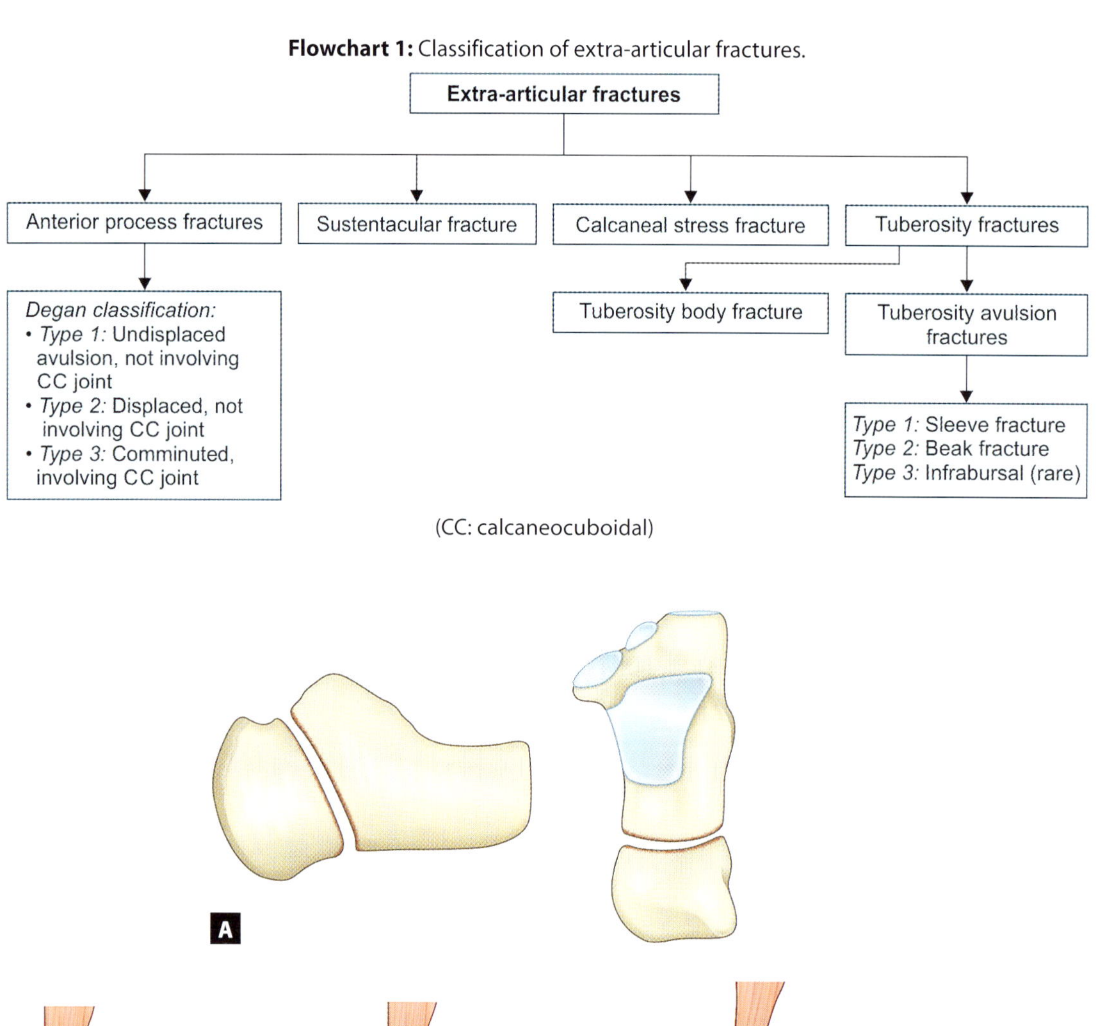

Figs. 1A to D: (A) Tuberosity body fracture; (B to D) Various types of tuberosity avulsion fractures: (B) Type I; (C) Type II; (D) Type III.

and posterior calcaneal (tuberosity and medial tubercle) fractures.[17]

The tuberosity fractures (**Figs. 1A to D**) are usually avulsion fractures and of the following types:

- *Type I:* "Sleeve fracture"—represents a sleeve of posterior tuberosity that has been avulsed from the pull of the gastrocnemius muscle.
- *Type II:* "Beak fracture"—with avulsion of the entire posterosuperior part of the tuberosity. Type II fracture is also referred to as the "extreme tongue-type" fracture[18] (**Fig. 2**).

- *Type III:* "Infrabursal avulsion fracture"—has been recently described as an infrabursal avulsion fracture of the middle third of the posterior tuberosity.[19]

The common denominator of these fractures apart from the mechanism of injury is that they occur in elderly osteopenic patients.[19] Furthermore, an extra-articular avulsion fracture that happens in the neuropathic Charcot foot has been well described in the literature.[13,20,21]

The sustentaculum is considered an extra-articular fracture (**Figs. 3A and B**), although it includes the middle facet of the subtalar joint.[22] Its incidence is 26% of all calcaneal

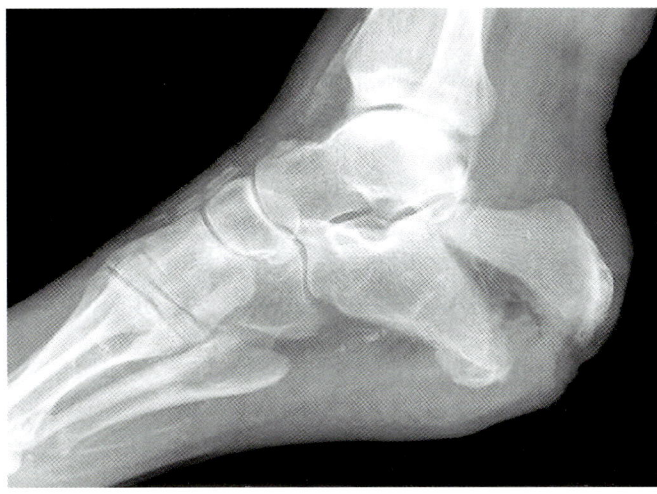

Fig. 2: Lateral radiograph demonstrating the so-called beak fracture. This type of fracture is notorious for skin complications if left untreated.

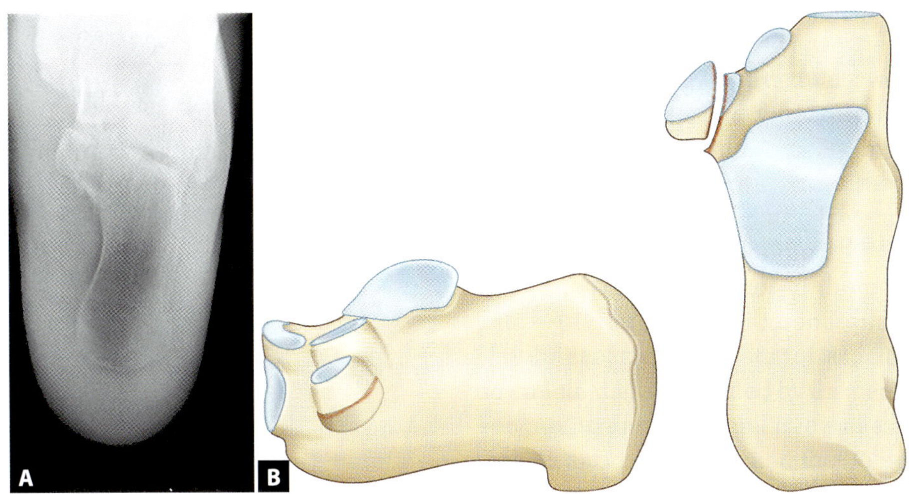

Figs. 3A and B: (A) Axial radiograph (Harris view) image shows an isolated sustentaculum fracture; (B) Line diagram depicting the fracture.

fractures, and it seems to be higher than previously thought.[3] Rowe included fractures of sustentaculum, anterior process, and tuberosity in one category.[23] It probably represents a high-energy injury that occurs with other varus loaded hindfoot and ankle trauma, and usually a talus fracture.[22,23]

Calcaneus stress fractures **(Fig. 4)** are also extra-articular fractures, and a detailed discussion of stress fractures is provided in Chapter 26.

The anterior process can fail either in compression or in avulsion and its fracture is accompanied by other foot injuries or preexisting deformities (calcaneonavicular coalition).[13] The Degan classification **(Figs. 5A to C)** describes three types according to the percentage of area

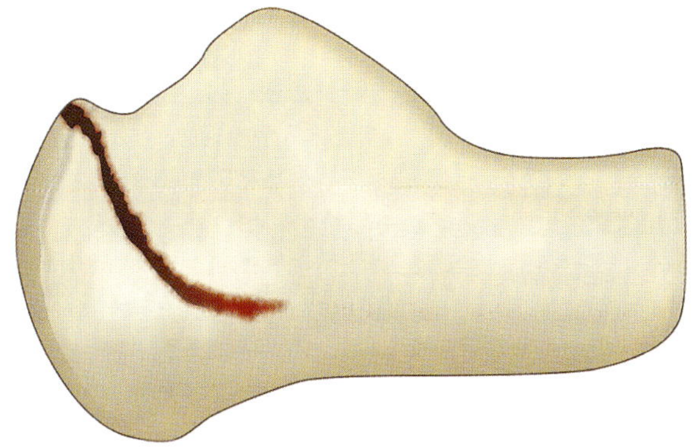

Fig. 4: Stress fracture of calcaneus, which is usually limited to the tuberosity and is often not seen on initial X-rays.

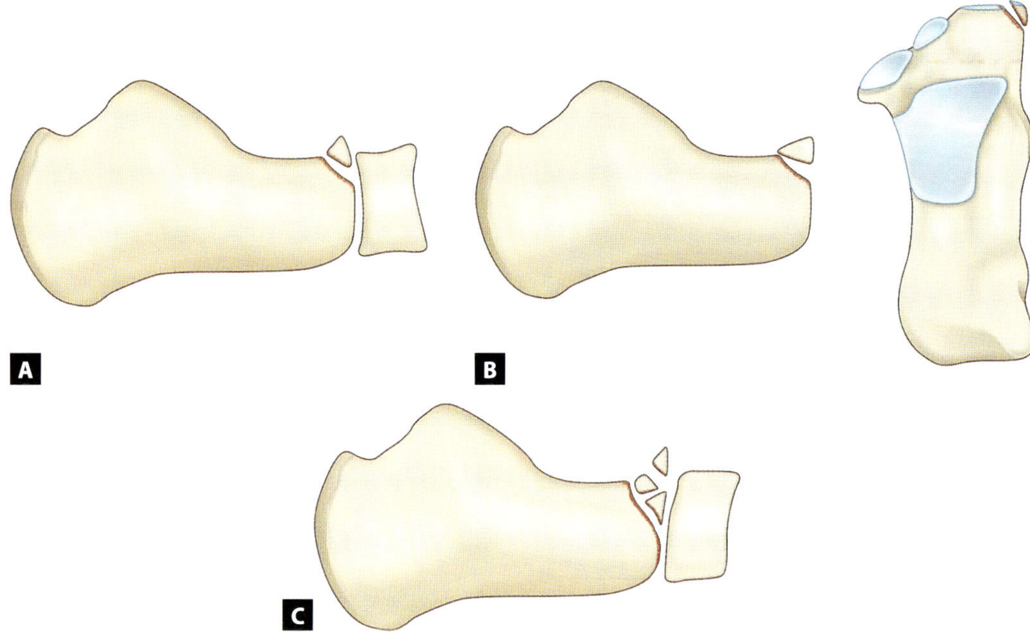

Figs. 5A to C: Degan classification showing the types of anterior process fractures: (A) Degan type I; (B) Degan type II; (C) Degan type III.

and displacement of the fractured anterior process and involvement of the calcaneocuboid joint.[24] A distinct type of injury that is not an anterior process fracture is the anterior avulsion fracture, which represents an avulsion of digitorum brevis muscle from the dorsolateral surface of the calcaneus and is commonly misdiagnosed as an ankle sprain.

■ BÖHLER CLASSIFICATION

In 1931, Dr Lorenz Böhler from Austria described the mechanism and the pathoanatomy of calcaneus fractures.[8] He did not describe the pattern of primary and secondary fracture lines that we currently appreciate as the typical pattern of fracture configuration, but he reported two fracture lines that split the bone in the longitudinal axis, leaving the sustentaculum in its place. He also recognized the lateral wall blowout and the consequent direction of major displacement. He was then able to describe the primary clinical deformity seen after these fractures, which is loss of height and broadening of the os calcis as well as the fragmentation and proximal displacement of the tuberosity that is usually seen. One of the major contributions of Dr Böhler's work in calcaneal fractures is the description of the so-called "tuber-joint angle", which is now known as the "Böhler's angle". In addition, he appreciated the fact that in these fractures, this angle can be measured as smaller, flat, or even reversed, a fact that is currently known to be an indirect measurement of the energy absorbed from the bone at the time of injury, a predictor of the outcome in displaced intra-articular calcaneal fractures, and also a tool for

selecting patients for operative treatment.[25,26] The amount of depression of Böhler's angle is currently used to classify the displaced intra-articular calcaneal fractures as those with an angle of <0° and those with an angle of >15°. Angles that are closer to normal (25–40°) have a more favorable outcome.[27]

■ ESSEX-LOPRESTI CLASSIFICATION

The work of Mr Essex-Lopresti, which was published in 1952,[16] greatly contributed to our understanding of the pathoanatomy and the mechanism of calcaneus fracture and offered a classification that is still a valuable tool for orthopedic trauma surgeons. Essex-Lopresti acknowledged the data available from previous works, mainly from Palmer[9] and Böhler,[8] and created a new classification scheme that discriminates extra-articular (not involving the "subtaloid" joint) from intra-articular fractures.

For intra-articular fractures, he proposed a mechanism that explains the displacement of major fragments and he classified the subsequent deformity. The momentum of force during a fall from a height is transmitted from the tibia to talus and consequently to calcaneus through two "routes". The "outer route" creates the primary fracture line through the crucial angle of Gissane. According to Essex-Lopresti, the remaining force is transmitted through the "inner route" and creates a constant sustentaculum fracture that is usually connected to a great part of the subtalar joint (posterior facet). Depending upon the amount of the energy absorbed and the position of the foot, a second fracture line or lines are created. Two distinct types of displacement can then occur according to the secondary fracture line configuration. In the so-called tongue-type fracture, the secondary line runs from the crucial angle of Gissane to the posterior surface of the tuberosity, and subsequently, a part of the posterior facet is attached to the posterior tuberosity. The talus, which is then driven into the calcaneus through the anterior part of the tongue, separates the sustentaculum from the rest of calcaneus through the primary fracture line. In the more common "joint depression-type" fracture, the secondary fracture line exits just behind the posterior facet **(Figs. 6 and 7)**. Based upon this classification scheme, Essex-Lopresti was able to make suggestions for treatment, prognosis, and outcome.

Original Essex-Lopresti classification:
- *Type I:* Subtalar joint intact
  - *Type I.A:* Calcaneal tuberosity fracture
    - *Type I.A1:* Beak type (Boyer)
    - *Type I.A2:* Medial border avulsion fracture
    - *Type I.A3:* Vertical fracture
    - *Type I.A4:* Horizontal fracture
  - *Type I.B:* Calcaneocuboid joint involved
    - *Type I.B1:* Parrot nose type
    - *Type I.B2:* Various other types
- *Type II:* Fractures involving the subtalar joint
  - *Type II.A:* Tongue-type fracture
  - *Type II.B:* Joint depression-type fracture

■ ZWIPP CLASSIFICATION

The Zwipp classification **(Fig. 8)** was developed in 1989[28] and is one of the first CT-based classifications. It differentiates calcaneal fractures into two to five fracture fragments (sustentaculum, tuberosity, subtalar joint, anterior process,

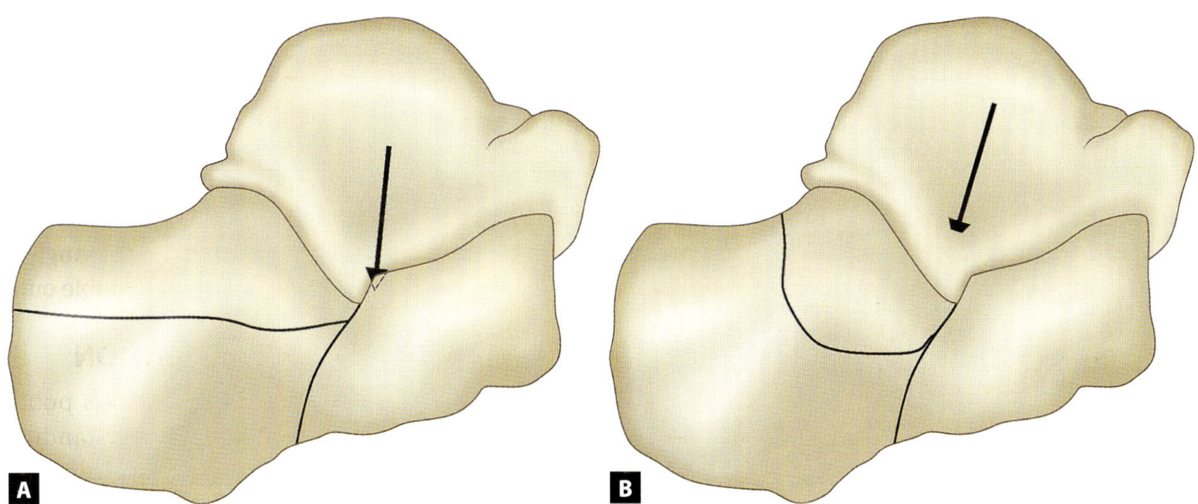

Figs. 6A and B: Essex-Lopresti classification. (A) Tongue-type fracture; (B) Joint depression-type fracture.
Source: Reprinted with permission.

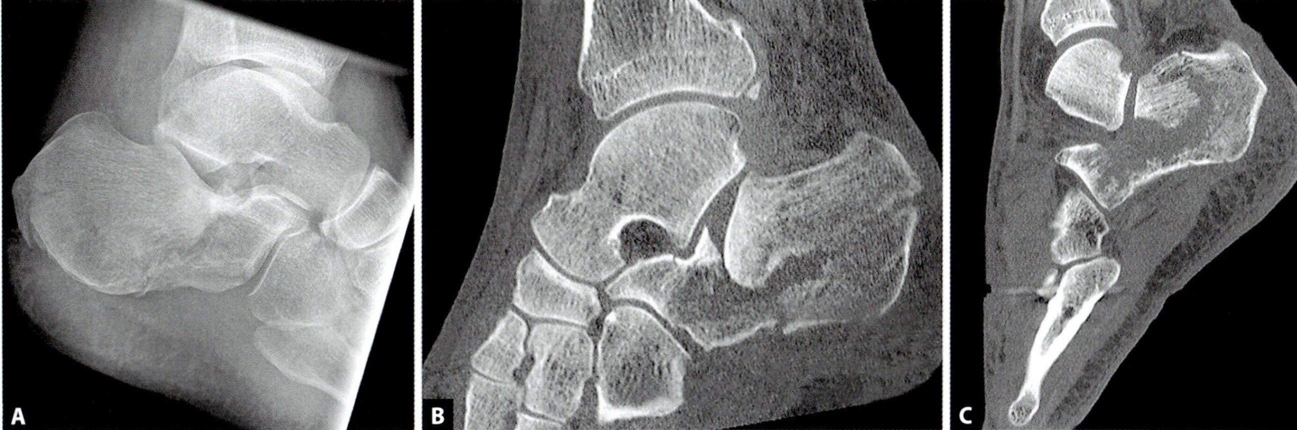

Figs. 7A to C: (A) Lateral radiograph; (B) Sagittal computed tomography (CT) image demonstrating a tongue-type intra-articular calcaneus fracture; (C) Sagittal CT image showing a joint depression-type intra-articular calcaneus fracture.

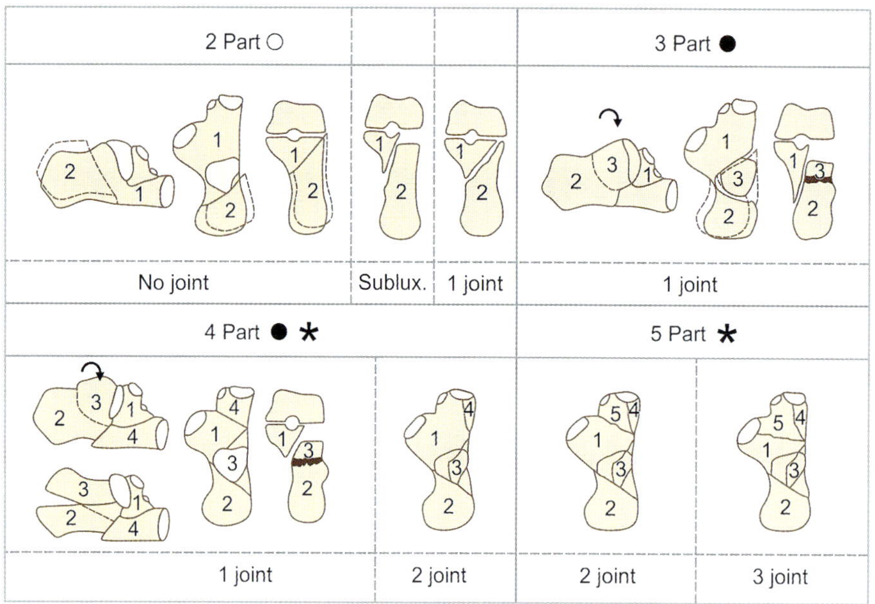

Fig. 8: Zwipp classification.
Source: Reprinted with permission.

and anterior subtalar joint fragment) and into the number of joints involved (posterior subtalar, calcaneocuboid, and anterior subtalar joint). A score is given to each fracture by adding the number of fracture fragments to the number of joints involved. Additional points are given for open fractures and the involvement of other tarsal bones. The maximum score that can be achieved with this classification is 12. The most severe "blowout" fracture is characterized as a five-fragment/three-joint fracture.[29]

CROSBY–FITZGIBBONS CLASSIFICATION

The Crosby and Fitzgibbons classification was developed in 1990.[30] It is a CT-based system that classifies the intra-articular fractures into three types:
1. *Type I:* Slightly or undisplaced posterior facet fractures
2. *Type II:* Displaced posterior facet fractures
3. *Type III:* Comminuted posterior facet fracture

SANDERS CLASSIFICATION

The Sanders classification **(Fig. 9)**[31] belongs to the CT-based classifications, and according to one recent review article, it is the most commonly cited classification of calcaneus fractures in the current orthopedic literature.[10]

This classification refers to intra-articular fractures and was developed in 1993 after following 120 patients for a minimum of 1 year. It utilizes the axial and coronal hindfoot CT cuts. The planes of reconstruction are the semicoronal (perpendicular to posterior facet) and the axial (parallel to the sole of the foot). The cut showing the widest part of the undersurface of the posterior facet of the talus is taken into

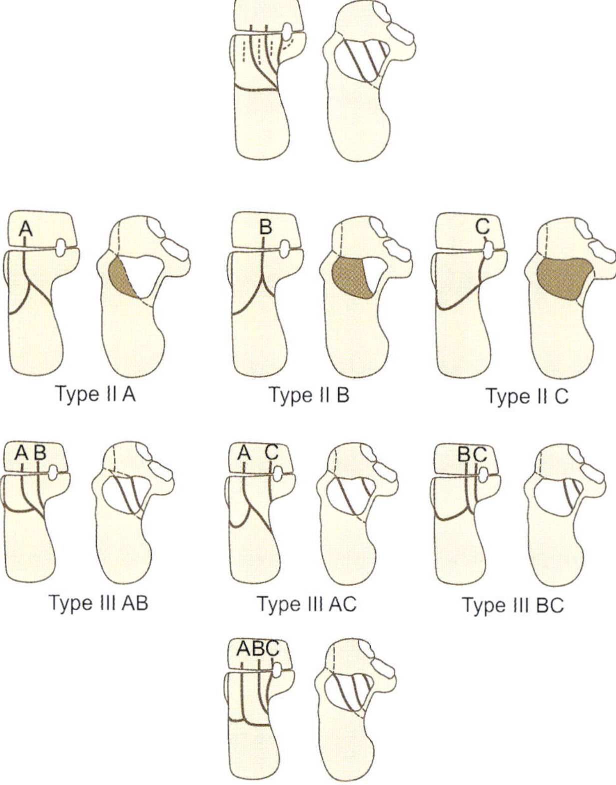

Fig. 9: Sanders classification system.
Source: Reprinted with permission.

consideration, and this is divided into three equal columns by two lines (A and B). Another line (C) that is drawn from the medial edge of the posterior facet of the talus divides the corresponding calcaneus from the sustentaculum. Thus, the entire calcaneus is divided in four segments: Lateral,

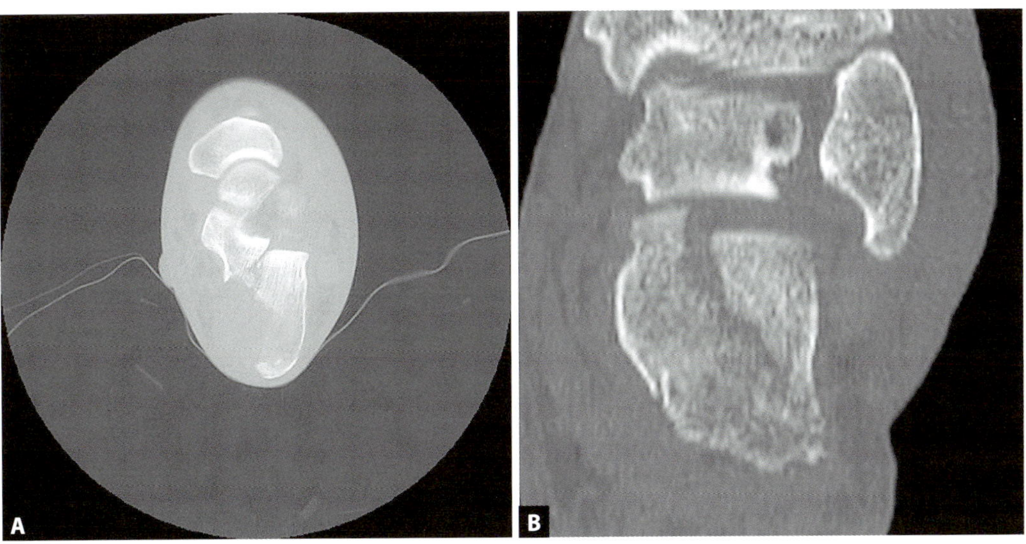

Figs. 10A and B: (A) Axial and (B) coronal computed tomography (CT) images of a Sanders type II calcaneus fracture.

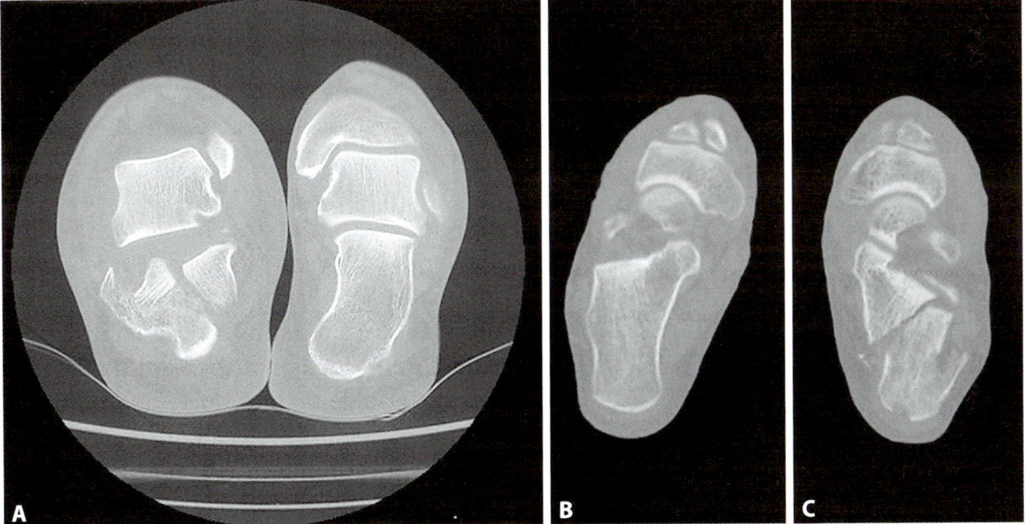

Figs. 11A to C: (A) Coronal computed tomography (CT) image showing a Sanders type IIIAB fracture; (B) Axial and (C) coronal CT images of a different patient.

central, medial, and sustentaculum segments. Four types of fractures are then described according to the number and the location of the fracture fragments. Type I fractures are truly nondisplaced intra-articular fractures. Type II fractures represent two-part fractures that can be subcategorized into IIA, IIB, and IIC subtypes **(Figs. 10A and B)**. Type III fractures **(Figs. 11A to C)**, which are subcategorized as IIIAB, IIIAC, and IIIBC, usually have a depressed articular segment. Type IV fracture represents a four-part or very comminuted fracture **(Figs. 12A and B)**:

1. *Type I:* All nondisplaced fractures regardless of the number of fracture lines
2. *Type II:* Two-part fractures of the posterior facet, displacement ≥2 mm
   - *Type IIA:* Fracture line lateral
   - *Type IIB:* Fracture line medial
   - *Type IIC:* Fracture line sustentaculum tali
3. *Type III:* Three-part fractures with a centrally depressed fragment; subtypes IIIAB, IIIAC, and IIIBC
4. *Type IV:* Four-part articular fractures; highly comminuted.

■ AO/OTA CLASSIFICATION

The comprehensive classification system that was developed by Maurice Müller and the AO Group[32] is a classification system for long bone fractures. It was later revised to include the fractures of the acetabulum, pelvis, and spine. The foot area was not included in this original scheme. Zwipp et al.[33] developed the integral classification for injuries (ICI) that is applicable to foot.

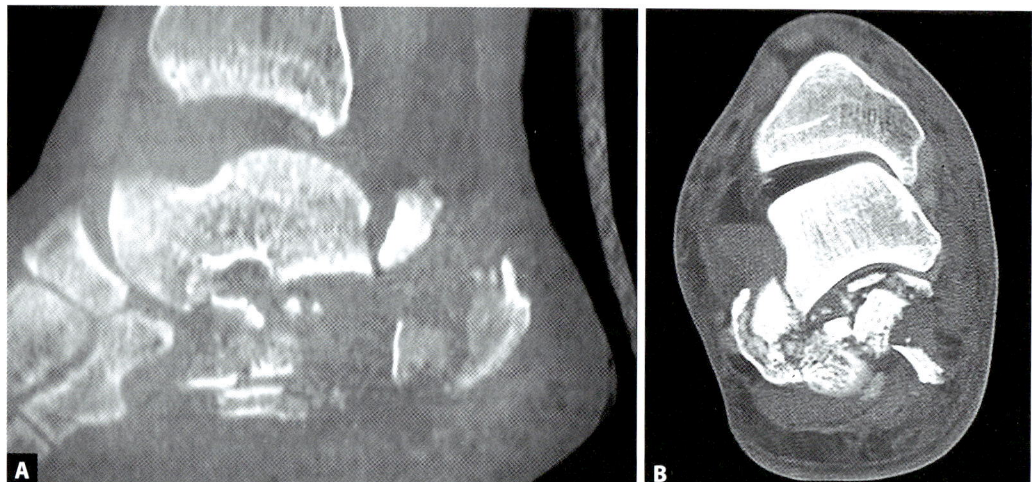

Figs. 12A and B: (A) Sagittal and (B) coronal computed tomography (CT) images showing a comminuted Sanders type IV calcaneus fracture.

The fracture and dislocations compendium of the Orthopedic Trauma Association (OTA) in 2007 revised the codes for some body areas, including the foot.[34] A new alphanumeric code was applied to every body area and is now in agreement with the AO classification (AO/OTA). The foot region is now given the number 8 and calcaneus is given the number 2. Avulsion fractures are type A, nonarticular body fractures are type B, and articular fractures involving the posterior facet are type C **(Fig. 13)**. This is the most common system used for documentation for publishing purposes.

- *Type A:* Avulsion or anterior process or tuberosity fractures
  - *Type A1:* Anterior process
    - *Type A1.1:* Noncomminuted fractures
    - *Type A1.2:* Comminuted fractures
  - *Type A2:* Medial, sustentaculum tali
    - *Type A2.1:* Noncomminuted fractures
    - *Type A2.2:* Comminuted fractures
  - *Type A3:* Tuberosity
    - *Type A3.1:* Noncomminuted fractures
    - *Type A3.2:* Comminuted fractures
- *Type B:* Nonarticular body fractures
  - *Type B1:* Noncomminuted fractures
  - *Type B2:* Comminuted fractures
- *Type C:* Articular fracture involving posterior facet
  - *Type C1:* Nondisplaced fractures
  - *Type C2:* Two-part fractures
  - *Type C3:* Three-part fractures
  - *Type C4:* Four or more parts fractures

(*Note: 82 has to be added before A, B, C; 8 = foot, 2 = calcaneus*)

■ DISCUSSION

Radiography versus CT-based classifications: The reality that CT-based classifications have gained acceptance over plain radiography-based classifications can be explained due to the complex anatomical structure of the calcaneus, with four articular surfaces and three articulations.[35] This makes CT an invaluable tool in assessing the complex distorted anatomy in the fracture setting and also aids significantly in preoperative planning. Despite this, a recent study[36] demonstrated that coronal CT scans might not accurately depict the amount of displacement. The authors argue that depression and rotation of the posterior facet fragment is commonly underestimated on coronal CT. They suggest coronal reconstruction images for better estimating the depression of fragment, and whenever this is not available, they recommend lateral radiographs for displacement evaluation.

Reliability and validity: The four most commonly used calcaneal fracture systems are the Essex-Lopresti, the Zwipp, the Crosby, and the Sanders classifications.[10] Reliability and validity are the two characteristics that make a classification system successful.[5] The variables that define the interobserver reliability are not clearly defined in the literature.[37] Nevertheless, there are several studies that have tested the interobserver reliability of calcaneus classification systems. Schepers et al. demonstrated moderate reliability and agreement among observers (orthopedic surgeons and radiologists) for the Crosby and Sanders classifications.[10] The Essex-Lopresti classification had higher reliability among orthopedic surgeons. Higher agreement was also observed among orthopedic surgeons compared

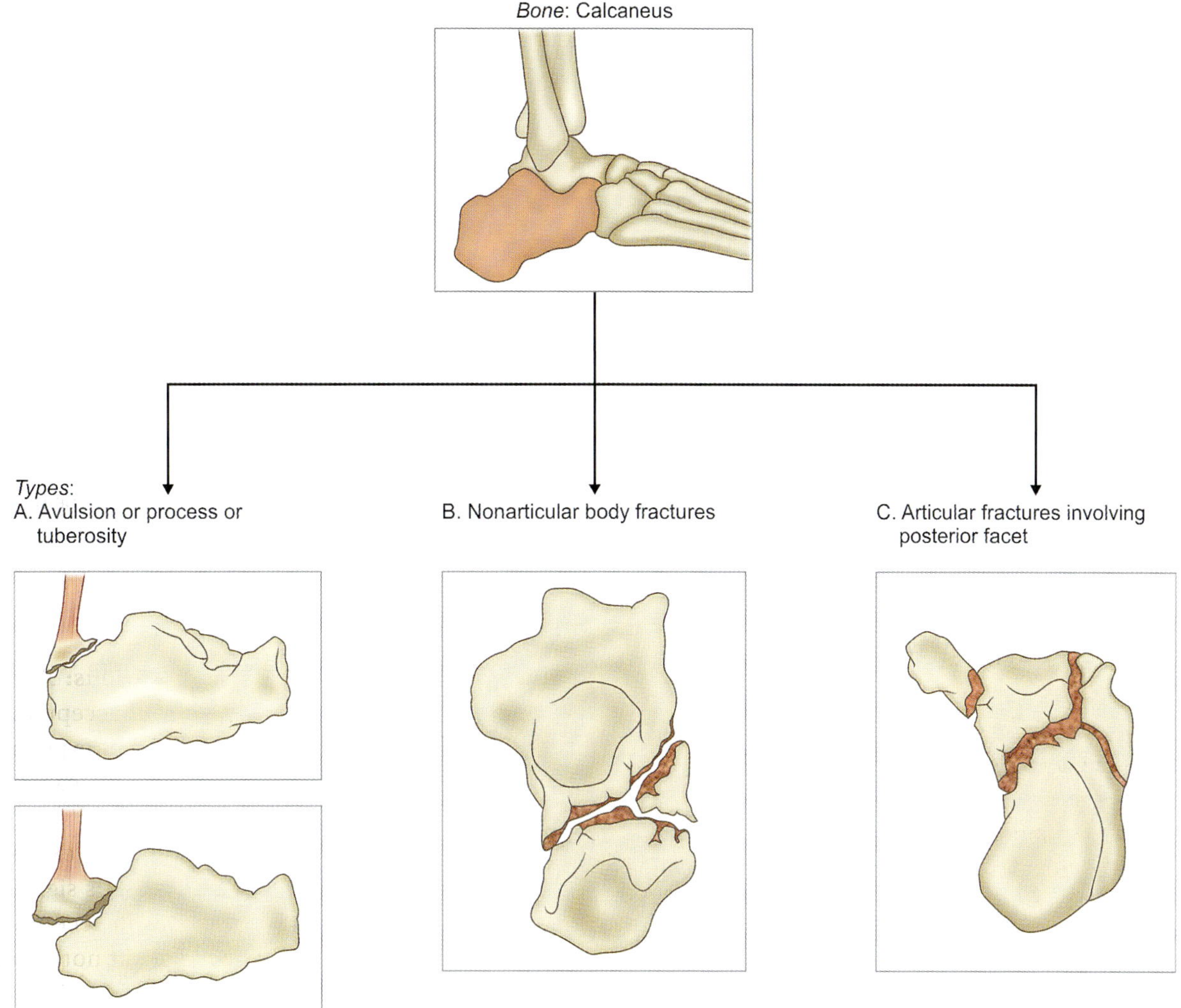

Fig. 13: AO/OTA classification.
Source: Reprinted with permission.

to radiologists when an acetabulum fracture classification, which is a complex three-dimensional (3D) structure such as the calcaneus, was tested in an animal model.[38] The authors attributed this to the operative experience of surgeons that allows them to acquire a 3D understanding of fracture patterns. Humphrey et al.[37] also tested the interobserver reliability of the Sanders classification. CT scan images as well as diagrammatic representations of the Sanders classification were given to experienced orthopedic trauma surgeons. Only moderate interobserver reliability was documented, leading the authors to suggest appreciation of every possible available piece of information (patient-related factors, injury factors, and full imaging studies) for treatment guidance and prognosis. Lauder et al.[39] after testing the Crosby–Fitzgibbons and Sanders classifications showed moderate interobserver reliability for both systems. The intraobserver reliability (validity) of the latter classification

was substantial. Additionally, Bhattacharya et al.[40] argued that both interobserver and intraobserver reliability of the Sanders system is only fair to moderate, thus suggesting caution in its usage and its interpretation. On the other hand, Furey et al.[41] concluded that with this classification system there was moderate agreement among the users, suggesting the system's consistency and uniformity.

Classification scheme guidance and prognostic value: Bhattacharya et al.[40] argued that a precise classification is not an absolute prerequisite in the management of calcaneal fractures. However, Sanders states that a detailed classification is needed for good management of these injuries.[42] In terms of treatment guidance and prognostic value of the most commonly used classification systems (i.e., construct validity),[43] Böhler's angle has been suggested to predict the long-term outcome of calcaneal fracture patients.[25] It has also been shown that patients with a flat angle have better outcomes after operative treatment than with nonoperative care.[26] The Essex-Lopresti system has been suggested to be of a prognostic value.[26] Andermahr et al.[44] compared the Zwipp and Sanders classifications and found that both systems are good prognostic tools, although the Zwipp system is more accurate and the Sanders classification is easier to use in everyday clinical practice. Furthermore, the Sanders classification has been shown to be predictive of outcome in various studies.[26,45] On the contrary, Lauder et al.[39] argued that neither the Crosby nor the Sanders classification system can be considered ideal for treatment suggestions and prognosis. Finally, Rubino et al.,[46] in a recent study aiming to identify the most predictive fracture classification and clinical outcome tool, compared the Essex-Lopresti, AO/OTA, and Sanders classifications. They concluded that CT-based classifications had higher predictive value than the conventional radiography-based classifications.

■ SUMMARY

None of the available classifications fulfills all the fundamental criteria for a perfect calcaneus fracture classification system. For the existing systems, reliability is usually moderate, and there is no direct association with treatment. On the other hand, it seems that there is sufficient correlation with the outcome.[10] The Crosby and Sanders classifications appear to fulfill most of the required criteria for good classification systems. The concept of testing the reliability and validity of fracture classifications is a new one, especially for the calcaneus as very little has been published to date. It is worth mentioning that in a study published in 2004 that evaluated the methodologies that were used up to that time for testing the reliability of various fracture classifications, no papers concerning foot injuries met the inclusion criteria.[43] Finally, there are very few studies that have tested the validity of foot and calcaneus classification systems. A 3D phase concept of development and validation of classification systems for calcaneal fractures has been proposed by Audige et al.[47] and is probably the best way to approach the problem. The development of a new or the revision of existing classification systems by clinical experts should be followed with a multicenter agreement study in clinical practice. The third step of a prospective clinical observational study should be the assessment of the prognostic value of such a new classification scheme.

■ REFERENCES

1. Court-Brown CM, Caesar B. Epidemiology of adult fractures: a review. Injury. 2006;37:691-7.
2. Tejwani NC, Pough K. Foot Injuries. Rosemont, IL: American Academy of Orthopaedic Surgeons; 2010.
3. Mitchell MJ, McKinley JC, Robinson CM. The epidemiology of calcaneal fractures. Foot (Edinb). 2009;19:197-200.
4. Brauer CA, Manns BJ, Ko M, Donaldson C, Buckley R. An economic evaluation of operative compared with nonoperative management of displaced intra-articular calcaneal fractures. J Bone Joint Surg Am. 2005;87:2741-9.
5. Garbuz DS, Masri BA, Esdaile J, Duncan CP. Classification systems in orthopaedics. J Am Acad Orthop Surg. 2002;10:290-7.
6. Eastwood DM, Gregg PJ, Atkins RM. Intra-articular fractures of the calcaneum. Part I: pathological anatomy and classification. J Bone Joint Surg Br. 1993;75:183-8.
7. Ostapowicz G, Sateri F, Wessel G. Results after fracture of the os calcis (author's transl). Arch Orthop Trauma Surg. 1978;91:11-8.
8. Bohler L. Diagnosis, pathology and treatment of fractures of the os calcis. J Bone Joint Surg (Am). 1931;13:75-89.
9. Palmer I. The mechanism and treatment of fractures of the calcaneus; open reduction with the use of cancellous grafts. J Bone Joint Surg Am. 1948;30A:2-8.
10. Schepers T, van Lieshout EMM, Ginai AZ, Mulder PGH, Heetveld MJ, Patka P. Calcaneal fracture classification: a comparative study. J Foot Ankle Surg. 2009;48:156-62.
11. Thoren O. Os calcis fractures. Acta Orthop Scand Suppl. 1964;70(Suppl. 70):1-116.
12. Carr JB, Hamilton JJ, Bear LS. Experimental intra-articular calcaneal fractures: anatomic basis for a new classification. Foot Ankle. 1989;10:81-7.
13. Schepers T, Ginai AZ, Van Lieshout EMM, Patka P. Demographics of extra-articular calcaneal fractures: including a review of the literature on treatment and outcome. Arch Orthop Trauma Surg. 2008;128:1099-106.
14. Squires B, Allen PE, Livingstone J, Atkins RM. Fractures of the tuberosity of the calcaneus. J Bone Joint Surg (Br). 2001;83:55-61.
15. Atkins RM, Allen PE, Livingstone JA. Demographic features of intra-articular fractures of the calcaneum. Foot Ankle Surg. 2001;7:77-84.
16. Essex-Lopresti P. The mechanism, reduction technique, and results in fractures of the os calcis. Br J Surg. 1952;39:395-419.
17. Fitzgibbons T, McMullen ST, Mormino MA. Fractures and Dislocations of the Calcaneus. Philadelphia, PA: Lippincott Williams & Wilkins; 2001.
18. Buckley R, Sands A. Calcaneus—Diagnosis/Decision—AO Surgery Reference. 2011. [online] Available from https://surgeryreference.aofoundation.org/orthopedic-trauma/adult-trauma/calcaneous. [Last accessed April, 2023].
19. Beavis RC, Rourke K, Court-Brown C. Avulsion fracture of the calcaneal tuberosity: a case report and literature review. Foot Ankle Int. 2008;29:863-6.
20. Biehl 3rd WC, Morgan JM, Wagner Jr FW, Gabriel R. Neuropathic calcaneal tuberosity avulsion fractures. Clin Orthop Relat Res. 1993:8-13.
21. Levi N, Garde L, Kofoed H. Avulsion fracture of the calcaneus: report of a case using a new tension band technique. J Orthop Trauma. 1997;11:61-2.

22. Della Rocca GJ, Nork SE, Barei DP, Taitsman LA, Benirschke SK. Fractures of the sustentaculum tali: injury characteristics and surgical technique for reduction. Foot Ankle Int. 2009;30:1037-41.

23. Rowe CR, Sakellarides HT, Freeman PA, Sorbie C. Fractures of the os calcis: a long-term follow-up study of 146 patients. Jama. 1963;184(12):920-3.

24. Degan TJ, Morrey BF, Braun DP. Surgical excision for anterior-process fractures of the calcaneus. J Bone Joint Surg Am. 1982;64:519-24.

25. Loucks C, Buckley R. Bohler's angle: correlation with outcome in displaced intra-articular calcaneal fractures. J Orthop Trauma. 1999;13:554-8.

26. Buckley R, Tough S, McCormack R, Pate G, Leighton R, Petrie D, et al. Operative compared with nonoperative treatment of displaced intra-articular calcaneal fractures: a prospective, randomized, controlled multicenter trial. J Bone Joint Surg Am. 2002;84:1733-44.

27. Buckley RE, Tough S. Displaced intra-articular calcaneal fractures. J Am Acad Orthop Surg. 2004;12:172-8.

28. Zwipp H, Tscherne H, Wulker N, Grote R. Intra-articular fracture of the calcaneus. Classification, assessment and surgical procedures. Unfallchirurg. 1989;92:117-29.

29. Zwipp H, Tscherne H, Thermann H, Weber T. Osteosynthesis of displaced intraarticular fractures of the calcaneus. Results in 123 cases. Clin Orthop Relat Res. 1993;290:76-86.

30. Crosby LA, Fitzgibbons T. Computerized tomography scanning of acute intra-articular fractures of the calcaneus: a new classification system. J Bone Joint Surg Am. 1990;72:852-9.

31. Sanders R, Fortin P, DiPasquale T, Walling A. Operative treatment in 120 displaced intraarticular calcaneal fractures. Results using a prognostic computed tomography scan classification. Clin Orthop Relat Res. 1993;87-95.

32. Müller ME, Nazarian S, Schatzker J. CCF Comprehensive Classification of Fractures: Pamphlets I and II. Bern: ME Müller Foundation; 1996.

33. Zwipp H, Baumgart F, Cronier P, Jorda E, Klaue K, Sands AK, et al. Integral classification of injuries (ICI) to the bones, joints, and ligaments—application to injuries of the foot. Injury. 2004;35(Suppl. 2):SB3-9.

34. Marsh JL, Slongo TF, Agel J, Broderick JS, Creevey W, DeCoster TA, et al. Fracture and dislocation classification compendium—2007: Orthopaedic Trauma Association classification, database and outcomes committee. J Orthop Trauma. 2007;21:S1-133.

35. Keener BJ, Sizensky JA. The anatomy of the calcaneus and surrounding structures. Foot Ankle Clin. 2005;10:413-24.

36. Ogawa BK, Charlton TP, Thordarson DB. Radiography versus computed tomography for displacement assessment in calcaneal fractures. Foot Ankle Int. 2009;30:1005-10.

37. Humphrey CA, Dirschl DR, Ellis TJ. Interobserver reliability of a CT-based fracture classification system. J Orthop Trauma. 2005;19:616-22.

38. Kickuth R, Laufer U, Hartung G, Gruening C, Stueckle C, Kirchner J. 3D CT versus axial helical CT versus conventional tomography in the classification of acetabular fractures: a ROC analysis. Clin Radiol. 2002;57:140-5.

39. Lauder AJ, Inda DJ, Bott AM, Clare MP, Fitzgibbons TC, Mormino MA. Interobserver and intraobserver reliability of two classification systems for intra-articular calcaneal fractures. Foot Ankle Int. 2006;27:251-5.

40. Bhattacharya R, Vassan UT, Finn P, Port A. Sanders classification of fractures of the os calcis. An analysis of inter- and intra-observer variability. J Bone Joint Surg Br. 2005;87:205-8.

41. Furey A, Stone C, Squire D, Harnett J. Os calcis fractures: analysis of interobserver variability in using Sanders classification. J Foot Ankle Surg. 2003;42:21-3.

42. Sanders R. Displaced intra-articular fractures of the calcaneus. J Bone Joint Surg Am. 2000;82:225-50.

43. Audige L, Bhandari M, Kellam J. How reliable are reliability studies of fracture classifications? A systematic review of their methodologies. Acta Orthop Scand. 2004;75:184-94.

44. Andermahr J, Jesch AB, Helling HJ, Jubel A, Fischbach R, Rehm KE. CT morphometry for calcaneal fractures and comparison of the Zwipp and Sanders classifications. Z Orthop Ihre Grenzgeb. 2002;140:339-46.

45. Csizy M, Buckley R, Tough S, Leighton R, Smith J, McCormack R, et al. Displaced intra-articular calcaneal fractures: variables predicting late subtalar fusion. J Orthop Trauma. 2003;17:106-12.

46. Rubino R, Valderrabano V, Sutter PM, Regazzoni P. Prognostic value of four classifications of calcaneal fractures. Foot Ankle Int. 2009;30:229-38.

47. Audige L, Bhandari M, Hanson B, Kellam J. A concept for the validation of fracture classifications. J Orthop Trauma. 2005;19:401-6.

Nonoperative Management of Calcaneal Fractures

Mandeep S Dhillon, Karthick Rangasamy

"All types of conservative treatments have advantages and disadvantages".
–Augusto Sarmiento et al, JBJS, 1977

"It takes five years to learn when to operate and twenty years to learn when not to".
–Anonymous

■ INTRODUCTION

Fractures of the calcaneum remain a challenging problem for orthopedic surgeons. Although Malgaigne[1] first described calcaneal fractures in 1843, they were routinely diagnosed following the advent of radiography in the latter half of the 18th century.[2,3] Even though modern surgical techniques have improved the outcomes of calcaneal fractures, there exists controversy concerning nonoperative management of calcaneal fractures since a significant correlation has not been established between the restoration of the anatomy, and functional outcomes and surgical complications are frequently encountered. Additionally, some surgeons do not have access to expertise, training, or equipment and implants that would allow them to operate on calcaneal fractures routinely.

HISTORICAL PERSPECTIVE REGARDING NONOPERATIVE MANAGEMENT OF CALCANEAL FRACTURES

Petit and DeSault first gave the treatment principles for calcaneus fractures in France in the year 1720.[4] They proposed "rest until the fragments consolidated." Until the 1900s, rest and elevation remained the mainstay of conservative management. Cotton[3] first advocated closed manipulation with the help of a hammer for calcaneal fractures in 1908 and condemned attempts at internal fixation. In 1935, Conn[5] looked at the varying and often disappointing outcomes of these injuries and proposed that the best preferred management would be delayed triple arthrodesis. Cotton also abandoned the technique of closed reduction in the late 1920s and started treating healed fractures when they presented with malunion. Böhler described the use of pin traction and clamps for the restoration of normal anatomy and introduced some modifications in the methodology. He laid emphasis on the restoration of Böhler's tuber angle. In 1931, Böhler[2] also started advocating open reduction and internal fixation (ORIF) for calcaneal fractures; however, forcible, closed methods with hammers and tongs, or traction and subsequent closed manipulation and casting, remained the principal protocols of his era. All these came about due to the frequent complications associated with the rudimentary techniques of surgery for calcaneal fractures prevalent in that era.

The first description of internal fixation of calcaneal fractures was given by Leriche[6] in 1922. During the 1950s, operative treatment of calcaneal fractures regained some favor,[7,8] and subsequently once again fell into disfavor, since several surgeons advocated nonoperative management in the 1960s and 1970s owing to the frequently encountered surgical complications.[9-12] Omoto and Nakamura[13] described a closed reduction technique in 2001 for displaced intra-articular fractures. They reported a successful reduction in 92 cases out of 102 cases. In their procedure, the patient is placed prone under regional or general anesthesia, and the knee is flexed to 90°. The thigh is supported by an assistant, while at the foot end, mediolateral pressure over the heel is applied by the surgeon. This is followed by a strong, in-line longitudinal traction by the surgeon. The tuberosity is manipulated, and the heel varus/valgus is rectified. Finally, a below-knee cast or compression bandage is applied **(Fig. 1)**.

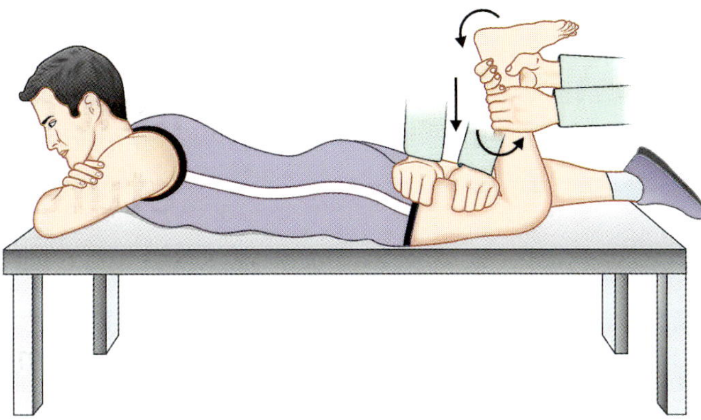

Fig. 1: Omoto technique for calcaneal fracture closed reduction.

INDICATIONS FOR NONOPERATIVE TREATMENT[14]

- Undisplaced or minimally displaced extra-articular fractures **(Fig. 2)**
- Minimally displaced intra-articular fractures or with step-off <2 mm **(Figs. 3A and B)**
- Undisplaced/type 1 or 2 anterior process fracture with congruent calcaneocuboid joint[15] **(Fig. 4)**
- Systemic disorders that include severe neurovascular insufficiency, poor glycemic control in insulin-dependent diabetes mellitus (DM), noncompliance (substance abuse), and disorders with immunodeficiency[16]
- Surgery prohibited by other medical comorbidities **(Figs. 5A and B)**
- Elderly patients who are household ambulators
- Lack of surgical expertise or equipment (maybe applicable in some areas)

HOW TO GIVE NONOPERATIVE TREATMENT?

The initial treatment strategy includes RICE (rest, ice, compression, and elevation) regimen plus appropriate and adequate supportive splintage. Once the swelling subsides, to prevent an equinus contracture, the ankle is locked in neutral flexion with the aid of a prefabricated fracture boot, and to reduce the edema, an elastic compression stocking is applied. Subtalar and ankle range of motion (ROM) exercises are commenced as early as feasible, and weight-bearing is restricted for a period of 10–12 weeks till the radiographic union is confirmed.[14] Nonsteroidal anti-inflammatory drugs (NSAIDs) can also be used to control pain in the early period. Some authors also use some enzymatic preparations to decrease edema; however, there is no definite evidence supporting their role in edema control. After 3 months, gradual and progressive weight-bearing is initiated as per the tolerance of the patient.

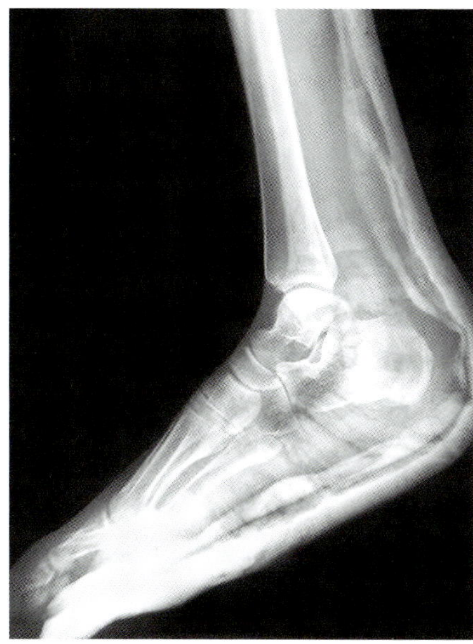

Fig. 2: Undisplaced extra-articular fracture being treated in splint in the initial stages.

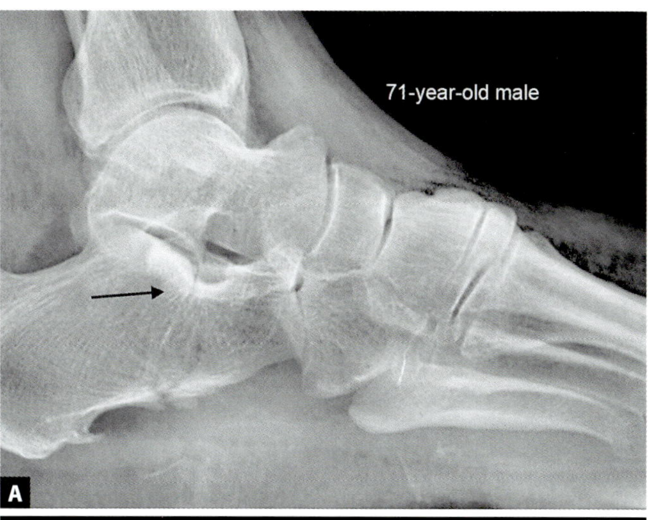

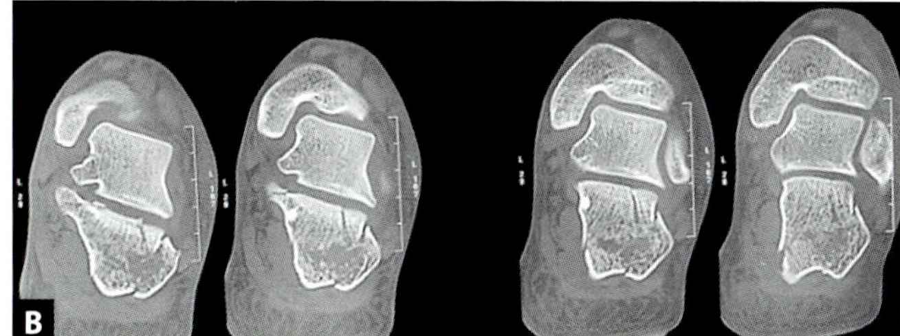

Figs. 3A and B: Undisplaced fracture (intra-articular) in an elderly male, which can be treated nonoperatively.

NONOPERATIVE TREATMENT FOR PEDIATRIC CALCANEAL FRACTURES

In the pediatric population, calcaneal fractures are rare, and the incidence amounts to 0.005–0.41%.[17,18] The actual

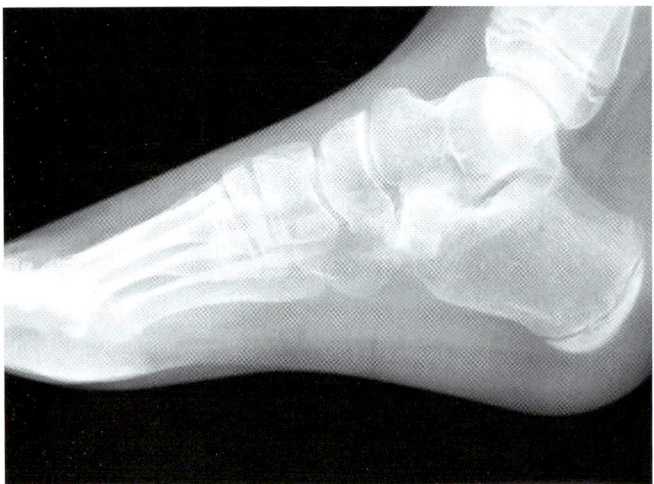

Fig. 4: Anterior process fracture in a 16-year-old girl which can be treated nonoperatively.

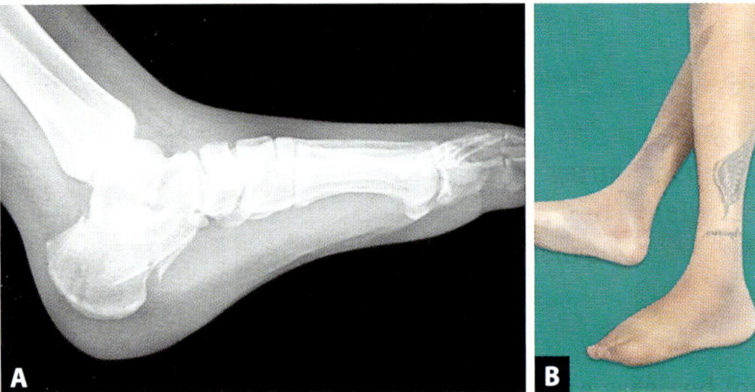

Figs. 5A and B: Bilateral case of displaced calcaneal fracture with a spinal injury and complete paraplegia. This could be an indication for nonoperative treatment.

incidence may be more, and the underreporting is because of missed diagnosis or occult fractures. Usually, the cause is low-velocity trauma, and the comminution is less frequent than in adults. These fractures are titled the "toddlers" fracture of the calcaneus in children between 9 months and 3 years of age.

Most studies on pediatric calcaneal fractures have reported excellent outcome with nonoperative treatment.[19-22] The choice of conservative strategy for the management of both intra- and extra-articular calcaneal fractures has no reported dysfunction in the available literatrure.[19-24] Fourteen intra-articular fractures were managed conservatively by Brunet,[19] and on follow-up, the children could walk flat on the ground with no significant difficulties. Mora et al.[25] observed that, in the intra-articular joint depression types, the posterior facet appeared to be intact, and this favorable outcome is a consequence of immense growth and remodeling potential of the immature calcaneus and talus. The involvement of low-velocity trauma and the enormous

reparative potential of the soft tissues also contributed significantly.

Nevertheless, the treatment of displaced intra-articular calcaneal fractures (DIACFs) in children is controversial and recent studies favor surgery via percutaneous or minimally invasive approaches. Schneidmuller et al.[26] suggested surgical intervention for the restoration of the articular surface to prevent the early onset of arthritis and the reestablishment of the width and length of the calcaneus to reinstate the anatomical arch of the foot. With the advent of minimally invasive sinus tarsi approaches, Xia et al.[27] and Tong et al.[28] were able to get good results with shorter surgical time and lower wound complications in DIACFs.

Nonoperative treatment is advised if the disruption of the three articular facets is <4 mm, no subluxation of subtalar joint due to widening, no fibular impingement from the lateral calcaneal cortex, posterior gap in tongue-type fracture is <1 cm, and no significant shortening of the Achilles tendon due to proximal pull of the fragment.[29]

NONOPERATIVE TREATMENT FOR GERIATRIC CALCANEAL FRACTURES

Geriatric calcaneal fractures are treated on the same lines as in adults. However, as mentioned above, some fractures may have to be managed conservatively if they are only household ambulators or have associated medical comorbidities, which preclude anesthesia in this population.[14] Greater age of the patient is not a contraindication for operative management because appreciable outcomes can still be achieved in physically and physiologically active individuals >65 years old. Treatment is rather fashioned to meet the functional demands and compliance and address the comorbidities of the patients.[16]

Special Situations

In certain special situations where fractures present with massive edema subsequently leading to the development of blisters, open and large wounds, or life-threatening injuries, or in patients with severe peripheral microangiopathy or uncontrolled diabetes, nonoperative treatment is preferred.[14] Some authors have also suggested bilateral calcaneal fractures as a relative indication for nonoperative management.[30]

OPERATIVE VERSUS NONOPERATIVE MANAGEMENT FOR CALCANEAL FRACTURES

Crosby and Fitzgibbons[31] managed calcaneal fractures with casting without reduction. They assessed the fracture morphology involving the posterior facet using a computed tomography (CT) classification and showed good outcomes with closed management in all undisplaced fractures. Kitaoka et al.[32] assessed the gait outcomes in 16 of 27 patients managed without reduction and casting. There was an alteration in the gait patterns in several patients, especially on uneven surfaces. This confirms the fact that nonoperative treatment of displaced fractures led to some degree of dysfunction.

O'Farrell et al.[33] compared operative versus nonoperative treatment in a quasi-randomized controlled trial of 24 patients with displaced intra-articular fractures. Better outcomes were noted in the operative group with respect to difficulties with footwear, greater pain-free walking distance, Böhler's angle, ROM at the subtalar joint, and return to daily work. A similar comparison was done in 1993 by Parmar et al.,[34] where 31 patients were managed conservatively and received ice packs, limb elevation, early foot movement, and physiotherapy, and 25 patients were managed surgically by open reduction plus Kirschner wire fixation. This was followed by 6 weeks' duration of cast immobilization. At 6–8 weeks, weight-bearing was allowed. The patients were assessed for pain, use of analgesics, ankle, and subtalar joint ROM, ability to walk, return to daily work and recreational activities, and use of footwear. The outcomes between the two groups at 1-year follow-up were not statistically significant.

Another study by Thordarson and Krieger[35] compared the same in 30 patients with displaced intra-articular fractures. The patients were assessed using a new functional outcome assessment questionnaire, with scores between 0 and 100. The parameters included pain (30 points), work (20 points), walking (20 points), exercise (10 points), shoe wear (10 points), and limitations of daily activity (10 points). Böhler's tuber angle was also taken into consideration. The operative treatment group showed statistically significant results.

Buckley et al.[36] reported that without group stratification, the functional results after both nonoperative and operative management of displaced intra-articular fractures were comparable. However, following the removal of individuals who were beneficiaries of workers' compensation and unmasking the data, the results were significantly better in certain groups of surgically managed patients.

Howard et al.[37] assessed complications in displaced intra-articular fractures managed surgically, which significantly contributed to morbidity. Among the 424 patients (459 fractures) included in the study, 218 patients (233 fractures) were managed nonoperatively, and the remainder 206 (226 fractures) were managed surgically with ORIF using a standard lateral approach. The operative group showed complications to a greater extent. Barla et al.[38] specifically studied the long-term results of displaced intra-articular fractures in 41 women (43 fractures), where 21 were managed nonoperatively and 20 underwent ORIF. The SF-36 and visual analog scale (VAS) scores showed a better picture in the operative group. The improvement of Böhler's angles in the operative group was also statistically significant ($p = 0.001$). Finally, over a 2–8-year follow-up, O'Brien et al.[39] reported the patients' individual satisfaction with gait. This study analyzed how patient demographics, fracture morphology, and treatment strategy influenced satisfaction with gait following displaced intra-articular fractures. The study included 319 patients (351 fractures) randomized to either nonoperative or operative treatment, and the individual gait satisfaction scores between the two groups were not significantly different.

In 2000, Randle et al.[40] performed a meta-analysis inferring the clinical and functional outcomes in displaced intra-articular fractures managed either operatively or nonoperatively with a minimum follow-up of 12 months. Different surgical techniques were implemented in the six studies chosen by Randle et al.,[40] from the use of Kirschner wires alone to the use of a sole bone screw, screws, and plate fixation with/without the augmentation with bone graft. It was inferred that there was an inclination toward better outcomes in the operative groups with respect to pain, gait abnormalities, return to daily work, and radiological findings. However, no treatment recommendations could be made for displaced fractures based on the studies included in the meta-analysis.

A large multicentric trial, the *"UK Heel trial"* by Griffin et al.,[41] comparing operative versus nonoperative management for DIACFs, found no significant differences in the functional outcome measures. But the trial was subjected to severe criticism by researchers for the use of faulty research methodology, namely selection bias (representation of a meager 7.5% of all the calcaneal fractures presented to the centers included in the study). Even a recent meta-analysis comparing nonoperative versus operative strategies for the management of DIACFs failed to produce clear recommendations in treatment (insufficient evidence to support operative treatment), although operative treatment is a slightly favorable option if anatomical reduction can be achieved by experienced surgeons.[42,43]

Recent literature also reports no difference in outcomes between operative and nonoperative groups. A balance between good functional results and reduced complications may be achieved with improved surgical techniques; however, no evidence exists that can establish a "gold standard" protocol for these fractures.[44]

■ SUMMARY

To summarize, both intra- and extra-articular calcaneal fractures can be managed nonoperatively with sustainable functional outcomes. This is also an economical choice, especially in centers with sparse resources and surgical facilities. Also, in given indications, it remains the method of choice with an acceptable outcome.

■ REFERENCES

1. Malgaigne JF. Operative Surgery: Based on Normal and Pathological Anatomy. Philadelphia: Blanchard and Lea. [Frederick Brittan, translator; 1851].
2. Böhler L. Diagnosis, pathology, and treatment of fractures of the os calcis. J Bone Joint Surg. 1931;13:75-89.
3. Cotton FJ, Wilson LT. Fractures of the os calcis. Boston Med Surg J. 1908;159:559-65.
4. Crosby LA, Kamins P. The history of the calcaneal fracture. Orthop Rev. 1991;20:501-9.
5. Conn HR. The treatment of fractures of the os calcis. J Bone Joint Surg. 1935;17:392-405.
6. Leriche R. Osteosynthese pour fracture par ecrasement du calcaneum a sept fragments. Lyon Chir. 1922;19:559.
7. Gissane W. Discussion on "Fractures of the os calcis" (Proceedings of the British Orthopaedic Association). J Bone Joint Surg. 1947;29:254-5.
8. Palmer I. The mechanism and treatment of fractures of the calcaneus; open reduction with the use of cancellous grafts. J Bone Joint Surg Am. 1948;30A:2-8.
9. Aitken AP. Fractures of the os calcis—treatment by closed reduction. Clin Orthop Relat Res. 1963;30:67-75.
10. Cave EF. Fracture of the os calcis—the problem in general. Clin Orthop Relat Res. 1963;30:64-6.
11. Lance EM, Carey Jr EJ, Wade PA. Fractures of the os calcis. Treatment by early mobilization. Clin Orthop Relat Res. 1963;30:76-90.
12. McLaughlin HL. Treatment of late complications after os calcis fractures. Clin Orthop Relat Res. 1963;30:111-5.
13. Omoto H, Nakamura K. Method for manual reduction of displaced intra-articular fracture of the calcaneus: technique, indications and limitations. Foot Ankle Int. 2001;22(11):874-9.
14. Sanders RW, Clare MP. Fractures of the calcaneus. In: Bucholz RW, Heckman JD, Court-Brown CM (Eds). Rockwood and Green's Fractures in Adults, 6th edition. Philadelphia: Lippincott Williams & Wilkins; 2006.
15. Dhinsa BS, Latif A, Walker R, Abbasian A, Back D, Singh S. Fractures of the anterior process of the calcaneum; a review and proposed treatment algorithm. Foot Ankle Surg. 2019;25(3):258-63.
16. Rammelt S, Sangeorzan BJ, Swords MP. Calcaneal fractures—should we or should we not operate? Indian J Orthop. 2018;52(3):220-30.
17. van Frank E, Ward JC, Engelhardt P. Bilateral calcaneal fracture in childhood. Case report and review of the literature. Arch Orthop Trauma Surg. 1998;118:111-2.
18. Landin LA. Epidemiology of children's fractures. J Pediatr Orthop B. 1997;6:79-83.
19. Brunet JA. Calcaneal fractures in children. Long-term results of treatment. J Bone Joint Surg Br. 2000;82:211-6.
20. Schantz K, Rasmussen F. Good prognosis after calcaneal fracture in childhood. Acta Orthop Scand. 1988;59:560-3.
21. Inokuchi S, Usami N, Hiraishi E, Hashimoto T. Calcaneal fractures in children. J Pediatr Orthop. 1998;18:469-74.
22. Wiley JJ, Profitt A. Fractures of the os calcis in children. Clin Orthop Relat Res. 1984;(188):131-8.
23. Schmidt TL, Weiner DS. Calcaneal fractures in children. An evaluation of the nature of the injury in 56 children. Clin Orthop Relat Res. 1982;(171):150-5.
24. Schindler A, Mason DE, Allington NJ. Occult fracture of the calcaneus in toddlers. J Pediatr Orthop. 1996;16:201-5.
25. Mora S, Thordarson DB, Zionts LE, Reynolds RA. Pediatric calcaneal fractures. Foot Ankle Int. 2001;22:471-7.
26. Schneidmueller D, Dietz HG, Kraus R, Marzi I. Calcaneal fractures in childhood: a retrospective survey and literature review. Unfallchirurg. 2007;110:939-45.
27. Xia S, Lu Y, Wang H, Wu Z, Wang Z. Open reduction and internal fixation with conventional plate via L-shaped lateral approach versus internal fixation with percutaneous plate via a sinus tarsi approach for calcaneal fractures—a randomized controlled trial. Int J Surg. 2014;12:475-80.
28. Tong L, Li M, Li F, Xu J, Hu T. A minimally invasive (sinus tarsi) approach with percutaneous K-wires fixation for intra-articular calcaneal fractures in children. J Pediatr Orthop B. 2018;27(6):556-62.
29. Jarvis JG, Moroz PJ. Fractures and dislocations of the foot. In: Beaty JH, Kasser JR (Eds). Rockwood and Wilkins' Fractures in Children, 6th edition. Philadelphia: Lippincott Williams & Wilkins; 2005.
30. Dooley P, Buckley R, Tough S, McCormack B, Pate G, Leighton R, et al. Bilateral calcaneal fractures: operative versus nonoperative treatment. Foot Ankle Int. 2004;25(2):47-52.
31. Crosby LA, Fitzgibbons T. Computerized tomography scanning of acute intra-articular fractures of the calcaneus. A new classification system. J Bone Joint Surg. 1990;72:852-9.
32. Kitaoka HB, Schaap EJ, Chao EY, An KN. Displaced intra-articular fractures of the calcaneus treated non-operatively. Clinical results and analysis of motion and ground-reaction and temporal forces. J Bone Joint Surg Am. 1994;76:1531-40.
33. O'Farrell DA, O'Byrne JM, McCabe JP, Stephens MM. Fractures of the os calcis: improved results with internal fixation. Injury. 1993;24:263-5.
34. Parmar HV, Triffitt PD, Gregg PJ. Intra-articular fractures of the calcaneum treated operatively or conservatively. A prospective study. J Bone Joint Surg Br. 1993;75:932-7.
35. Thordarson DB, Krieger LE. Operative vs. nonoperative treatment of intra-articular fractures of the calcaneus: a prospective randomized trial. Foot Ankle Int. 1996;17:2-9.
36. Buckley R, Tough S, McCormack R, Pate G, Leighton R, Petrie D, et al. Operative compared with nonoperative treatment of displaced intra-articular calcaneal fractures: a prospective, randomized, controlled multicenter trial. J Bone Joint Surg Am. 2002;84(10):1733-44.
37. Howard JL, Buckley R, McCormack R, Pate G, Leighton R, Petrie D, et al. Complications following management of displaced intra-articular calcaneal fractures: a prospective

randomized trial comparing open reduction internal fixation with nonoperative management. J Orthop Trauma. 2003;17:241-9.

38. Barla J, Buckley R, McCormack R, Pate G, Leighton R, Petrie D, et al. Displaced intraarticular calcaneal fractures: long-term outcome in women. Foot Ankle Int. 2004;25:853-6.

39. O'Brien J, Buckley R, McCormack R, Pate G, Leighton R, Petrie D, et al. Personal gait satisfaction after displaced intraarticular calcaneal fractures: a 2-8 year followup. Foot Ankle Int. 2004;25:657-65.

40. Randle JA, Kreder HJ, Stephen D, Williams J, Jaglal S, Hu R. Should calcaneal fractures be treated surgically? A meta-analysis. Clin Orthop Relat Res. 2000;(377):217-27.

41. Griffin D, Parsons N, Shaw E, Kulikov Y, Hutchinson C, Thorogood M, et al. Operative versus non-operative treatment for closed, displaced, intra-articular fractures of the calcaneus: randomised controlled trial. BMJ. 2014;349:g4483.

42. Luo X, Li Q, He S, He S. Operative versus nonoperative treatment for displaced intra-articular calcaneal fractures: a meta-analysis of randomized controlled trials. J Foot Ankle Surg. 2016;55(4):821-8.

43. Dhillon MS, Prabhakar S. Treatment of displaced intra-articular calcaneus fractures: a current concepts review. SICOT J. 2017;3:59.

44. Razik A, Harris M, Trompeter A. Calcaneal fractures: where are we now? Strategies Trauma Limb Reconstr. 2018;13(1):1-11.

Operative Management: Surgical Approaches

SS Suresh, Mandeep S Dhillon

"Vision is the art of seeing what is invisible to the others".

–Jonathan Swift

INTRODUCTION

Open reduction remains the gold standard treatment for displaced fractures of the calcaneus since it restores the congruity of the subtalar joint and restores the normal anatomy of the bone. Various surgical techniques have been described, with the extended lateral approach being the most common; however, the technique used depends on the personality of the fracture and the training and competence of the surgeon. Open surgical fixation of the fracture is attendant with the risk of wound-related complications which occur in around 30% of the patients. Breakdown of lateral calcaneal skin flap is a major concern with an extended lateral approach. The extended lateral approach gives adequate exposure of the lateral wall of the calcaneus and permits the surgeon to fix a lateral plate. In addition, a lag screw can be passed into the medial sustentacular fragment. However, the lateral calcaneal flap which is supplied by the lateral calcaneal artery (LCA) is at risk with this approach.

Calcaneal fracture is considered a soft-tissue injury with rapid onset of swelling and ecchymosis, with onset of fracture blisters. Respect for the soft tissues and proper timing and approaches determines the outcomes.

The wound complications with the extensile lateral approach made people think of minimally invasive techniques. However, limited approaches in this area demand a thorough knowledge of the anatomy and the reduction techniques.

PALMER APPROACH (LIMITED LATERAL SINUS TARSI APPROACH)

The exposure is done with the patient in the prone position. A curved incision 6 cm in length follows the course of the peroneal tendons. Care is taken in isolating and protecting the sural nerve. The peroneal tendons are displaced anteriorly after incising the sheath. The calcaneocuboid joint is opened after dividing the calcaneofibular ligament (CFL). A Kirschner wire (K-wire) is passed into the posterior aspect of the calcaneum to facilitate reduction and for better visualization of the calcaneocuboid joint. The articular surfaces can now be identified for reduction and stabilization.

Comminuted fragments along the lateral wall can now be brought back to normal position by compressing with the hand.

Some authors have reported excellent to very good results in 70% of the patients operated by this technique.[1-3]

SINUS TARSI APPROACH (LIMITED LATERAL APPROACH)

In a systematic review of the literature, the authors found that the sinus tarsi approach gave similar results compared to the extended lateral approach. The authors found an overall good to excellent result in over 75% of cases, with a wound complication rate of 48%.

Weber et al. found no statistical difference in the wound complications when comparing limited lateral and extended lateral approaches;[4] however, sural nerve injuries were significantly higher in the extended lateral approach.[3] The sural nerve is at risk in both the proximal and distal ends of the extended lateral approach **(Fig. 1)**.[5]

The sinus tarsi approach is useful in a selected group of patients who are prone to getting wound complications if the extended lateral approach is used.

SMALL LATERAL APPROACH (LIMITED SINUS TARSI APPROACH)

In the operating room, the patient is placed in the semilateral position.

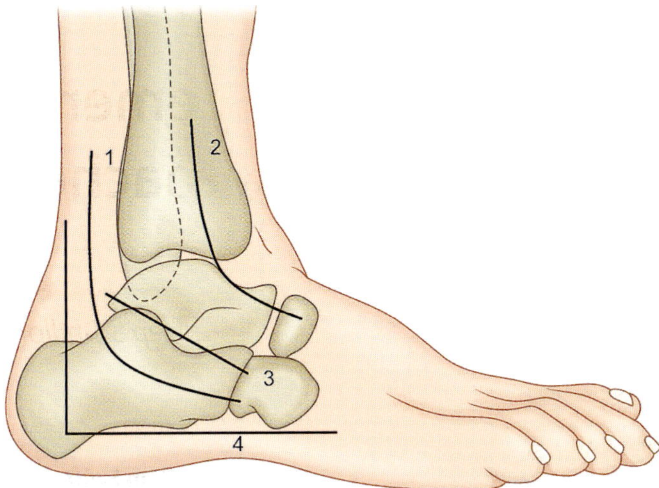

Fig. 1: Extended lateral approach versus sinus tarsi approach. Line diagram showing approaches and nerves: (1) Sural nerve, (2) superficial peroneal nerve, (3) sinus tarsi approach, and (4) extended lateral approach.

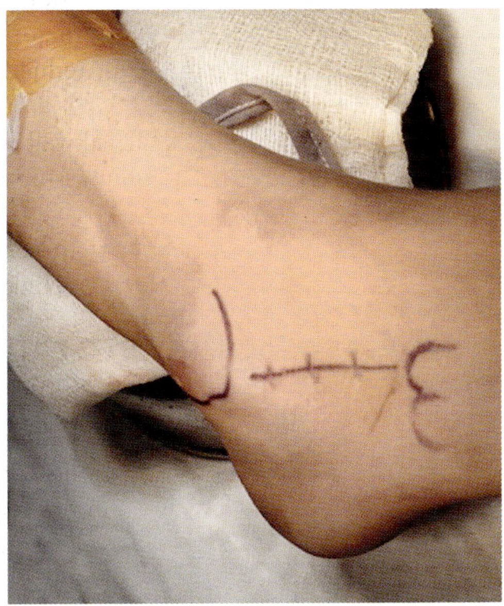

Fig. 2: The skin incision marked for the sinus tarsi approach.

The lateral incision is 5–6 cm long, beginning from the anterolateral corner of the calcaneocuboid joint, and extends posteriorly in a straight line to the ankle up to 1–2 cm anterior to the tendo calcaneus **(Fig. 2)**.

The incision is carried down to the sheath of the peroneal tendons. The sural nerve and the short saphenous vein are isolated and protected. The sheath of the peroneal tendons is now opened, where it meets the inferior extensor retinaculum. This exposes the anterolateral border of the sinus tarsi. The extensor digitorum brevis (EDB) is elevated distally to expose the calcaneocuboid joint.

The sinus tarsi is dissected only to the extent necessary for exposure **(Figs. 3A and B)**. By sharp dissection, the lateral wall of the calcaneum is exposed. At the posterior border, the CFL and the lateral talocalcaneal ligament are excised en bloc. These ligaments along with the sheath of the peroneal tendons are now retracted to get more exposure of the posterior aspect of the subtalar joint. The lateral wall along with the overlying tissues are retracted as a trap door. The posterior articular facet can now be inspected. The depressed fragments are now elevated and fixed. The tuberosity fragments are now realigned using K-wires as joysticks passed from posterior calcaneus.

It is technically difficult to visualize medial fractures of the posterior facet and to reduce the medial wall fracture, which are done under imaging and in a closed manner.[6,7]

■ EXTENSILE SINUS TARSI APPROACH

This approach is especially suitable for patients who are at risk of wound complications such as smokers.[8]

The patient is positioned in full lateral or semilateral position with the help of sandbags. A longitudinal incision is made, beginning 3 cm above the tip of the lateral malleolus, along the posterior border of the distal fibula. From the tip of the fibula, the incision is directed toward the base of the fourth metatarsal and continued toward the calcaneocuboid joint. The incision lies in the internervous plane of the superficial peroneal nerve and the sural nerve **(Fig. 4)**.

The sinus tarsi fat pad is mobilized dorsally. Now, the intermediate part of the inferior extensor retinaculum is released to get exposure of the fracture line passing obliquely through the angle of Gissane. The EDB muscle is elevated off of the lateral process and is reflected distally and dorsally.

At this moment, the peroneal tendons are retracted and the inferior peroneal retinaculum is released to expose the lateral calcaneal wall. The sural nerve remains uninjured as the tissues over the peroneal tendons are undisturbed. The tissues over the lateral wall of the calcaneus up to the tuberosity are elevated in a retrograde manner subperiosteally. The CFL is incised and elevated with the entire lateral calcaneal flap. This may be reattached once the fixation is over. The superior peroneal retinaculum (SPR) may be opened if there is a need to inspect the peroneal tendons. The floor of the SPR is left undisturbed, thereby protecting the LCA, which passes 2 mm of the superior border of the floor of the SPR at the middle of the peroneal sheath. Dividing the interosseous talocalcaneal ligament brings into view the medial articular fragment by giving varus stress to the foot. This ligament being a primary stabilizer of the subtalar joint is transected only when absolutely necessary. At this moment, the fracture can be mobilized with a Schanz pin

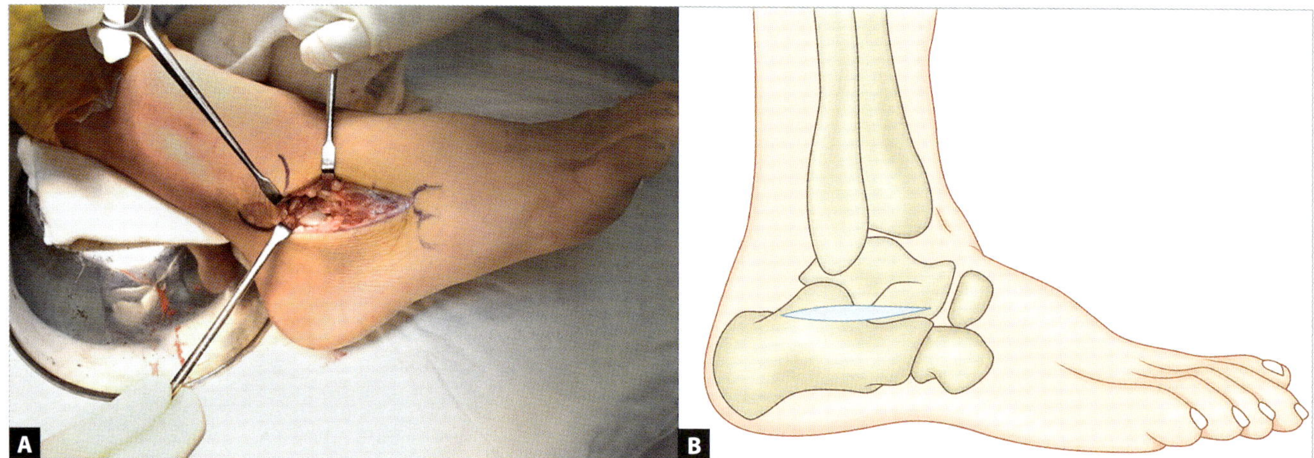

Figs. 3A and B: Minimal dissection exposes the calcaneus and subtalar joint.

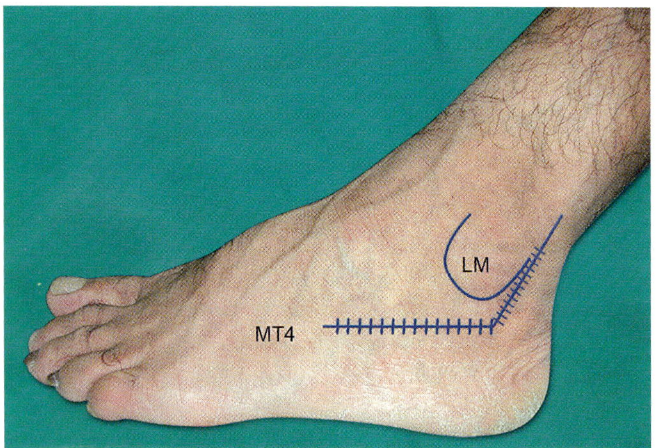

Fig. 4: The lateral aspect of the foot with the incision marked for extended sinus tarsi approach. (LM: lateral malleolus; MT4: fourth metatarsal bone)

through the tuberosity, and provisional reduction and temporary stabilization can be done with K-wires. Firstly, the anterior fragment is reduced and pinned to the sustentacular fragment, and then the lateral articular fragments are reduced and pinned. The tuberosity is then reduced and temporarily pinned from posteriorly into the sustentacular fragment or the anterior process.

Once the adequate reduction is observed with imaging, a lateral calcaneal plate is slid under the subperiosteally elevated soft-tissue flap and the plate is directed and fixed to the anterior fragments. After fixation of the anterior articular fragments, the screws for the tuberosity are inserted percutaneously. After the fixation, the EDB and the sinus tarsi fat pad are reduced and sutured back into their anatomic locations. If required, the CFL may be repaired back.

The advantage of this approach is preservation of the blood supply to the lateral calcaneal skin flap by avoiding

dissection through the deep portion of the superficial peroneal retinaculum.

The LCA runs parallel to the small saphenous vein in the space between the tendo-Achilles and the lateral malleolus.

The lateral arch of the foot is formed by the LCA, a branch of the anterior tibial artery, and the lateral tarsal artery, a branch of the dorsalis pedis artery or the anterior tibial artery.[9]

■ GEEL AND FLEMISTER APPROACH

Geel and Flemister used a curved linear incision posteriorly and parallel to the sural nerve without any sharp angulation in order to avoid the wound healing complications **(Figs. 5A and B)**.[10]

The approach follows the Langer's lines, starting anterior to the tendo-Achilles, 2 cm superior to the tip of the lateral malleolus. It then extends obliquely to the tuberosity of the calcaneus, inferior to the peroneal tendons to the level of the anterior process. The incision is deepened and the sural nerve is isolated and protected. The incision is deepened directly to the bone and the full-thickness flap, which includes the peroneal tendons in its sheath, is elevated anteriorly. The fracture is reduced and temporarily stabilized with K-wires, and then to definitive fixation. Authors reported only one superficial wound infection out of the 33 cases operated, and none of the patients developed sural nerve injury.[10]

■ POSTEROPLANTAR APPROACH[11]

The advantage of this approach is that it is done through internervous and intervascular planes, thereby helping in developing a well-vascularized soft-tissue flap **(Fig. 6)**.

Surgery is done in the prone position with the feet hanging over the end of the operating table. The incision starts

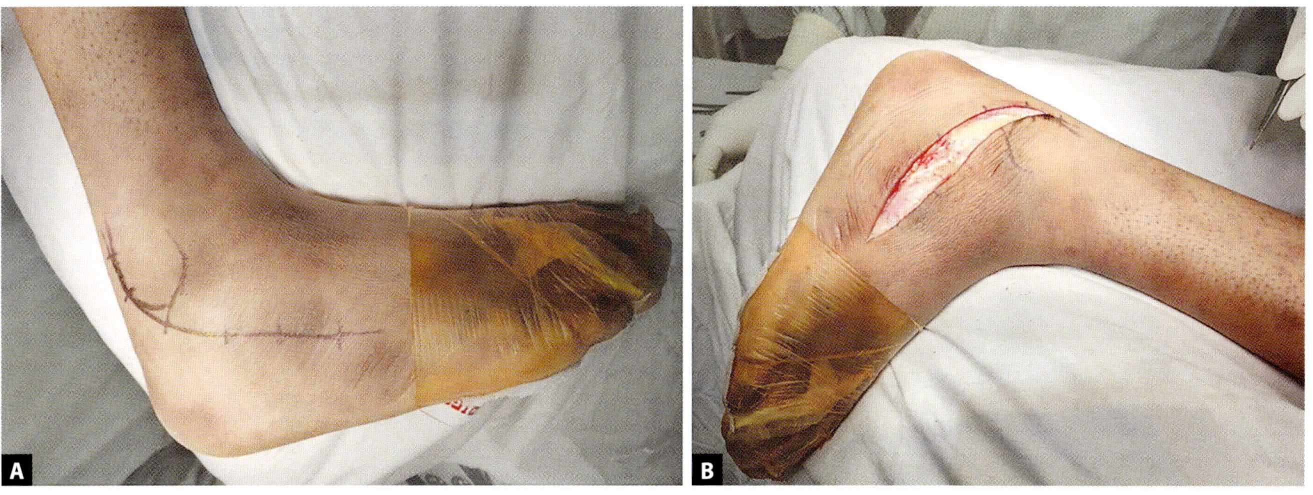

Figs. 5A and B: Geel and Flemister approach.

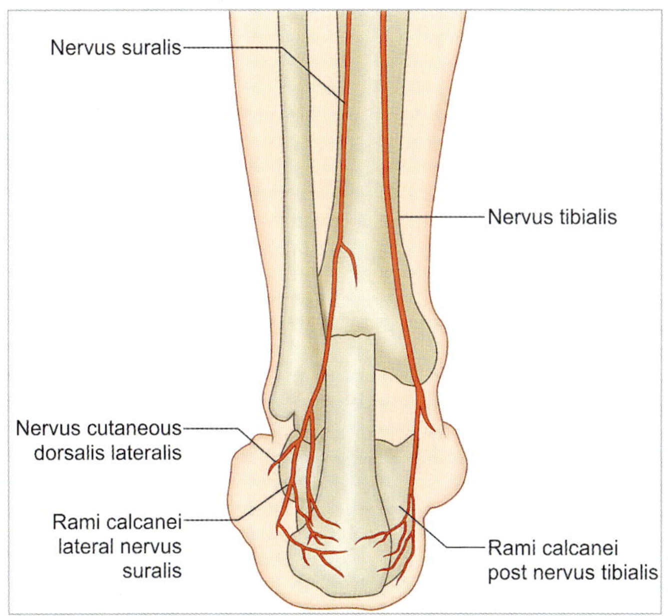

Fig. 6: Course of nerves visualized from the posterior aspect of the foot and ankle.

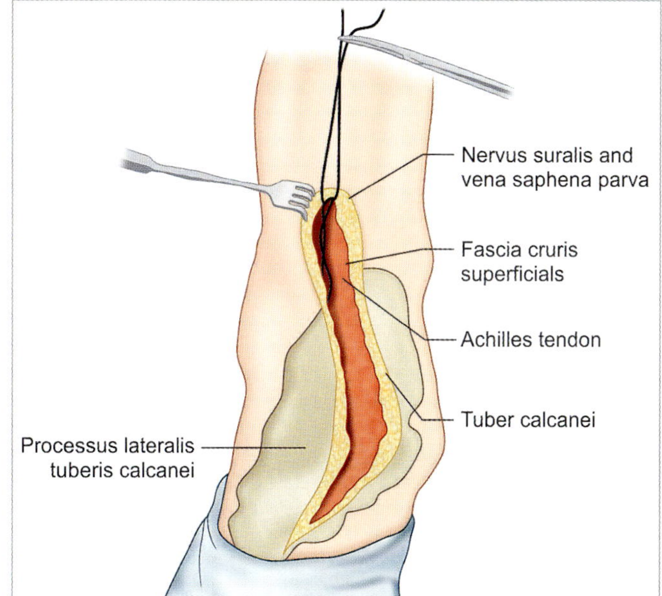

Fig. 7: Posterior plantar approach through the internervous and intervascular planes. The sural nerve is protected with loops.

8–10 cm proximal to the tuberosity of the calcaneus along the lateral side of the tendo-Achilles. This leads to the middle of the heel to the sole where it turns to the tuberosity of the fifth metatarsal. The sural nerve can be visualized in the proximal part of the incision and is isolated and protected with loops **(Fig. 7)**. The incision goes right down to the tuberosity of the os calcis, plantar aponeurosis, and the tuberosity of the fifth metatarsal.

The peroneus longus tendon crosses just proximal to the end of the incision. Dissection along the peroneal tendon and its sheath leads to the lateral wall of the calcaneus.

Thus, a skin and subcutaneous flap is raised. The plantar aponeurosis, the tendons of abductor digiti quinti, flexor hallucis longus (FHL), and flexor digitorum brevis muscles are incised close to their origins exposing the plantar aspect of the calcaneus. The medial side is mobilized as a medial flap containing the skin, subcutaneous tissue, and all short plantar muscles down to the tendon of the FHL. Now, almost the entire calcaneus is visible **(Fig. 8)**.

After the procedure, the foot muscles and the plantar aponeurosis are returned to their original position and sutured back. Skin is sutured with wide skin sutures 15–20 cm apart.

The advantage mentioned by Patnaik et al. is that the scar retracts inside, leaving no problem with weight-bearing.[12] Though the author mentions good functional results in

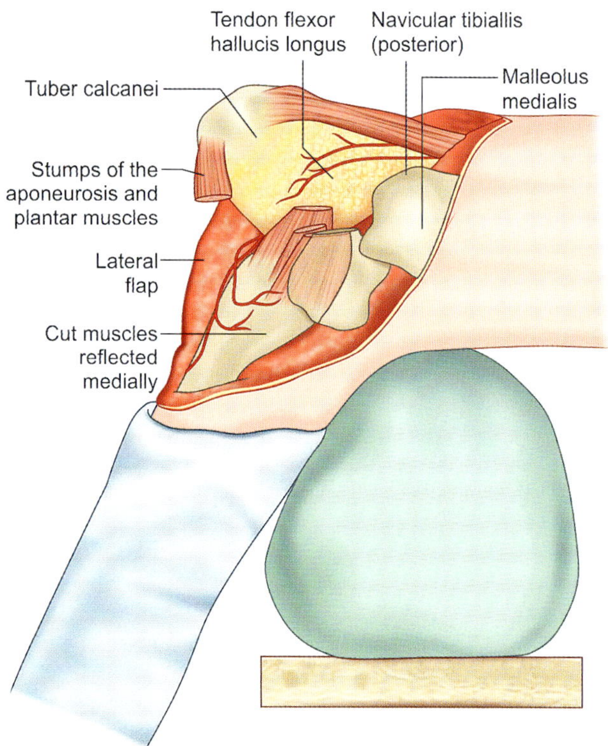

Fig. 8: Posterior plantar approach, showing the exposure of the os calcis. Extension to the medial side is shown.

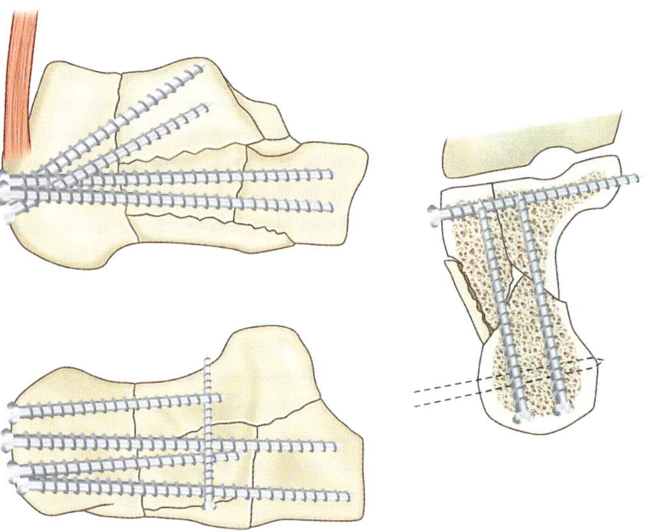

Fig. 9: Fixation with multiple screws.

the 15 cases operated, which included open reduction of fractures, damage to the plantar fat pad is of concern.[12] The procedure has not become popular and there are no reports of osteosynthesis of the calcaneus through this approach.

STRAIGHT LATERAL SUBTALAR APPROACH

The patient is positioned lateral and a 5 mm Schanz screw is inserted into the posterolateral tuberosity of the calcaneum. Closed reduction of the fracture is done by distraction valgus–varus levering using the Schanz screw as the joystick.

If reduction is not obtained, another Schanz pin is inserted into the anterolateral aspect of the distal tibia and connected to a distractor. An incision of 4–5 cm long is made from the tip of the lateral malleolus to the calcaneocuboid joint toward the base of the fourth metatarsal. The interval between the peroneal tendons and the sinus fat pad is dissected. Distally, the fascia of EDB is incised and the muscle is split in line with its fibers as far as the calcaneocuboid joint. At this moment, the posterior facet, the anterior process, and the calcaneocuboid joint are accessible. The fragments are cleaned off soft tissues, and the impacted posterolateral fragment is elevated and everted to access the impacted medial wall. Reduction of the fragments is now possible, and they are fixed temporarily with K-wires. Now, continue the dissection along the angle of Gissane to the

anterior facet and its cuboid facet. Definitive fixation can now be done with a lateral plate, fixing the posterior joint block to the anterior process. Now the tuberosity fragment is levered into its position. Multiple screws can now be introduced through a transverse incision at the posterior part of the heel distal to the insertion of the tendo-Achilles **(Fig. 9)**. Weber et al. used two parallel screws directed upward so that they end in the posteromedial and posterolateral fragments. They then used two additional screws into the dorsal portion of the anterior process of the calcaneus. If there is bulge in the lateral wall, that is now reduced and a screw is used if necessary.

EXTENDED LATERAL TRANSCALCANEAL APPROACH

Surgery is done with the patient in the lateral position. The incision starts about 5 cm proximal to the lateral malleolus almost in the posterior midline, and extends distally anterior to the tendo-Achilles along the posterior edge of the heel. It then curves anteriorly along the edge of the foot to the base of the fifth metatarsal. The incision passes posterior to the sural nerve which is elevated with the anterior flap **(Fig. 10)**.

The incision is deepened to the bone. Anteriorly, the calcaneocuboid joint is exposed by splitting the abductor muscles along its fibers. A thick subperiosteal flap is raised till the subtalar joint by sharp dissection. The peroneal tendons along with its sheath are elevated along with this flap. By placing a level into the talar neck, the soft tissues are retracted exposing the posterior aspect of the subtalar joint. Sometimes an osteotomy may be required on the lateral

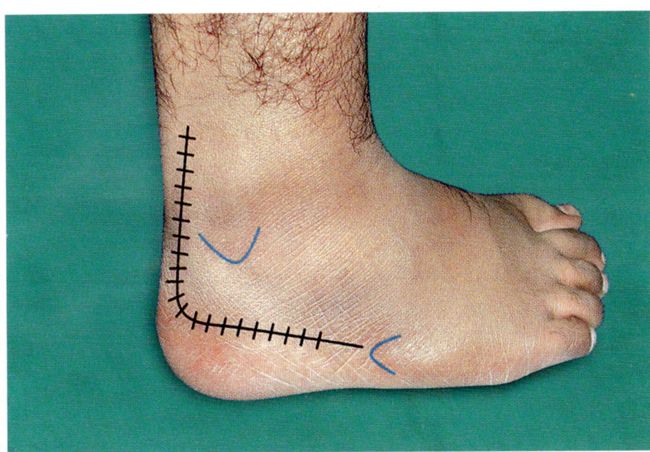

Fig. 10: Skin marking for the extended lateral transcalcaneal approach.

wall, and the fragment turned down to visualize the lateral joint fragment.

Once the fragment is lifted off, the medial side of the calcaneum can be seen, with the sustentacular fragment above and the body fragment below. Varus deformity of these fragments is reduced with bone leverage with a periosteal elevator. Reduction is now held with K-wires. Lateral joint fragment is now reduced to the sustentacular fragment and congruity of the posterior subtalar joint facet is restored. This reduction is also held with K-wires **(Figs. 11A to E)**.

Weber et al. used an AO 3.5 Y-shaped plate for the lateral fixation.[4]

SUSTENTACULAR APPROACH[13]

The sustentacular approach is ideal for isolated fractures of the sustentaculum tali. This may also be combined with the extended lateral approach if there is comminution of the sustentaculum tali and its medial joint facet. A 3–5 cm horizontal incision is made directly over the sustentaculum tali, which lies 2 cm below and 1 cm anterior to the tip of the medial malleolus. Fixation is usually done with long 3.5 mm compression screws **(Figs. 11A to E)**.

MEDIAL APPROACH[13]

With this approach, there is no control of the joint congruity of the posterior facet, and only indirect reduction of the fracture fragments is possible. In such cases, an additional lateral incision is mandatory.

The incision is made horizontally or as a lazy S cut, 8–10 cm long, midway between the tip of the medial malleolus and the sole. The incision begins 2.5 cm anterior and 4 cm distal to the medial malleolus and directed to the tendo-Achilles. The neurovascular bundle is identified and protected. The interval between the FHL and the posterior

tibial nerve is developed. The abductor hallucis muscle is retracted to expose the medial surface of the calcaneal body.

The bump felt immediately above the FHL tendon is the sustentaculum tali. The fragment can be temporarily fixed with K-wires and definitive fixation is done with screws.

CARR'S MODIFICATION OF THE MEDIAL APPROACH[7]

The major obstacle of the medial approach described by Rammelt and Zwipp is the medial neurovascular bundle. Carr modified the medial approach to avoid injury to the medial neurovascular structures and providing enough exposure to fix a small plate **(Figs. 12A to C)**.[14] If more exposure of the tuberosity is required, the incision can be extended proximally. The incision is made obliquely two finger-breadths posterior to the medial malleolus **(Fig. 13)**.

GILLIE'S APPROACH[15]

The incision is 2.5 inches along the lateral side of the tendo-Achilles to the os calcis **(Fig. 14)**. The incision is deepened and the plane between the gastrosoleus complex and the long toe flexors is developed. Little bit of fat lying between the tendo-Achilles and the subtalar joint is excised for better visualization. If necessary, this can be converted to the extended lateral approach.

CINCINNATI UNIVERSITY APPROACH

The patient is positioned prone, with the leg supported on a sandbag. A lateral and medial approach is made as in classical approaches to the calcaneum. This is then connected below the insertion of the tendo-Achilles with a transverse posterior incision **(Fig. 15)**. Subperiosteally dissect to create a U-shaped flap consisting of skin, fatty heel pad, and plantar fascia. This approach is particularly useful in children's fractures.[16]

The Cincinnati university approach is used to approach the entire plantar surface of the calcaneus.

COMBINED MEDIAL AND LATERAL APPROACHES[17]

The lateral surface is approached through a modified Kocher approach. The incision which is 10–12 cm long begins proximal and posterior to the tip of the fibula and curves at the level of the floor of the sinus tarsi to reach the calcaneocuboid joint. The incision is carried down to the sheath of the peroneal tendons. The sural nerve is identified and protected. The anterior flap is retracted above the sheath of the peroneal tendons. The peroneal tendons are retracted anteriorly. The CFL is identified and the

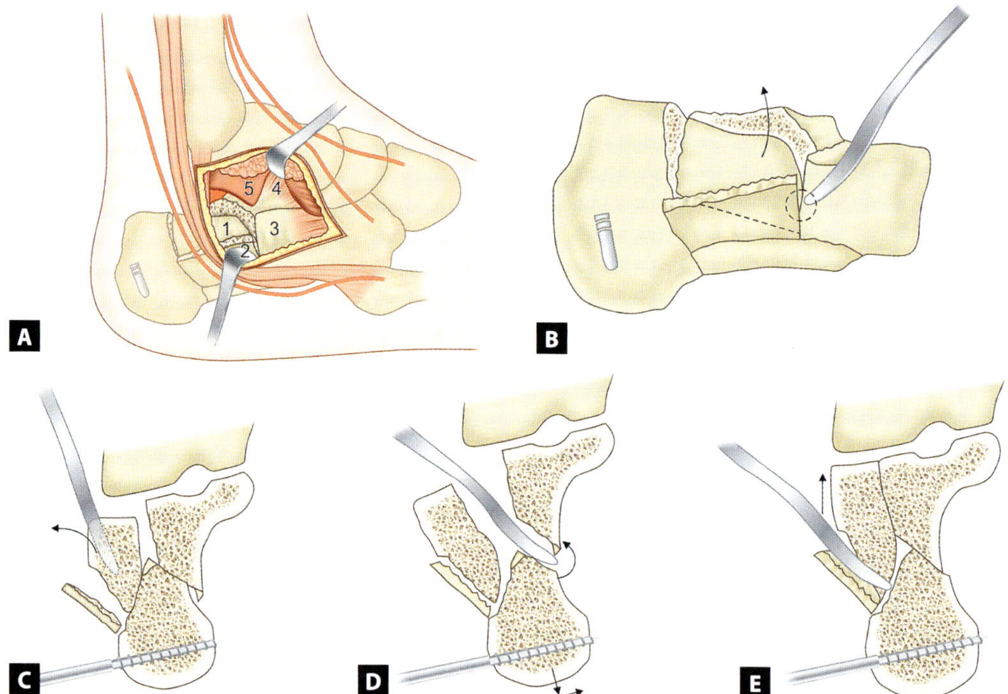

Figs. 11A to E: (A) Artworks showing steps of calcaneus reduction: (1) Impacted facet fragment, (2) lateral wall fragment, (3) anterior process, (4) interosseous ligament, and (5) lateral process of talus; (B and C) Removing lateral wall and facet fragment; (D and E) Reduction of tuberosity and facet fragment. Opening lateral wall with extended lateral approach.

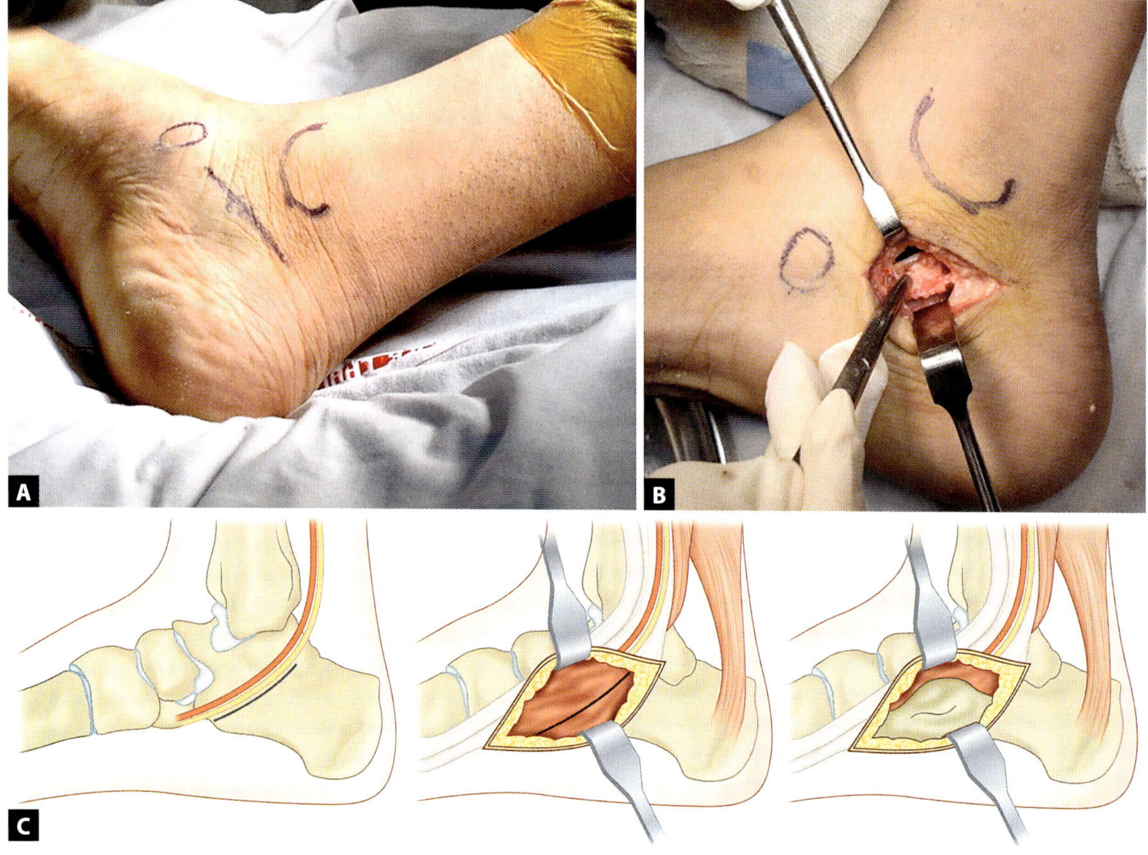

Figs. 12A to C: Medial approach to the sustentaculum.

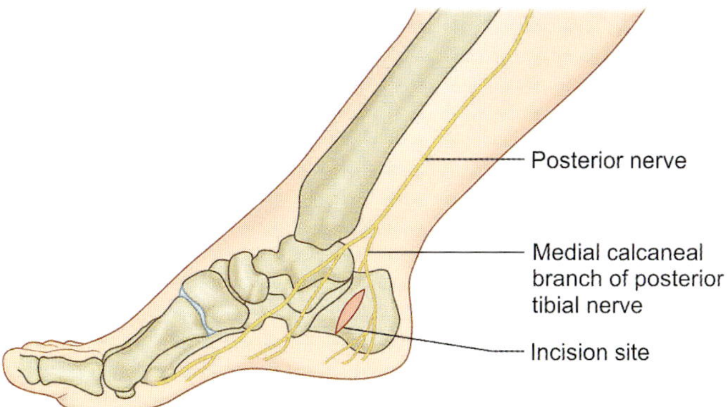

Fig. 13: Limited medial approach two finger-breadths posterior to the medial malleolus.

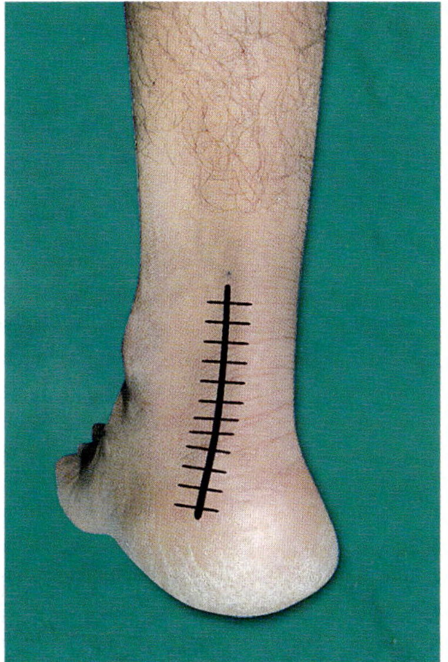

Fig. 14: Skin marking of Gillie's approach on the lateral side of the tendo-Achilles.

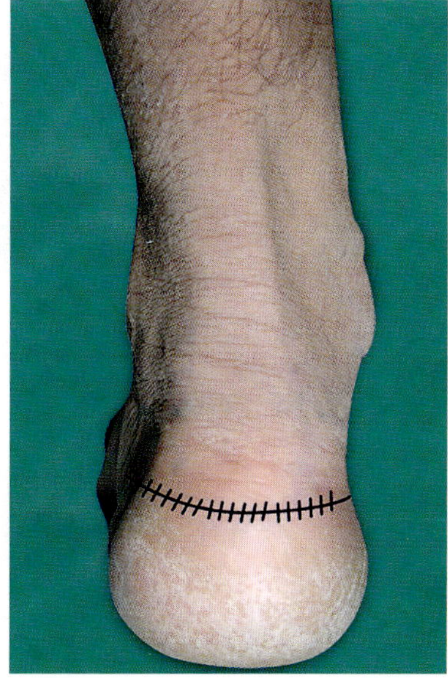

Fig. 15: Skin marking of Cincinnati University approach.

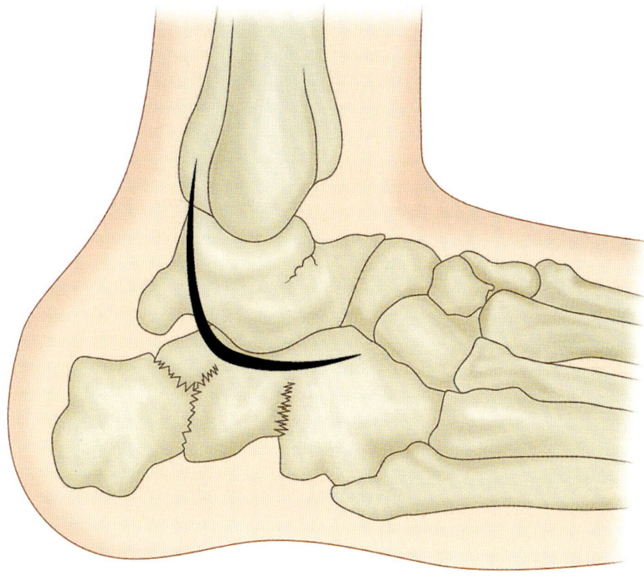

Fig. 16: Medial incision in combined medial and lateral approaches.

talocalcaneal ligament anterior to it is excised. The lateral wall of the calcaneus is denuded of soft tissue. Now the distal end of the CFL is detached. This ligament along with the fibulotalocalcaneal ligament and the sheath of the peroneal tendons is retracted superiorly. The entire lateral wall of the calcaneus is now visible. The fracture is reduced and temporarily held with K-wires. If the imaging does not show congruent reduction of the medial side, a medial approach is made **(Fig. 16)**.

A finger is passed through the dorsal surface of the calcaneum from the lateral incision, posterior to the posterior facet, until the skin on the medial side is tented. A vertical incision of 6–8 cm is now made extending from the tip of the finger to the edge of the fat pad of the heel. The flexor retinaculum is now incised. The neurovascular bundle is retracted anteriorly and the abductor hallucis muscle is retracted inferiorly to expose the fracture surfaces. The tuberosity can now be grasped with reduction forceps.

The fragments are now reduced and held with K-wires before definitive fixation.

Accurate reduction of the tuberosity relative to the superomedial fragment is possible through the medial approach and through the lateral approach the posterior facet.

◼ OLLIER APPROACH

Incision begins over the dorsolateral aspect of the talonavicular joint and continues inferoposteriorly and obliquely to end 1 cm inferior to the lateral malleolus **(Fig. 17)**. The long extensors of the toes are exposed and

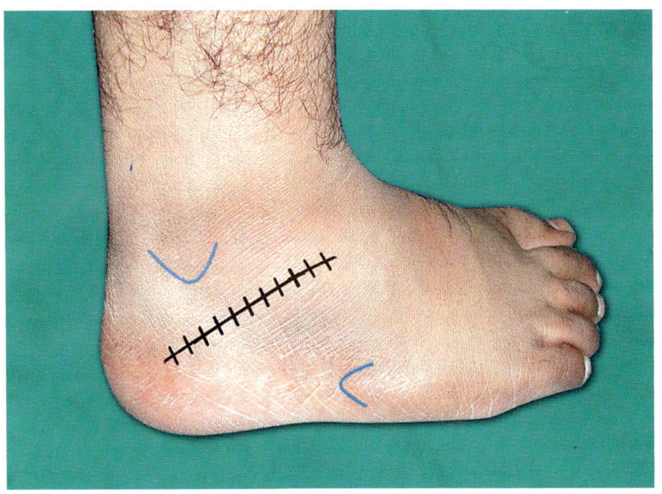

Fig. 17: Skin marking on the lateral side for Ollier approach.

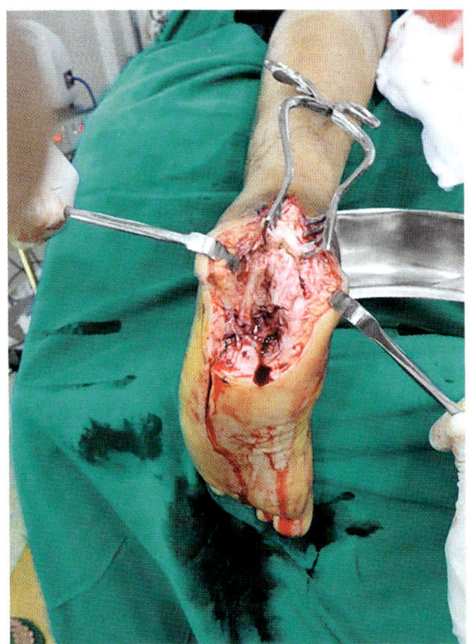

Fig. 18: Split calcaneus after Gaenslen's approach.

retracted superiorly. Inferiorly, the peroneal tendons are exposed and retracted.

The origin of the EDB is divided and retracted distally. The sinus tarsi are now exposed. The incision is ideal for a subtalar arthrodesis.

■ HEEL SPLITTING APPROACH

First described by Gaenslen in 1931, *the split heel approach is an excellent and safe way of management for chronic osteomyelitis of calcaneum, especially when there is a central ulcer or soft-tissue defect.*

The incision starts on the plantar surface of the foot, below tuberosity of the fifth metatarsal bone, on a line bisecting the heel and the middle toe. It then extends over the heel and ends after splitting the tendo-Achilles for about 3 cm. The cut is through the skin and plantar aponeurosis, in between abductor digiti quinti and flexor digitorum brevis. The quadratus plantae fibers were exposed and split longitudinally. The calcaneum can be divided from posterior to anterior with a broad osteotome and split into two halves to expose the interior of the bone **(Fig. 18)**.[18,19]

■ REFERENCES

1. Maxfield JE, McDermott FJ. Experiences with the Palmer open reduction of fractures of the calcaneus. J Bone Joint Surg Am. 1955;37A:99-106.
2. Palmer I. The mechanism and treatment of fractures of the calcaneus: open reduction with the use of cancellous grafts. J Bone Joint Surg Am. 1948;30A:2-8.
3. Chan S, Ip FK. Open reduction and internal fixation for displaced intra-articular fractures of the os calcis. Injury. 1995;26:111-5.
4. Weber M, Lehmann O, Sagesser D, Krause F. Limited open reduction and internal fixation of displaced intra-articular fractures of the calcaneum. J Bone Joint Surg Br. 2008;90(12):1608-16.
5. Schepers T. The sinus tarsi approach in displaced intra-articular calcaneal fractures: a systematic review. Int Orthop. 2011;35:697-703.
6. Mostafa MF, El-Adl G, Hassanin EY, Abdellatif MS. Surgical treatment of displaced intra-articular calcaneal fracture using a single small lateral approach. Strateg Trauma Limb Reconstr. 2010;5:87-95.
7. Carr JB. Surgical treatment of intra-articular calcaneal fractures: a review of small incision approaches. J Orthop Trauma. 2005;19:109-17.
8. Femino JE, Vaseenon T, Levin DA, Yian EH. Modification of the sinus tarsi approach for open reduction and plate fixation of intra-articular calcaneus fractures: the limits of proximal extension based upon the vascular anatomy of the lateral calcaneal artery. Iowa Orthop J. 2010;30:161-7.
9. Andermahr J, Helling HJ, Landwehr P, Fischbach R, Koebke J, Rehm KE. The lateral calcaneal artery. Surg Radiol Anat. 1998;20:419-23.
10. Geel CW, Flemister Jr AS. Standardized treatment of intra-articular calcaneal fractures using an oblique lateral incision and no bone graft. J Trauma. 2001;50:1083-9.
11. Poigenfürst J. The postero-plantar approach to the os calcis. Orthop Traumatol. 1993;2:44-54.
12. Patnaik VVG, Singla RK, Gupta PN. Surgical incisions—their anatomic basis, part III—lower limb. J Anat Soc India. 2001;50:48-58.
13. Rammelt S, Zwipp H. Calcaneus fractures: facts, controversies and recent developments. Injury. 2004;35:443-61.
14. Eastwood DM, Langkamer VG, Atkins RM. Intra-articular fractures of the calcaneum. Part II: Open reduction and

internal fixation by the extended lateral transcalcaneal approach. J Bone Joint Surg Br. 1993;75(2):189-95.

15. Gallie WE. Subastragalar arthrodesis in fractures of the os calcis. J Bone Joint Surg. 1943;25:731-6.

16. Van Frank E, Ward JC, Engelhardt P. Bilateral calcaneal fracture in childhood: case report and review of the literature. Arch Orthop Trauma Surg. 1998;118:111-2.

17. Stephenson JR. Treatment of displaced intra-articular fractures of the calcaneus using medial and lateral approaches, internal fixation, and early motion. J Bone Joint Surg Am. 1987;69(1):115-30.

18. Gaenslen FJ. Split-heel approach in osteomyelitis of os calcis. J Bone Joint Surg. 1931;13(4):759-72.

19. Horwitz T. Partial resection of the os calcis and primary closure in the treatment of resistant large ulcers of the heel, with or without osteomyelitis of the os calcis. Clin Orthop Relat Res. 1972;84:149-53.

8

Percutaneous Reduction and Fixation of Calcaneal Fractures

Tim Schepers

"Methods mean nothing unless they are applied intelligently and are adapted to the case in hand".
–Paul Magnuson, 1938

■ INTRODUCTION

Probably, the oldest surgical technique for calcaneal fractures is percutaneous reduction and fixation. In 1855, Clark published his method to reduce a displaced calcaneus fracture (or dislocation) with some form of pulley system, predating the first radiograph about 40 years.[1]

The percutaneous (or minimally invasive) approaches were commonly used before open reduction and internal fixation (ORIF) was established. In times when ORIF was associated with a too high complication rate or adequate fixation systems (e.g., anatomic plates) were lacking.[2] After the introduction of preoperative antibiotics and an increased understanding of the fracture anatomy with the rise of the computed tomography (CT) scans in the mid-1980s, open reduction (via the extended lateral approach) became the new gold standard. However, many still use the percutaneous techniques (or turned to other less invasive procedures such as the sinus tarsi approach) to date.

■ PRINCIPLES OF MANAGEMENT

The surgical management of calcaneal fractures is aimed at restoring the overall anatomy and reducing the articular surface of the posterior facet.

Any procedure for displaced intra-articular calcaneal fractures (DIACF) should:
- Restore the height and length of calcaneum
- Correct the varus/valgus malalignment
- Correct the heel widening at the tuberosity
- Anatomical reduction of the posterior facet fragments.

Percutaneous reduction of DIACF is based on the principle of ligamentotaxis to achieve the above stated goals **(Figs. 1A to C)**. It relies on the presence of the strong

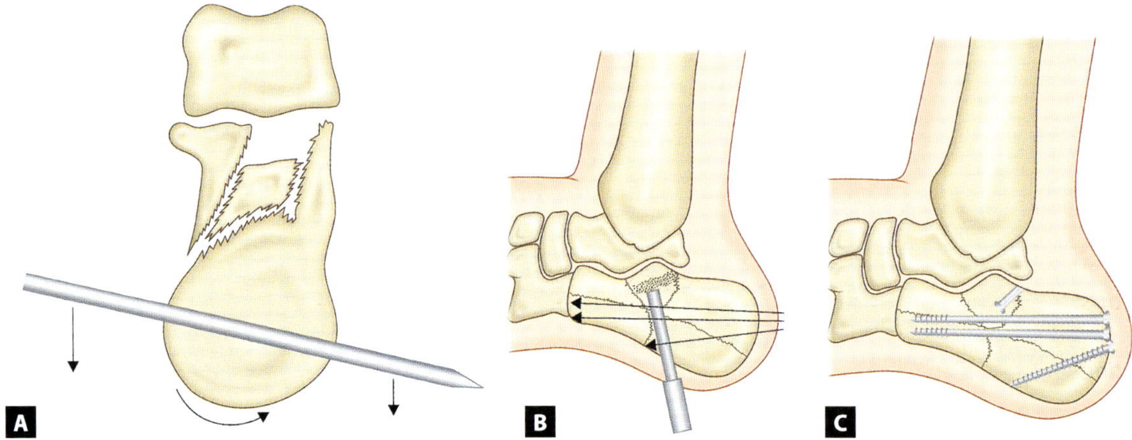

Figs. 1A to C: (A) A thick Kirschner wire (K-wire) or a Steinmann pin is placed into the calcaneal tuberosity to give traction and correct the height and length of the calcaneus. The varus angulation can also be corrected by pulling this pin at an angle toward the lateral side. (B) A bone punch is inserted below the depressed region of the posterior facet, which is lifted up with gentle push. The articular congruity of the posterior facet thus regained is verified under an image intensifier. K-wires are then placed to maintain the reduction. (C) After achieving reduction, screws are placed to maintain the length, height, and the posterior facet articular congruity.

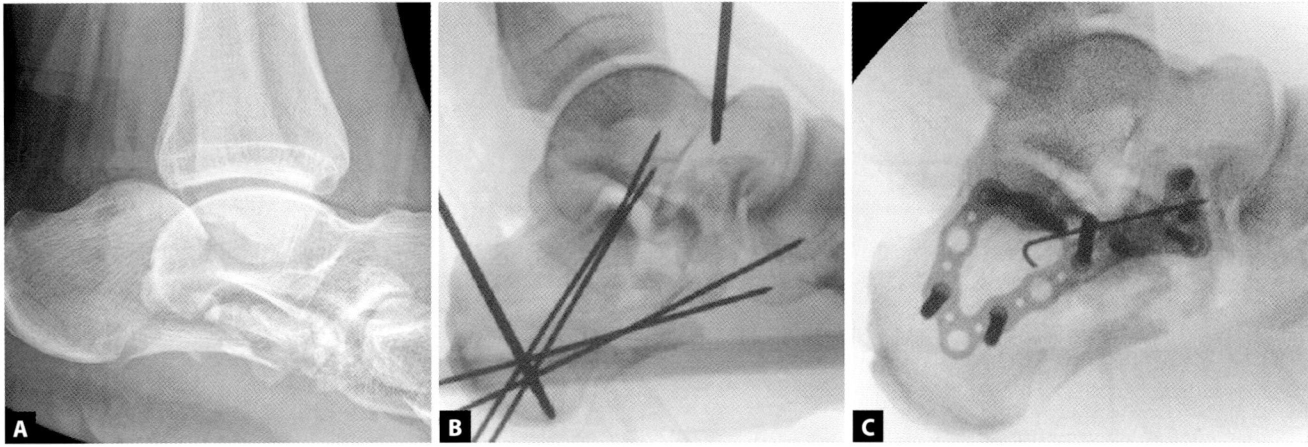

Figs. 2A to C: (A) Grade-2 open fracture of the calcaneus with subtalar dislocation; (B) Reduction with Schanz pin (removed) and small distractor and temporary fixation with Kirschner wire; (C) Definitive open reduction and internal fixation via extended lateral approach.

joint capsule and various ligaments that surround and stabilize the calcaneum. The ligaments include, among others, the talocalcaneal ligament in between the subtalar joint, the calcaneofibular ligament on the lateral side, and the tibiocalcaneal ligaments on the medial side, besides assisting in the reduction of the bony fragments attached to these specific ligaments. Fragments that are not attached to ligaments (e.g., central joint fragments) should be reduced by leverage with Kirschner wires (K-wires) inserted in the fragment or using a blunt punch inserted from the plantar side of the foot.

Following the reduction, a percutaneous fixation with screws, K-wires, or an external frame is performed. The fixation method should preferably allow for early full range of motion exercises.

The percutaneous techniques are well suited for less complex fractures (e.g., Sanders type II). In poor soft tissues such as open fractures or in less fit patients with a high risk of complications, the percutaneous techniques are a viable option.[3,4] In addition, percutaneous reduction can be used as an emergency procedure as a bridge to definitive surgery in either open fractures or severe tongue-type fractures with skin at risk for ischemic injury **(Figs. 2A to C)**.

■ DIFFERENT TECHNIQUES

Percutaneous techniques can be divided into different groups:
- *Distraction or ligamentotaxis:*
  - Single-point distraction
  - Two-point (linear) distraction
  - Triple-point (triangular) distraction
- K-wire leveraging (without distraction forces)
- *External fixation:*
  - Unilateral frame

- Bilateral frame
- Circular frame
- Arthroscopically assisted procedures
- Balloon-kyphoplasty technique.

Ligamentotaxis

Single-point Distraction

The earliest percutaneous technique utilized a Steinmann pin just above the calcaneus in front of the Achilles tendon.[2] Later, the pin was drilled through the tuberosity **(Fig. 3A)**. By applying traction, the arch of the foot could be restored by reducing the upward displacement of the tuberosity. Some performed a percutaneous Achilles tenotomy prior to traction and applied a cast while continuing the traction.[1]

Others applied elaborate contraptions to maintain the traction. The chances over time in these techniques are shown nicely in the review by Goff from 1938.[2]

More recently, this single-point distraction is still in use to aid in the reduction of calcaneal fractures.[5] However, especially the single-point distraction is rarely used in solitude. Additional maneuvers are required to realign the calcaneus.

Two-point Distraction

Two-point distraction (linear) involves traction on the tuberosity of the calcaneus with countertraction being provided at the talar neck[6] or tibia shaft[1] **(Fig. 3B)**. Lorenz Böhler is most famous for this technique; however, he fine-tuned his practice several times over the years. Many have followed his advice with or without modifications.[1] Following reduction by traction, the widening of the heel was addressed using a screw vise as compression clamp. After radiographs showed satisfactory reduction, a cast was applied embedding both traction pins.

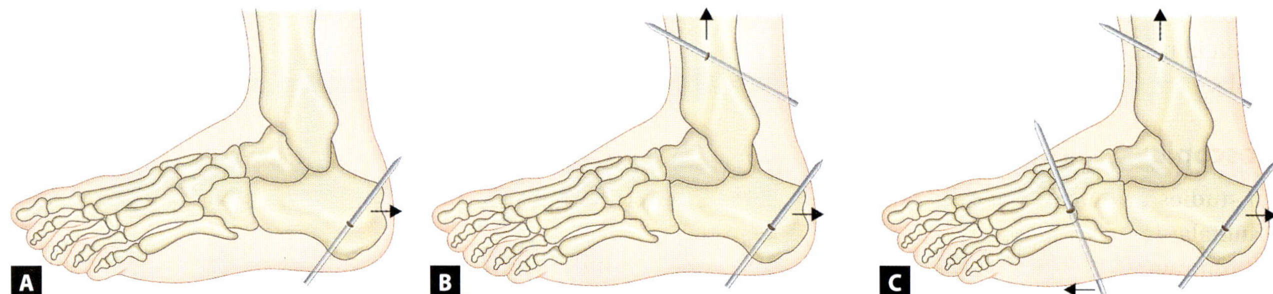

Figs. 3A to C: (A) Traction is given at the calcaneal tuberosity to correct the height and varus in the single-point distraction method; (B) Two-point distraction consists of traction and countertraction through the calcaneus and the tibia or talar neck; (C) Three-point distraction consists of giving traction through the tibia, tibia and also at the forefoot or cuboid. This helps in achieving the correct height, length, and axis in calcaneal fractures.

Three-point Distraction

The use of three-point (triangular) distraction was published by both McBride and Gill in 1944 and later popularized by Forgon and Zadravecz.[7] Traction is applied to the calcaneal tuber, talus, or tibia and cuboid bone or the forefoot to achieve the distraction **(Fig. 3C)**.[1] These three points of distraction provide forces opposite to those that caused the fracture, thus helping in reduction of the fracture and reorientation of the anatomy in all three planes.[8,9]

Kirschner Wire Leveraging

Indirect fracture reduction by K-wire or axial pin leverage is often named after Peter Essex-Lopresti.[10] It was, however, introduced by Westhues in 1934 and modified with the use of a specially designed spike by Gissane in 1941. Others quickly adopted this technique as well, stating that it was most suited for tongue-type fractures.[11] After inserting the pin (Steinmann, Schanz, or Gissane) from the posterior superior lateral joint fragment, it is used as a lever to realign the joint fragment by elevation of the fragment and pulling the tuber out of varus. The maneuver has a role in tongue-type fractures, particularly Sanders type IIC, in which this fragment contains the whole posterior facet, displaced in entirety. However, it can also be used in type IIB as well as more complex fractures, with or without additional maneuvers. The lateral wall is then squeezed inward to diminish the widening of the calcaneus. In the older descriptions, this was followed by applying a plaster slipper or lower leg cast that incorporated the pin. Later studies used either K-wires or (cannulated) screws for stabilization of the reduction.[11-13] For joint-depression-type fractures, the reduction maneuvers can be more elaborate.

External Fixator

The use of external fixation suits two purposes: First to aid in the reduction, especially height and axis, and second, to maintain reduction. Overall, four different ways of external fixation are described in the literature.

Unilateral External Fixation

Following percutaneous reduction, one could use external fixation to maintain the position of the fragments. Special, calcaneal fracture-specific, unilateral external fixation devices have been used by Magnan et al. and later by others.[14] The reduction is partially done with the frame; however, additional techniques as described above may be applied as well.

Bilateral External Fixation

Bilateral frames are placed on both sides of the foot. This allows for more controlled distraction and correction of the axis by distracting one side more than the opposite side. The pins for the external fixation can be placed solely on the calcaneus (proximal and distal fragments of tongue-type fracture, from calcaneal tuberosity to the tibia shaft, from calcaneal tuberosity to the talar neck, or in a triangular delta-shape fashion on the tuber calcaneus, tibia shaft, and either fore/midfoot or talar neck).

Circular (Ilizarov) Frame

The Ilizarov frame, initially used for the treatment of nonunions and malunions, is also known as the (fine wire) circular frame.[15] The treatment of displaced calcaneal fractures using the Ilizarov frame is directed at lowering the complication rates associated with the open approaches. It usually consists of one or two rings at the level of tibia shaft connected to a footplate that is attached to the calcaneus with fine wires or a ring at the calcaneus and around the talus. The frame is used as a reduction tool using ligamento-taxis via two- or three-point distraction. Some authors used the Ilizarov frame in combination with a sinus tarsi approach or Ollier approach. Others used fully percutaneous techniques to reduce the posterior facet.[16] The frame is usually left in place for 6–12 weeks, but early weight-bearing is possible.[15]

Arthroscopically Assisted Procedure

Several studies have shown that an anatomical reduction of the subtalar joint, with a step-off of <2 mm, is associated with an improved outcome.[17] The percutaneous reduction fully relies on the fluoroscopic imaging to assess the subtalar joint, making the identification of small step-offs difficult. To obtain the best possible percutaneous reduction, without fully opening the joint, arthroscopy has been described first in 2002.[18] Using a posterolateral and anterolateral portal, the subtalar joint is evaluated following percutaneous reduction. The reduction techniques are similar to those described above. This technique is preferably used in Sanders type II fractures.[18]

Balloon-kyphoplasty Technique

Probably the latest addition to the percutaneous armament is the balloon-assisted reduction, also known as kyphoplasty or stentoplasty.[19] By inflating a balloon underneath the subtalar joint, it pushes the subtalar joint back in place. By subsequently injecting cement (usually calcium phosphate or polymethylmethacrylate) in the cavity, the reduction of subtalar joint is supported. To guide the vector of compression and prevent blow-out of the plantar cortex, K-wires can be inserted at the bottom of the tuberosity. To aid in reduction of the height and axis, single-point traction can be used. Most authors subsequently refrain from further fixation; some use cannulated screws following cement injection or temporary K-wires. The additional benefit of this technique, in addition to the low wound complication rate, is the early return to full weight-bearing.[19]

Even though all the abovementioned techniques look unique in their own way, they have much overlap. They represent a continuous evolution of the percutaneous treatment of DIACF. No single technique has a satisfactory result in all cases. Therefore, various different techniques are often combined to obtain the best possible reduction and maintain it.[1]

■ FRACTURE FIXATION

The fixation of percutaneously treated calcaneal fractures initially consisted of retaining the reduction pin (Steinmann or Schanz) and embedding it in a cast.[10]

Kirschner wires are still often used as a quick and cheap alternative. The K-wires can either be inserted just underneath the joint (subchondral), transarticular, or in a bundle to stabilize the fracture.[20] Currently, cannulated or noncannulated screws are mostly preferred or specifically designed nails may be used.[21] Internal fixation reduces the need for implant removal (obligatory in K-wires) and the occurrence of pin-tract infection with subsequent osteomyelitis (see "Complications"). The fracture fixation can be additionally stabilized using injectable supplements.[22]

■ PERCUTANEOUS TREATMENT JOINT DEPRESSION TYPE

A case example of percutaneous treatment of joint-depression-type fracture is shown in **Figures 4A to E**.

■ PERCUTANEOUS TREATMENT TONGUE TYPE

A case example of percutaneous treatment of tongue-type fracture is shown in **Figures 5A to D**.

■ POSTOPERATIVE TREATMENT

The postoperative treatment is dependent on the techniques used. In case of external fixation, the pins should be taken care of adequately.

Preferably, the patient is allowed and urged to start full range of motion exercises as soon as possible. Especially in the first 2 weeks, the leg should be elevated to prevent edema-related complaints. A light compression stockinette may be used to counteract the swelling. If K-wires are used for fixation, they are removed at about 6–8 weeks. Prior to removal, the tips of the K-wires may be covered with short pieces of drain-tube. An above-ankle cast postoperatively is less preferable and may be used only in cases with diminished compliance. Weight-bearing is started depending on the comminution of the fracture and the stability of the fixation. Usually, after 8 weeks, there is sufficient fracture healing to start protected weight-bearing with crutches. If guidance is needed in postoperative exercises or gradually building up weight-bearing physiotherapy may be indicated.

■ RESULTS OF PERCUTANEOUS TREATMENT

Albeit some have tried to pool data on all forms of less invasive and percutaneous techniques,[23] this might be less desirable because of the heterogeneity in the literature on percutaneous treatment of calcaneal fractures. Not only because of differences in reduction and fixation techniques but also in the inclusion of specific fracture patterns, e.g., solely tongue-type fractures or severe open injuries, or in the exclusion of more comminuted fractures (e.g., Sanders type IV).[13,18,24] It may be a better idea to present combined results per treatment modality. The literature was searched for review articles pooling data for the results of

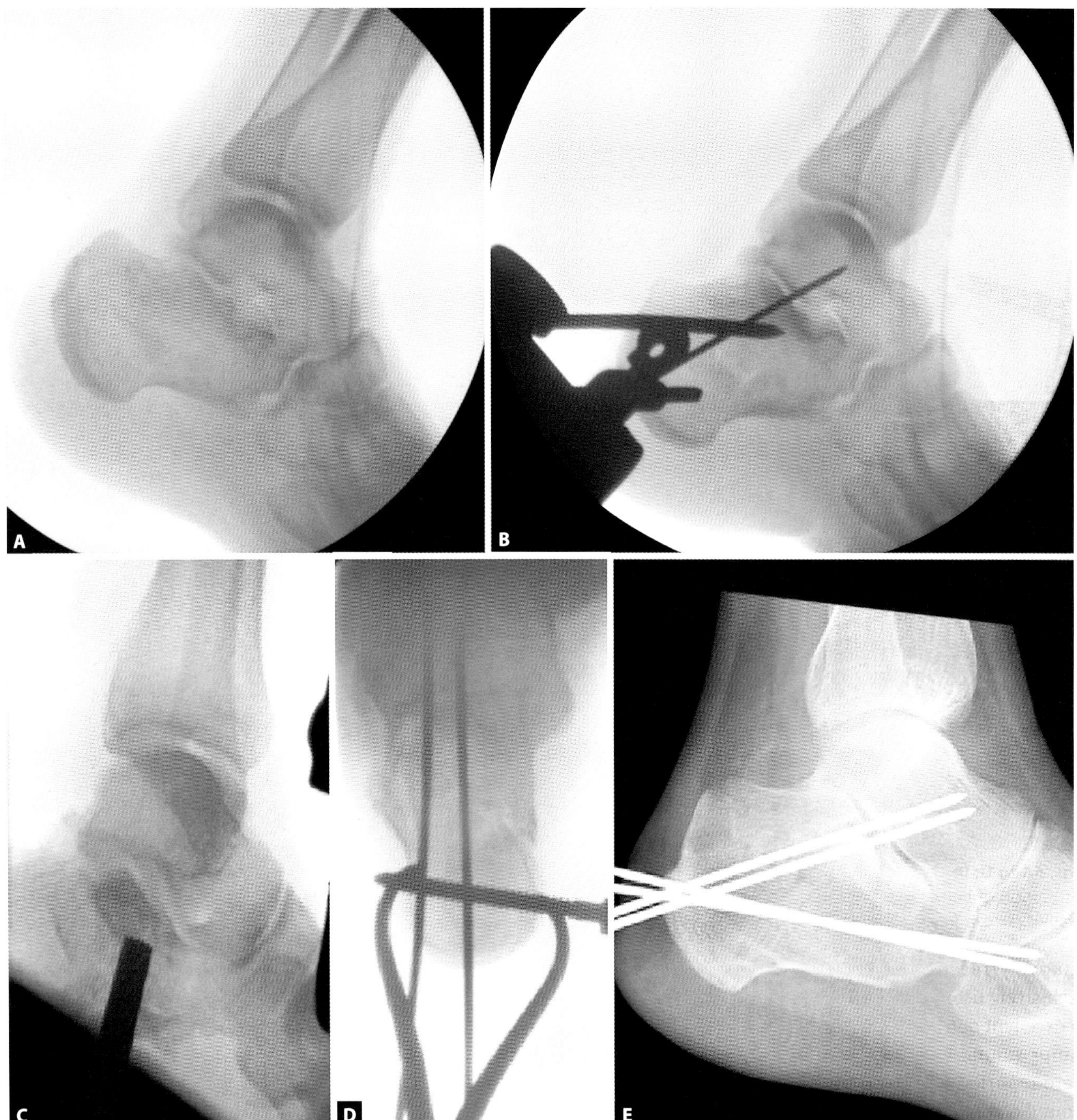

Figs. 4A to E: (A) Joint-depression-type calcaneal fracture; (B) Placement of femoral distractor on medial tibia shaft and calcaneal tuberosity, reduction aided using Steinmann pin; (C) Alternative reduction maneuver (different case) using blunt punch; (D) Correction of varus using large Weber clamp; (E) Definitive fixation using Kirschner wires.

ligamentotaxis, K-wire leveraging, and external fixation for DIACF. Narrative reviews were not included.

Schepers and Patka reviewed the literature regarding the treatment using ligamentotaxis. A total of eight studies were included, which were published from 1990 to 2008.[1] Good to excellent results were seen in 61–90% of patients.

Wound complications occurred between 2 and 30%, loss of reduction between 4 and 67%, and secondary fusion was reported between 2 and 15%. The highest rate of wound complications was seen in a series using external fixation.

No dedicated systematic review could be identified concerning the Westhues/Essex-Lopresti method. Three

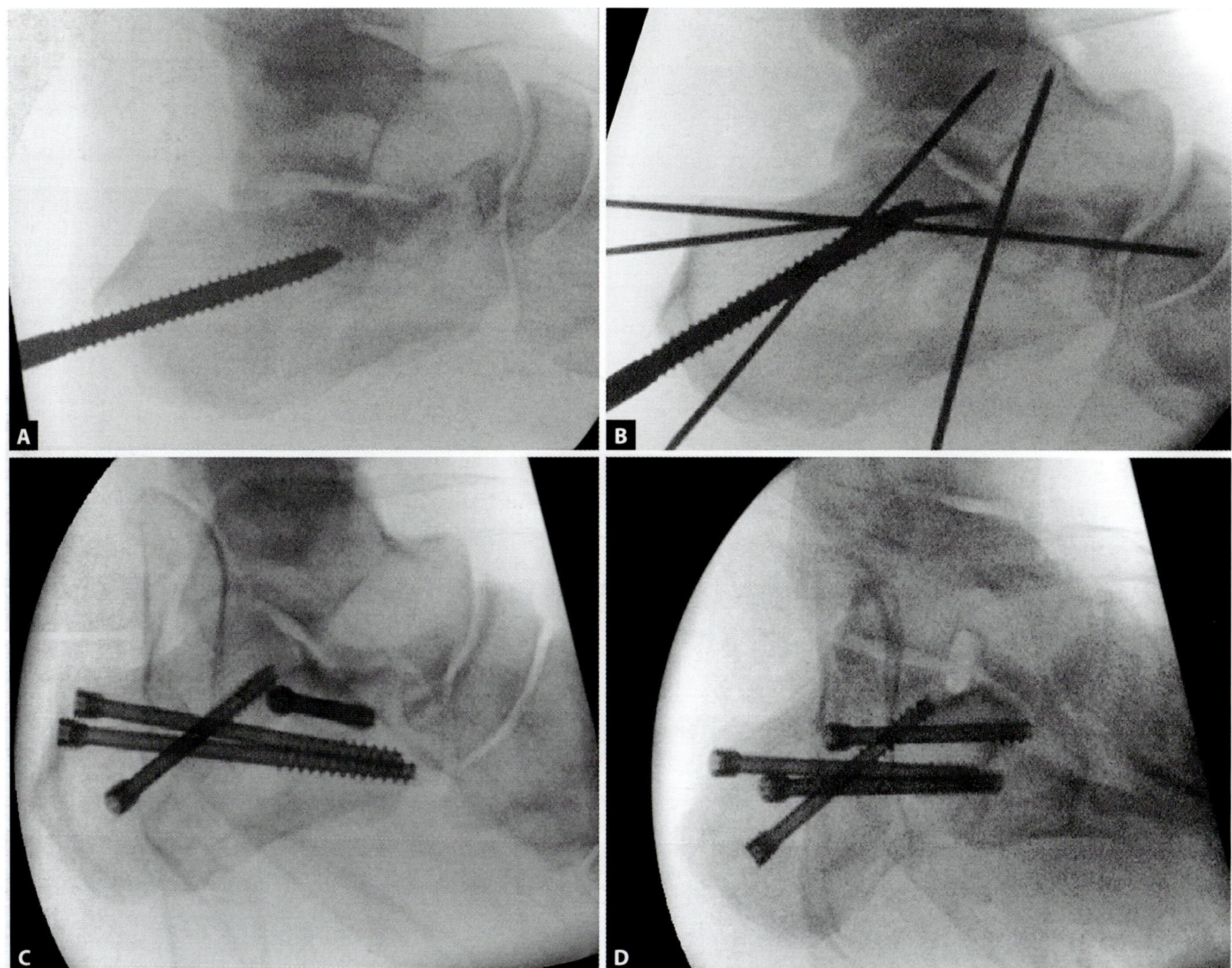

Figs. 5A to D: (A) Tongue-type calcaneal fracture prior to reduction with Schanz pin according to Westhues/Essex-Lopresti; (B) Following restoration of height, width, axis, and subtalar joint congruity and provisional fixation with Kirschner wires; (C) Definitive fixation with headless screws (lateral view); (D) Definitive fixation with headless screws (Brodén view).

relatively recent studies reporting on patients treated exclusively using the Essex-Lopresti method reported good to excellent outcomes between 70 and 80%.[11-13] A total of six minor wound complications, mainly drainage from pins, were reported for which antibiotics were given. No major wound complications occurred.

The results from the literature of treatment using the Ilizarov frame were combined by Muir et al.[15] A total of 11 studies with 255 calcaneal fractures were included in their review. Four studies used a fully percutaneous technique, and the others included a limited approach to the subtalar joint. The American Orthopedic Foot and Ankle Society (AOFAS) score, reported in four studies, ranged from a mean of 66–88 points. Overall, 86% of patients reported a good to excellent outcome. Albeit pin-tract infections were common (22.6%), serious complications, including deep infection (0.8%) and wound infection (1.6%), were less likely to occur.

Five studies reported on arthritis, and moderate or severe subtalar joint pain was reported in 36.7%.[15]

Marouby et al. performed a review regarding the percutaneous arthroscopically assisted treatment of DIACF.[25] They included eight studies that were mostly retrospective in nature and had a low level of evidence. In this review, 152 patients with 155 fractures were included. One superficial postoperative wound infection occurred. The AOFAS score per study varied from 72.1 to 94.1 points. The conclusion of the study was that despite the steep learning curve, the arthroscopically assisted treatment is a viable option with low complication rates.[25]

■ COMPLICATIONS

Every percutaneous technique has its own specific limitations and subsequent complications.

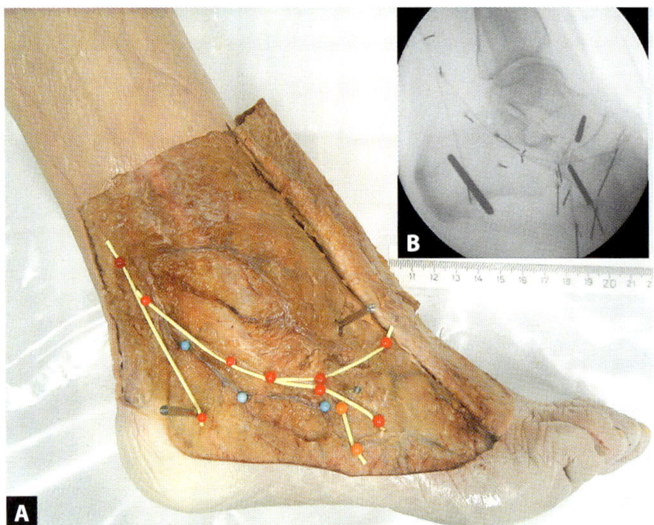

Figs. 6A and B: (A) Anatomical dissection showing the course of the sural nerve and vascular structures following the insertion of three distraction pins (calcaneal tuberosity, talar neck, and cuboid). (B) Fluoroscopy image showing the close relationship of the lateral calcaneal branch of the sural nerve.

The insertion of the distraction or external fixator pins should be done carefully, and not cause harm to any essential structure **(Figs. 6A and B)**.[26,27]

The use of K-wires for fracture fixation or external fixation pins may lead to pin-tract infection, and the use of large diameter headed screws may lead to painful implants that may need removal at a later stage. The use of cement [especially if polymethyl methacrylate (PMMA) is used] in the kyphoplasty technique may interfere with screw placement in the future in case a subtalar arthrodesis is needed.

The number of wound complications has a wide range from 0 to 15%.[1,9,28] Comparative studies of all levels of evidence comparing wound complication rates between open reduction (extended lateral approach) and percutaneous treatment show significantly lower complication rates (three to five times lower on average) in the percutaneous group.[22,28,29] The rate of complications in the sinus tarsi approach is somewhat in the middle.

The rate of implant removal ranges from 0 to 46–66%.[30] The high rates of implant removal in some studies may be due to the use of large-diameter screws with bulky screwheads. Several studies have since then advocated the use of headless screws.

The main complication in all percutaneous techniques, except perhaps for the arthroscopically assisted percutaneous procedures, is the difficulty of obtaining an anatomical result. In some less severe fractures, this may be possible; however, in complex fractures, this will most likely not be the case. This is, for example, reflected in the various images in articles with residual step-offs, gaps, insufficiently reduced height (low angle of Böhler), or persistent widening of the calcaneus. If percutaneous reduction fails, one should opt for conversion to an open technique.

The timing of the procedure is essential and should be performed preferably within the first week. Many studies perform the procedure within the first days following trauma. Waiting too long may cause partial consolidation of fracture fragments and the inability to perform an anatomical reduction.

In addition, a high rate of secondary fusions may be necessary in percutaneously treated patients, if follow-up is sufficiently long. As stated by Professor Zwipp in an expert-opinion comment on percutaneous reduction and fixation by DeWall et al., "Although it appears that percutaneous fixation may minimize postoperative infections and maintain subtalar motion, without expectation of anatomic joint reduction, I believe that the subtalar joint will deteriorate rapidly and require premature fusion".[28] This is backed up by the study by De Boer et al., where it was shown that out of 33 percutaneously treated patients, a total of 12 (36%) needed secondary subtalar arthrodesis at a median follow-up of 88 months.[30] However, none of the 27 patients treated by ORIF via an extended lateral approach with a median follow-up of 56 months needed a secondary fusion. The percutaneously treated patients also showed a lower rate of return to similar work and sports.[30] Studies on percutaneous reduction and fixation should include postoperative CT scans after surgery to assess the quality of the reduction.

In conclusion, the percutaneous reduction and fixation has several advantages over the ORIF. Mostly thanks to the significantly lower rates of surgical site infections and the early stage it can be performed. In less complex fractures, good reduction may be achieved; however, in more comminuted injuries, this will be less likely the case. Certain injuries in certain patients (open fractures or significant comorbidities) may benefit from a percutaneous procedure. In addition, the percutaneous reduction can be a valuable tool in a staged emergency procedure. Future research should focus on correlation between reduction parameters (height, width, axis, joint congruity) following percutaneous reduction and fixation and the functional outcome at sufficient follow-up (especially the need for secondary fusion). Using the arthroscope during the percutaneous procedure can aid in obtaining an improved reduction.

■ REFERENCES

1. Schepers T, Patka P. Treatment of displaced intra-articular calcaneal fractures by ligamentotaxis: current concepts' review. Arch Orthop Trauma Surg. 2009;129(12):1677-83.

2. Goff CW. Fresh fractures of the os calcis. Arch Surg. 1938;36:744-65.

3. Hammond AW, Crist BD. Percutaneous treatment of high-risk patients with intra-articular calcaneus fractures: a case series. Injury. 2013;44(11):1483-5.

4. Spierings KE, Min M, Nooijen LE, Swords MP, Schepers T. Managing the open calcaneal fracture: a systematic review. Foot Ankle Surg. 2019;25(6):707-13.

5. Stulik J, Stehlik J, Rysavy M, Wozniak A. Minimally-invasive treatment of intra-articular fractures of the calcaneum. J Bone Joint Surg Br. 2006;88(12):1634-41.

6. Frohlich P, Zakupszky Z, Csomor L. Experiences with closed screw placement in intra-articular fractures of the calcaneus. Surgical technique and outcome. Unfallchirurg. 1999;102(5):359-64.

7. Forgon M, Zadravecz G. Repositioning and retention problems of calcaneus fractures. Aktuelle Traumatol. 1983;13(6):239-46.

8. de Vroome SW, van der Linden FM. Cohort study on the percutaneous treatment of displaced intra-articular fractures of the calcaneus. Foot Ankle Int. 2014;35(2):156-62.

9. Schepers T, Schipper IB, Vogels LM, Ginai AZ, Mulder PGH, Heetveld MJ, et al. Percutaneous treatment of displaced intra-articular calcaneal fractures. J Orthop Sci. 2007;12(1):22-7.

10. Essex-Lopresti P. The mechanism, reduction technique, and results in fractures of the os calcis. Br J Surg. 1952;39(157):395-419.

11. Pillai A, Basappa P, Ehrendorfer S. Modified Essex-Lopresti/Westheus reduction for displaced intra-articular fractures of the calcaneus. Description of surgical technique and early outcomes. Acta Orthop Belg. 2007;73(1):83-7.

12. Shih JT, Kuo CL, Yeh TT, Shen HC, Pan RY, Wu CC. Modified Essex-Lopresti procedure with percutaneous calcaneoplasty for comminuted intra-articular calcaneal fractures: a retrospective case analysis. BMC Musculoskelet Disord. 2018;19(1):77.

13. Tornetta P 3rd. Percutaneous treatment of calcaneal fractures. Clin Orthop Relat Res. 2000;375:91-6.

14. Corina G, Mori C, Vicenti G, Galante VN, Conserva V, Speciale D, et al. Heel displaced intra-articular fractures treated with mini-calcaneal external fixator. Injury. 2014;45(Suppl. 6):S64-71.

15. Muir RL, Forrester R, Sharma H. Fine wire circular fixation for displaced intra-articular calcaneal fractures: a systematic review. J Foot Ankle Surg. 2019;58(4):755-61.

16. McGarvey WC, Burris MW, Clanton TO, Melissinos EG. Calcaneal fractures: indirect reduction and external fixation. Foot Ankle Int. 2006;27(7):494-9.

17. Rammelt S, Sangeorzan BJ, Swords MP. Calcaneal fractures—should we or should we not operate? Indian J Orthop. 2018;52(3):220-30.

18. Rammelt S, Amlang M, Barthel S, Gavlik JM, Zwipp H. Percutaneous treatment of less severe intraarticular calcaneal fractures. Clin Orthop Relat Res. 2010;468(4):983-90.

19. Toro G, Langella F, Gison M, Toro G, Moretti A, Toro A, et al. Stentoplasty of calcaneal fractures: surgical technique and early outcomes. Injury. 2019;50(Suppl. 2):S70-4.

20. Golec P, Golec J. Evaluation of long-term quality of life using the foot and ankle outcome score (FAOS) questionnaire in patients treated by minimally invasive reduction and percutaneous stabilization of intra-articular calcaneal fractures. Med Sci Monit. 2020;26:e921602.

21. Schepers T. Sinus tarsi approach with screws-only fixation for displaced intra-articular calcaneal fractures. Clin Podiatr Med Surg. 2019;36(2):211-24.

22. Chen L, Zhang G, Hong J, Lu X, Yuan W. Comparison of percutaneous screw fixation and calcium sulfate cement grafting versus open treatment of displaced intra-articular calcaneal fractures. Foot Ankle Int. 2011;32(10):979-85.

23. van Hoeve S, Poeze M. Outcome of minimally invasive open and percutaneous techniques for repair of calcaneal fractures: a systematic review. J Foot Ankle Surg. 2016;55(6):1256-63.

24. Wallin KJ, Cozzetto D, Russell L, Hallare DA, Lee DK. Evidence-based rationale for percutaneous fixation technique of displaced intra-articular calcaneal fractures: a systematic review of clinical outcomes. J Foot Ankle Surg. 2014;53(6):740-3.

25. Marouby S, Cellier N, Mares O, Kouyoumdjian P, Coulomb R. Percutaneous arthroscopic calcaneal osteosynthesis for displaced intra-articular calcaneal fractures: systematic review and surgical technique. Foot Ankle Surg. 2020;26(5):503-8.

26. Mekhail AO, Ebraheim NA, Heck BE, Yeasting RA. Anatomic considerations for safe placement of calcaneal pins. Clin Orthop Relat Res. 1996(332):254-9.

27. Thomson CM, Esparon T, Rea PM, Jamal B. Monoaxial external fixation of the calcaneus: an anatomical study assessing the safety of monoaxial pin insertion. Injury. 2016;47(10):2091-6.

28. DeWall M, Henderson CE, McKinley TO, Phelps T, Dolan L, Marsh JL. Percutaneous reduction and fixation of displaced intra-articular calcaneus fractures. J Orthop Trauma. 2010;24(8):466-72.

29. Jin C, Weng D, Yang W, He W, Liang W, Qian Y. Minimally invasive percutaneous osteosynthesis versus ORIF for Sanders type II and III calcaneal fractures: a prospective, randomized intervention trial. J Orthop Surg Res. 2017;12(1):10.

30. De Boer AS, Van Lieshout EM, Den Hartog D, Weerts B, Verhofstad MH, Schepers T. Functional outcome and patient satisfaction after displaced intra-articular calcaneal fractures: a comparison among open, percutaneous, and nonoperative treatment. J Foot Ankle Surg. 2015;54(3):298-305.

Fixation by Extensile Lateral Approach

Richard E Buckley, Balvinder Rana

"Before undergoing a surgical operation, arrange your temporal affairs. You may live".

–Ambrose Bierce

■ INTRODUCTION

The extensile lateral approach to the calcaneus is the standard approach for surgical fixation of displaced intra-articular calcaneus fractures. It provides excellent exposure to the subtalar joint, anterior process, lateral wall, and calcaneal tuberosity. Adequate visualization of these structures facilitates the anatomic reduction of the articular surface and the restoration of normal calcaneal morphology. These are the primary goals of surgical treatment. Although it is commonly used and certainly the most utilitarian approach for treating these fractures, there can be catastrophic complications with open reduction and internal fixation, even, rarely, leading to amputation. The surgeon who wishes to operate on calcaneal fractures must have a healthy respect for the risk factors associated with poor outcomes and awareness of the indications and relative indications for nonoperative treatment and percutaneous techniques. Furthermore, issues of timing, positioning, imaging, and the associated complications must be thoroughly understood in order that an adequate surgical plan can be implemented. These issues are addressed in this chapter.

■ INDICATIONS

Calcaneus fracture management is a controversial subject, and when presented with a calcaneal fracture, the surgeon is faced with making decisions on treatment aspects, many of which are mired in controversy.

The first decision is to choose between operative or nonoperative treatment. Both patient factors and fracture characteristics must be considered together in this decision. Undisplaced and minimally displaced fractures can be successfully treated nonoperatively.[1] Careful measurements of Böhler's angle and the critical angle of Gissane in good lateral images give an objective measurement of the degree of disruption to the normal morphology. Harris views show changes in the width of the tuberosity, angulation of the tuberosity, and intra-articular fractures of the posterior and middle facets. Computed tomography (CT) scans have the highest yield as they reveal the precise location of the fracture lines and the degree of comminution present. Relevant patient factors include advanced age, medical comorbidities, diabetes, vascular disease, and smoking, which have all been shown to place the patient at a higher risk for wound complications and these patients should not undergo an open procedure without a cautious assessment of the risks and benefits.[1-4]

Percutaneous reduction techniques and combined percutaneous and mini-open procedures are also options which should be considered. Extra-articular fractures, tongue-type or beak fractures, and simple joint depression-type fractures may be addressed satisfactorily with percutaneous fixation with or without a small lateral incision to aid in reduction. Cases which have soft-tissue compromise or patient factors which are likely to lead to complications may also be better treated with this approach which minimizes the soft-tissue damage but still allows for some manipulation of fracture fragments and reduction maneuvers.[5]

Medial approaches are used in unusual specific instances such as fractures of the sustentaculum or when interposed medial structures cannot be removed from the fracture site from the lateral side. Open fractures of the calcaneus also occur more often on the medial side, necessitating a medial approach.

So, it is only after a judicious look at both the patient and the fracture and understanding of the options for treatment that the surgeon can proceed to plan an open lateral approach for a calcaneus fracture. If the surgical goals of anatomic reduction of the articular surface and restoration of calcaneal morphology can be obtained without an open approach or if patient factors put the extremity at risk with an open procedure, then it is not indicated. The best candidates to undergo fixation through an extensile lateral approach have a fracture pattern that is known to benefit from surgical treatment and patient factors which minimize the risks of infection. Younger, healthy, motivated, nonsmoking patients with a closed, displaced intra-articular fracture are most likely to have a good outcome after fixation through this approach.[1-4] Unfortunately, not all patients fit into the profile of ideal candidate and some degree of judgment must be applied in every case to decide who is reasonable enough to undergo this surgery. Most importantly, the risks and realistic outcomes must be discussed with and understood by the patient, who has the most at stake and likely the least understanding of this difficult fracture.

TIMING OF SURGERY

Calcaneus fractures are inherently high-energy injuries and there is almost universally a great deal of swelling of the foot and ankle with blistering of the skin. This soft-tissue damage is aggravated by the surgery and a difficult postoperative closure from skin edema greatly increases the risk of skin necrosis and infection. The sequelae of these problems can be devastating, requiring prolonged ... and potentially ... to wait ... lialized ... lling is ... inkles ... llexion ... ppears ... pected

regularly, and the findings documented prior to the surgery. Delaying >3 weeks greatly increases the difficulty of obtaining an acceptable reduction and potentially reduces the utility of an open procedure. It may be that the soft-tissue issues do not resolve in time to undergo a successful operation despite the relative indications. In these cases, as with delayed presentations of calcaneus fractures, limited surgical goals must be considered through percutaneous techniques or nonoperative treatment and the resulting malunions dealt with through reconstructive procedures when the fracture has fully healed.

POSITIONING

Proper positioning is important for both the surgeon and the patient. The lateral approach is most easily performed with the patient in a decubitus position on the contralateral side. The upper extremities should be positioned using arm boards and appropriate padding and straps taking care to leave anesthesia with easy access to the intravenous site. The nonoperative leg should be padded at the level of peroneal nerve, free of pressure areas, and anterior on the operating table. The operative limb is placed posterior to the nonoperative side and elevated with enough padding so that the limbs are clear of each other in both the anteroposterior (AP) and lateral planes to facilitate intraoperative imaging **(Figs. 2A to C)**. The leg is placed in an above-knee tourniquet for hemostasis and prepped and draped to the knee with a surgical glove over the toes. In this position, the surgeon can approach the fracture either sitting or standing from the foot of the operating table.

RELEVANT ANATOMICAL CONSIDERATIONS

The extensile lateral approach creates a full-thickness ...al flap which is elevated over the lateral side ...neus. This flap must be treated with great care ... the operation as severe complications may ...ft-tissue compromise, leading to skin necrosis, ...ardware, and infection.[6]

...nding the vascular anatomy of this flap is ...to minimizing complications. The skin on the ...e of the hindfoot is supplied by three arteries— ...caneal artery, (2) the lateral malleolar ...ateral tarsal artery. Borrelli and Lashgari's ...ed that the lateral calcaneal artery, a ...roneal artery, appeared to be responsible ... blood supply to the corner of the flap ...e lateral approach, and because of its ...rtical limb of the incision, an awareness ...portant to save it from injury **(Figs. 3A**

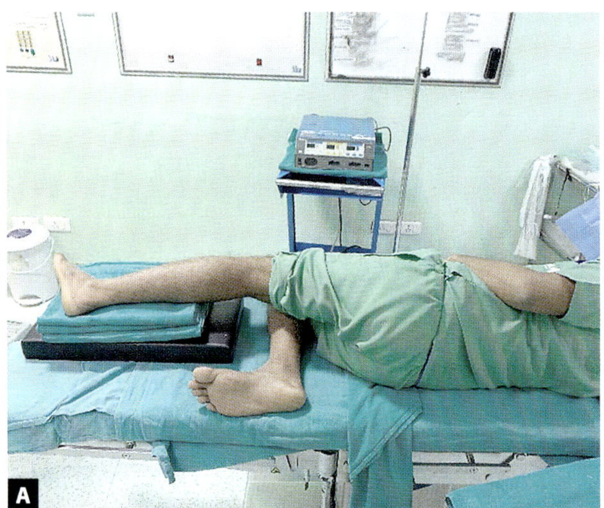

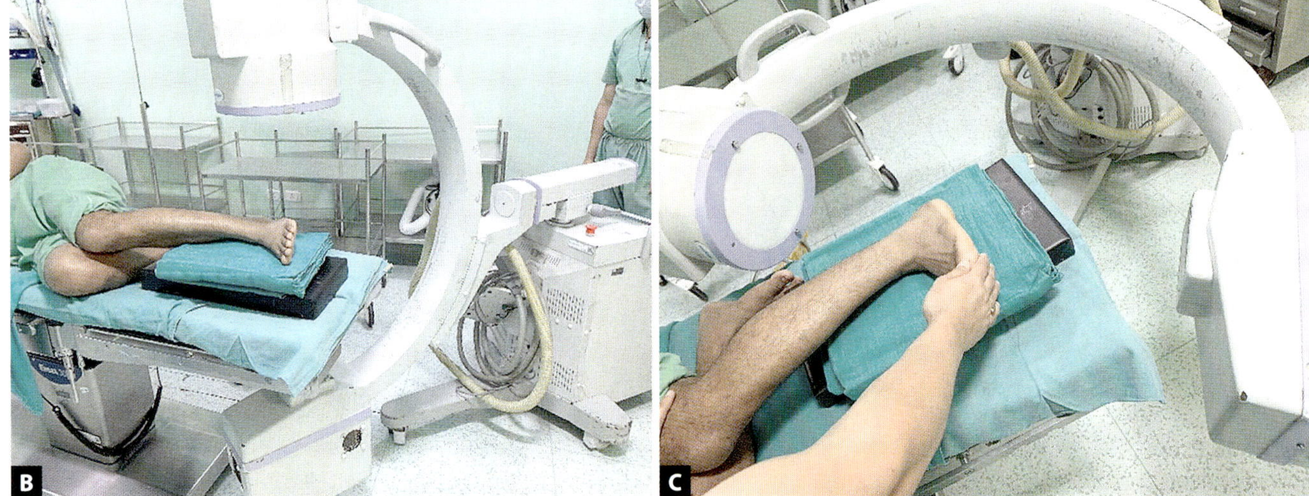

Figs. 2A to C: Lateral position: Leg, ankle, and foot supported on boards/sheets (A) and position of image intensifier for (B) lateral and (C) axial views (dummy patient).

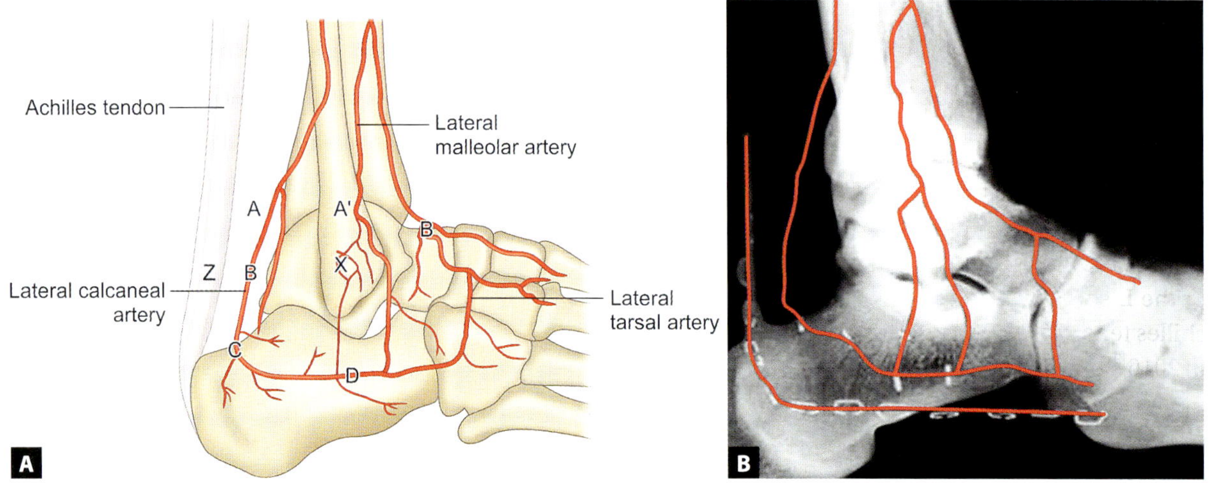

Figs. 3A and B: Circulation on the lateral surface of calcaneus showing lateral calcaneal branch of the peroneal artery, likely to be injured by the vertical limb of the extensile lateral approach. Keeping the vertical part of the incision posterior, close to the Achilles tendon (B), will save this vessel and may lead to lesser soft-tissue complications.
Source: Redrawn from Borrelli and Lashgari.[7]

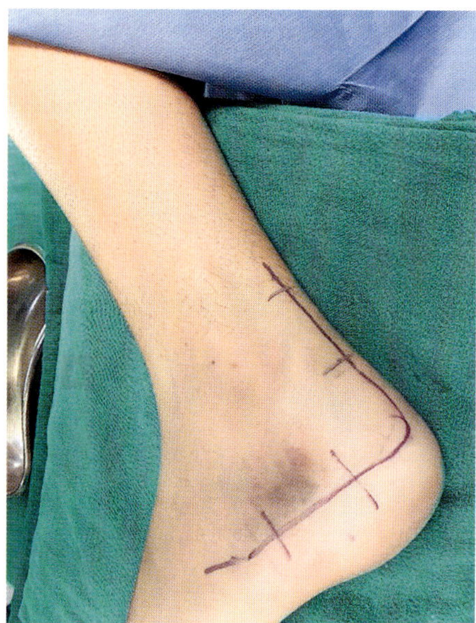

Fig. 5: The L-shaped incision with the vertical limb close to the lateral border of the Achilles tendon and the horizontal limb along the junction of the dorsal and plantar skin. The two limbs meet in a gentle curve.

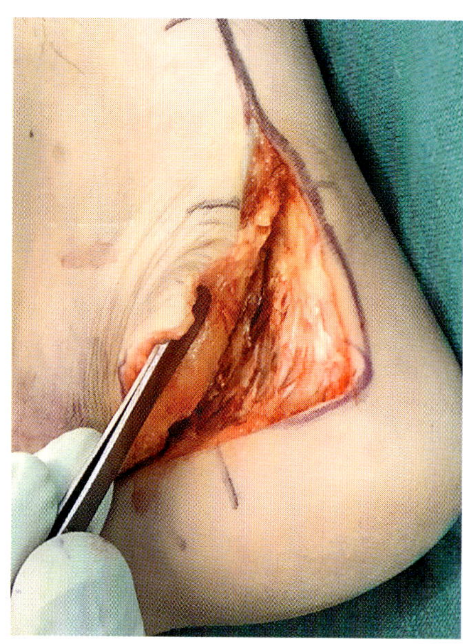

Fig. 6: Full-thickness subperiosteal flap started at the curve of the incision and dissected proximally from the lateral surface of the calcaneus.

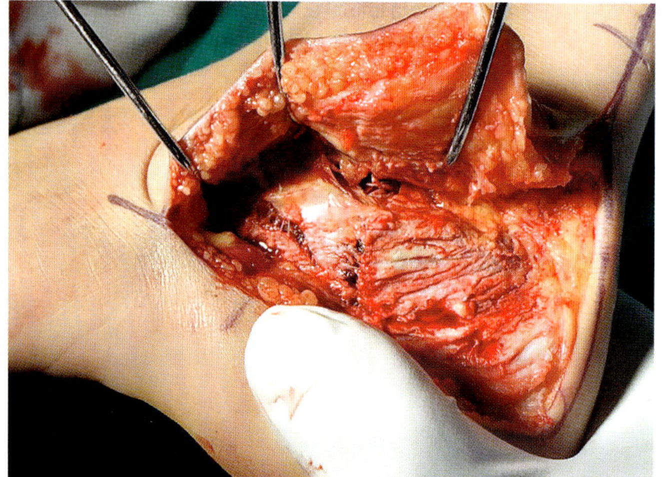

Fig. 7: Three K-wires used to retract the flap: The distal one in the cuboid, middle in the neck of talus, and proximal in the tip of lateral malleolus.

the sural nerve, which may be seen in the operative field at both ends of the incision. Distally, the abductor digiti minimi is present along the inferior lateral border of the calcaneus and should be protected to avoid unnecessary bleeding in the wound. The flap should be carefully raised proximally in the subperiosteal plane along the full length of the incision **(Figs. 6 and 7)**. The peroneal tendons are visualized as the flap is raised and should be carried superiorly together with their sheath and retinaculae toward the sinus tarsi in this full-thickness flap. Careless dissection with the blade can easily injure the skin or peroneal tendons. The exposure is

adequate when the anterior process, tuberosity, posterior facet, and the lateral process of the talus are visualized. At this point, the flap can be held in an elevated position by 2 mm K-wires placed as needed in any of the lateral process of the talus, talar neck, cuboid, or distal fibula and gently bent back to act as curved retractors **(Fig. 7)**.

Once this exposure is carried out, the surgeon can turn to the surgical plan and address the issues specific to that fracture. Generally speaking, the surgical goals address anatomic reduction of the articular surface of the posterior facet, restoration of Böhler's angle, return of calcaneal height and width in approximately 5° valgus alignment, and reconstruction of the critical angle of Gissane between the anterior process and the posterior facet. With the typical primary and secondary fracture lines seen in calcaneal fractures, a stepwise approach to this reconstruction generally starts anteriorly and medially and works posteriorly and laterally to complete the fixation. This involves first reducing the fracture fragments to the anteromedial or "constant" fragment **(Figs. 8 and 9)**. This "constant" fragment is critical to surgical fixation through the lateral approach. The strong medial deltoid ligaments and the nature of the pattern of injury in these fractures tend to cause this anteromedial fragment to remain in an anatomic position relative to the talus. As such, the "constant" fragment serves as a foundation for the fixation of the rest of the fracture. This functions as a foundation not only anatomically due to its stable anatomic location but also structurally as a point of fixation because of the relatively dense bone of the sustentaculum

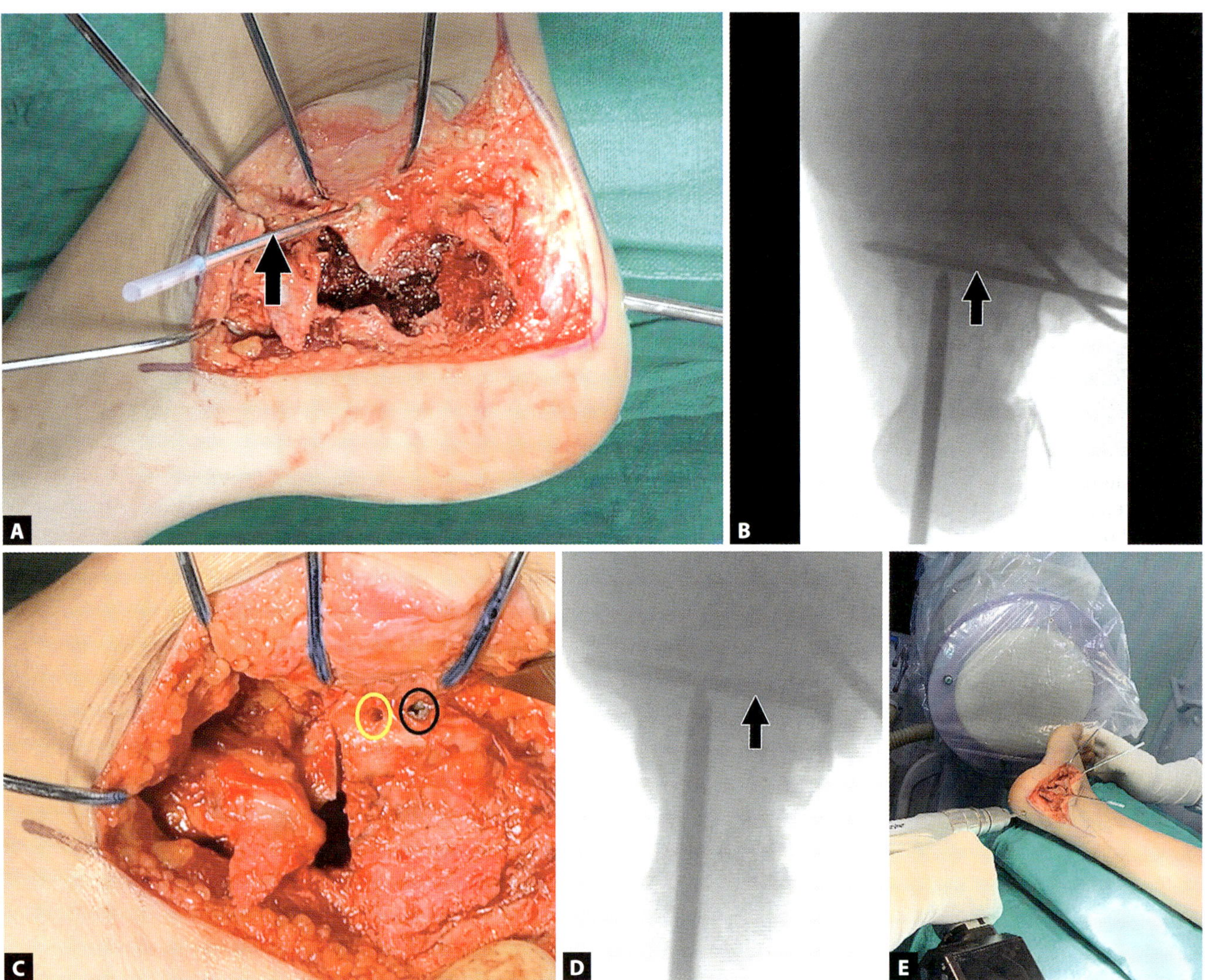

Figs. 11A to E: (A) Elevated lateral facet fragment fixed to medial constant fragment with a K-wire (black arrow). (B) The wire position confirmed as being in the sustentaculum medially and subchondral bone beneath the posterior facet in the axial images. (C) 3.5 mm fully threaded lag screw used to fix the lateral posterior facet to medial posterior facet constant fragment (black circle). Yellow circle shows the hole of removed K-wire which will be used to insert a second subchondral screw. (D) Axial C-arm image confirming correct screw position and length with Steinmann pin in place and (E) how to take an axial image in the operating theater.

unnecessary pressure on the soft tissues. The flap should be handled very gently, particularly around the apex, and the wound closed with careful dermis-to-dermis apposition of the skin edges under minimal tension using interrupted absorbable stitches subcutaneously and nylon stitches of the Allgöwer–Donati type in the skin **(Fig. 15)**. The leg should be placed into a splint, and 24 hours of antibiotics administered for infection prophylaxis.

◼ POSTOPERATIVE MANAGEMENT

Routine postoperative management should include removal of the drain after 24–48 hours, with dressing change and subtalar range of motion exercises to start at about 2 days. Nonweight-bearing with gentle range of motion of the affected limb should continue for 12 weeks with particular attention given to the wound apex. The blood supply to the tip of the flap is tenuous and frequently is a site of skin necrosis and wound breakdown. In these cases, it may be necessary to apply negative pressure dressings until the wound granulates in. If skin necrosis leads to infection and exposed hardware, it poses a serious problem that will require debridement and consultation from plastic surgery for soft-tissue care with possible flap coverage and skin grafting.

■ REFERENCES

1. Buckley R, Tough S, McCormack R, Pate G, Leighton R, Petrie D, et al. Operative compared with nonoperative treatment of displaced intra-articular calcaneal fractures: a prospective, randomized, controlled multicenter trial. J Bone Joint Surg Am. 2002;84:1733-44.
2. Bajammal S, Tornetta 3rd P, Sanders D, Bhandari M. Displaced intra-articular calcaneal fractures. J Orthop Trauma. 2005;19:360-4.
3. Buckley RE, Tough S. Displaced intra-articular calcaneal fractures. J Am Acad Orthop Surg. 2004;12:172-8.
4. Howard JL, Buckley R, McCormack R, Pate G, Leighton R, Petrie D, et al. Complications following management of displaced intra-articular calcaneal fractures: a prospective randomized trial comparing open reduction internal fixation with nonoperative management. J Orthop Trauma. 2003;17:241-9.
5. Tornetta P 3rd. The Essex-Lopresti reduction for calcaneal fractures revisited. J Orthop Trauma. 1998;12:469-73.
6. Hoppenfeld S, de Boer P, Buckley R. The ankle and foot. Surgical Exposures in Orthopaedics: The Anatomic Approach. Philadelphia: Lippincott Williams & Wilkins; 2009. [Chapter 12].
7. Borrelli J Jr, Lashgari C. Vascularity of the lateral calcaneal flap: a cadaveric injection study. J Orthop Trauma. 1999;13(2):73-7.
8. Sirisreetreerux N, Sa-Ngasoongsong P, Kulachote N, Apivatthakakul T. Location of vertical limb of extensile lateral calcaneal approach and risk of injury of the calcaneal branch of peroneal artery. Foot Ankle Int. 2019;40(2):224-30.
9. Kwon JY, Gonzalez T, Riedel MD, Nazarian A, Ghorbanhoseini M. Proximity of the lateral calcaneal artery with a modified extensile lateral approach compared to standard extensile approach. Foot Ankle Int. 2017;38(3):318-23.

the application of plates difficult **(Figs. 2A and B)** and also makes the reconstruction of the posterior facet, along with the regaining of Bohler's and Gissane's angles, a complex issue. Additionally, this has to be done without soft-tissue compromise.

With a better understanding of biomechanics, better metallurgy, and implant designs, the maximal evolution of calcaneal implants has occurred in the last three decades. Modern implants allow early mobilization after fixation, with their usage often individualized and dictated by the fracture type. Although an ideal implant for the calcaneus is yet to be devised, the available evidence for its use decides the usage of the implants. This, in turn, depends on individual clinical

expertise, patient expectations, and cost issues. Many times, local factors such as skin conditions or wounds dictate the choice of a particular implant for fixation.

■ SCREW FIXATION

Extra-articular avulsion fractures are relatively easy to stabilize and are best fixed with screws under compression.

Single or multiple screws can be used as required. Well-placed compression screws assure good outcomes and, if applied percutaneously, can be used with minimal surgical insult **(Fig. 3)**. One screw is usually insufficient, and at least two screws should be used.

■ WIRE FIXATION

The K-wires alone are inadequate for the definitive fixation of complex calcaneal fractures. In certain scenarios, such as undisplaced avulsion fractures,[6,7] or even undisplaced body fractures, judiciously applied K-wires allow percutaneous stabilization but would not allow early ambulation. These are ideal for temporary stabilization during fracture reconstruction **(Fig. 4)** and are not recommended as the definitive form of fixation. However, these are now being used more frequently along with external fixation **(Figs. 5A and B)** as a means to maintaining the fracture reduction of various fragments.

■ EXTERNAL FIXATORS

External fixators are now considered the best choice for any open fracture, and even in the calcaneus, these are now being more frequently employed. These can be used

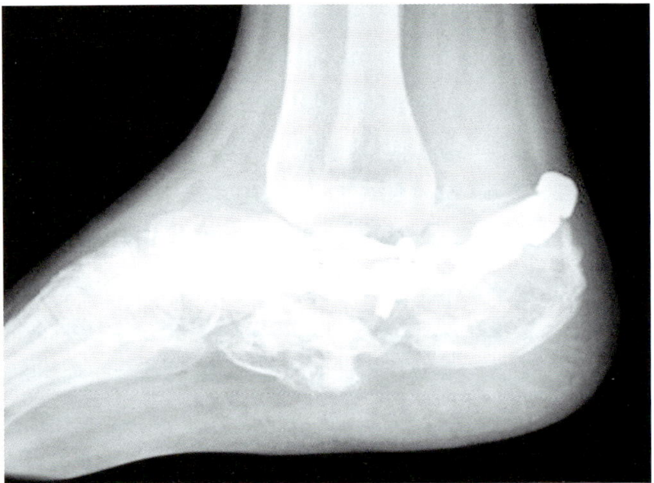

Fig. 1: Deformed calcaneus after attempted open reduction and internal fixation.

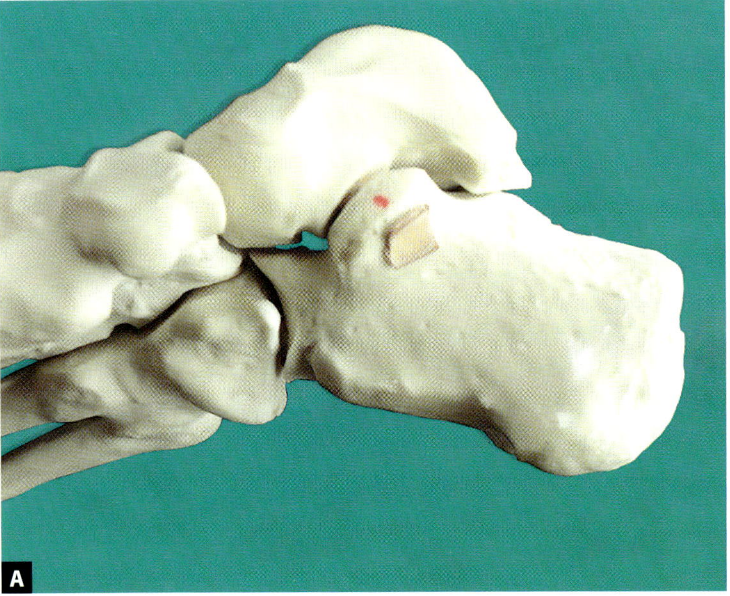

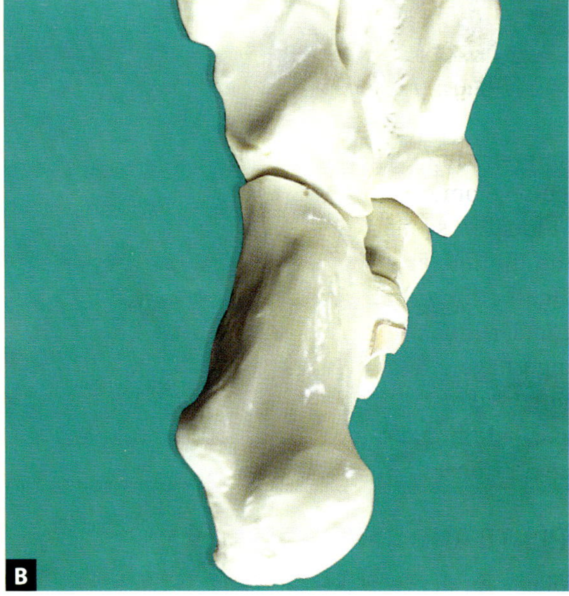

Figs. 2A and B: Odd shape of the calcaneus.

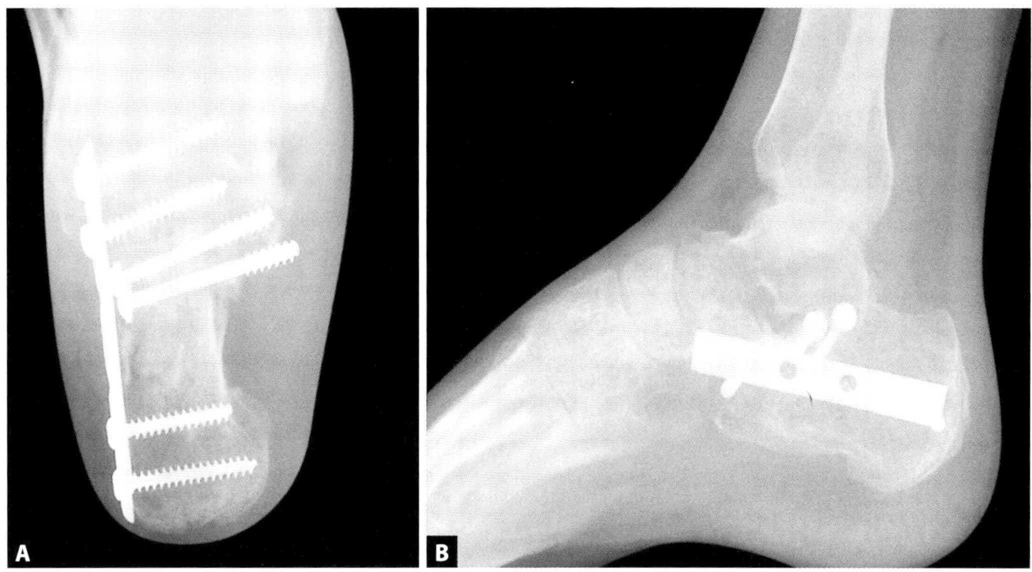

Figs. 6A and B: Fixation of calcaneal fracture with two screws in facet area and semitubular plate. Note excellent anatomical reconstitution of the bone.

This gave fairly good results when employed by surgeons having requisite experience, but deferred weight-bearing was the rule, and bone grafting was routinely employed.

However, there was poor maintenance of the elevated posterior facet, the late collapse of the fracture construct, and plate-related lateral complications **(Fig. 1)**. This led to further changes in the thought process, and implant evolution progressed further.

The 1990s saw an emergence of double plate configurations and the development of single-construct H- or Y-reconstruction plates. Extensive hardware was often used; Bezes used a second short straight plate in addition to a flat plate, forming a "Y" construct. Letournel employed the principles used in acetabular and pelvic fracture surgery, modifying them to develop the concept of a single "Y" plate and the anatomic reconstruction plates (with arms), which were made especially for calcaneus.

■ LOCKING PLATES

In the modern world of science, the emphasis shifted to low-profile, versatile implants, which also allowed stable fixation. Thus, the plate profile/thickness was reduced to minimize soft tissue breakdown. The plates were made less rigid for molding to irregular surfaces, and their complex structure allowed varied screw placement to ensure rigid support of the bone fragments at various levels. This led to the evolution of the thinner, single-construct calcaneal locking plates **(Figs. 7A and B)**. These also have better outcomes in comminuted fractures.

With the advent of the locking plate concept by Wagner and the AO group, the concept was extended for use in the foot and ankle.[8-14] Synthes Medical GmbH, Solothurn, Switzerland marketed a versatile locking calcaneal plate with 15 locking holes, allowing for multiple fracture pattern fixations. Bendable superior and inferior tabs provide support for the anterior process and plantar fragments **(Figs. 8A and B)**. Angled and ascending holes buttress the sustentaculum and provide better support to the calcaneotalar articular surface. The plate is applied through the lateral extensile approach, and molding is done with the help of special sleeve benders **(Figs. 8A and B)**; multiple locking screws or standard small fragment screws provide bicortical and/or unicortical fixation. The threaded locking holes offer a fixed-angle construct to buttress the articular surfaces of the calcaneus and permit multiple points of fixation to buttress small fragments. The locking holes provide 15° of angulation when using 2.7 mm cortex screws and 5° of angulation when using 3.5 mm cortex screws. This locking calcaneal plate is side specific, made of titanium, and comes in two sizes, 69 and 76 mm.

Variations of this concept have been marketed by different implant manufacturers. Stryker Corporation, USA, has modified the calcaneal plate design into two separate plates **(Figs. 9 and 10)**.

The standard laterally placed plate is somewhat thicker and has been modified somewhat to have two arms perpendicular to the main plate to allow tuberosity and anterior end stabilization.

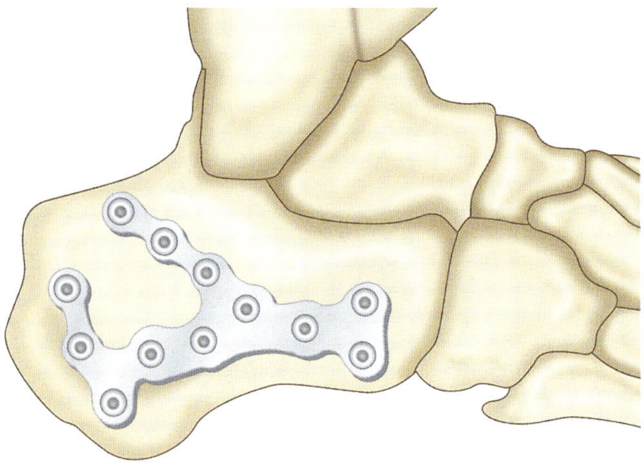

Fig. 9: Stryker two-arm plate.

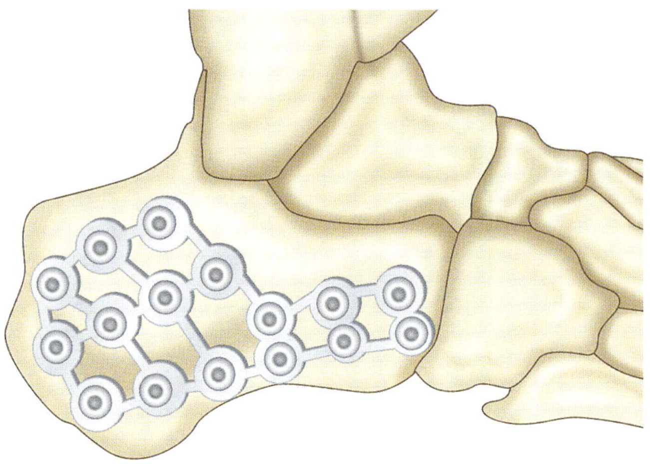

Fig. 10: Stryker mesh plate.

Variations of the plate construct have also led to the evolution of the so-called wave plate by Tornier Medical, Saint-Ismier Cedex, France. Designed to accommodate a less-invasive incision, this plate is in the form of a "wave" and is introduced almost percutaneously. The anatomic contour of the plate was developed after an extensive CT study of over 30 unique anatomies; the plate has a nonlocking apex hole, which allows for optimal lag reduction of the sustentaculum tali. Each additional hole allows for a locking or nonlocking screw option. It is made available with specific reduction instrumentation for tuberosity manipulation during fracture reduction.

As of now, the locking plates for comminuted calcaneus fractures seem to be the best available option.[17-19] However, cost and surgical expertise are two important factors, which have to be considered, as implant affordability and availability of technical expertise are often a problem in developing countries. It is important to comprehend that calcaneal fracture surgery using complex implants has a steep-learning curve.

MODIFICATIONS AND INNOVATIONS IN THE 21ST CENTURY

In the 21st century, there was a focus on developing and refining percutaneous and minimally invasive techniques. New plates are developed, which are relatively thinner in thickness **(Figs. 11 and 12)**, 1.35 mm, and have polyaxial locking screws availabile.[20,21] The plate itself does not have a thread but a lip, and the screw with extra thread in the head cut its thread into the plate at an angle determined by the surgeon. Due to increasing thread diameter, the screw locks in this position. Reshaping is possible as the plate and screw are made of titanium of different hardness grades, which are easy to insert below the skin, maintaining the principles of MIS. The plate has softer titanium than screws, and a special screwdriver is needed to tighten the screws and ensure that they cut a thread into the lip of the plate.[20,21]

BIOABSORBABLE IMPLANTS AND SCREWS

The evolution of bioabsorbable implants has made many authors think about their application in selected calcaneal fractures.[22-24] Plate-related irritability, high infection rates, and subsequent need for implant removal make this option theoretically attractive. Zhang et al.[25] have used bioscrews and prospectively compared them with plates in 97 randomized patients over 2 years; they found acceptable results at an average of 23 months' follow-up. We feel, however, that bioabsorbable implants may not be strong enough to withstand the stress of these displaced fractures, and their indications in complex calcaneal fractures are limited at the present moment. Min et al.[26] have described the surgical technique for using bioabsorbable pins; however, there is limited literature supporting these implants for calcaneal fractures at the present moment. The authors of this chapter think that the presently available implants have a limited application for depressed calcaneal fractures, and the stability afforded by them may be insufficient in displaced fractures.

To summarize, intra-articular calcaneus fractures are complex fractures, which are difficult to stabilize. The reason we get improved results following open reduction and internal fixation nowadays is the use of better surgical techniques and better implants. Locking calcaneus plates decreases the need for graft, allows early weight-bearing, and has better hold in osteoporotic bone, in addition to being moldable. However, the only disadvantages are their high cost and steep-learning curve.

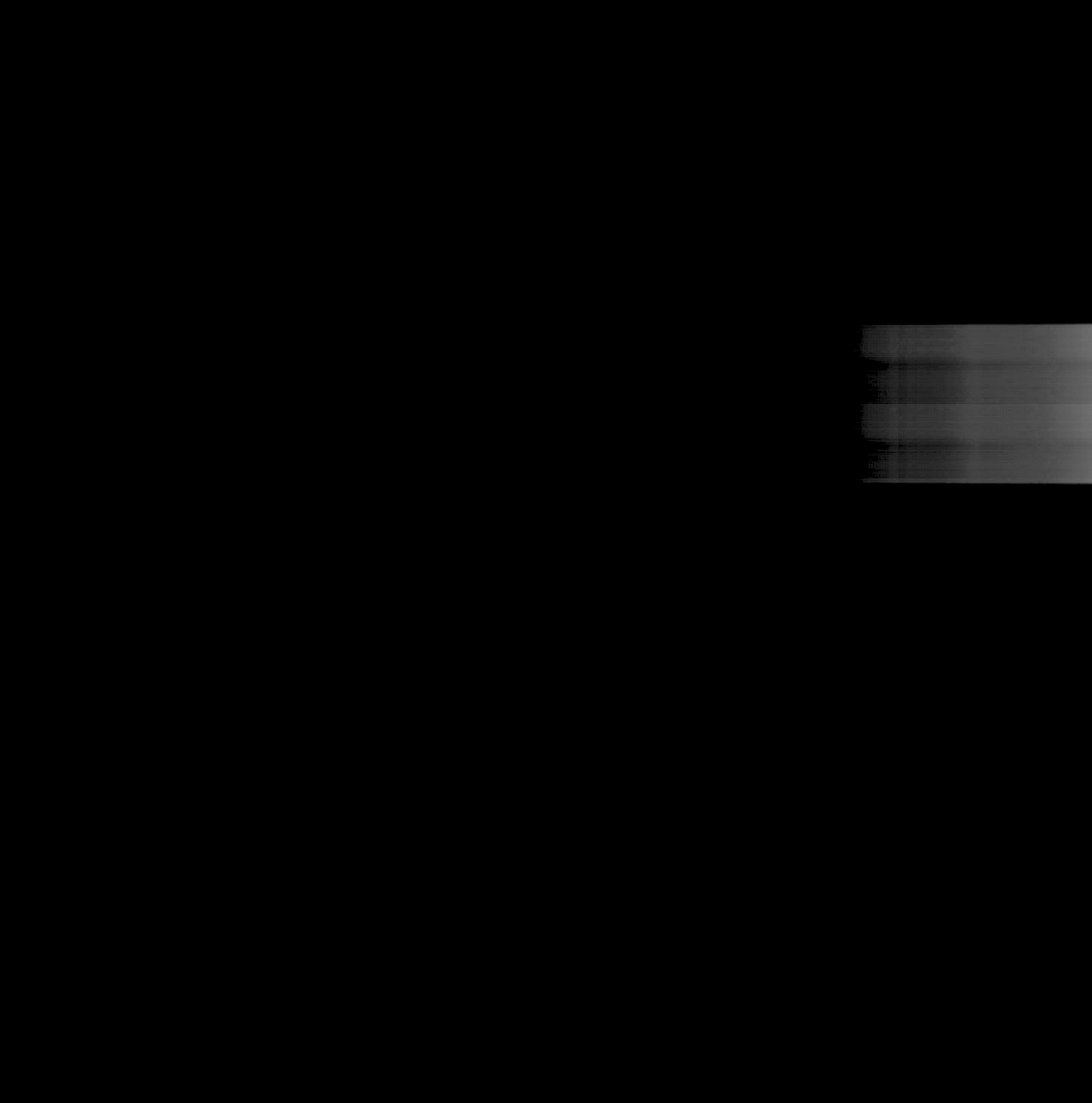

12. Stoffel K, Booth G, Rohrl SM, Kuster M. A comparison of conventional versus locking plates in intraarticular calcaneus fractures: a biomechanical study in human cadavers. Clin Biomech. 2007;22(1):100-5.

13. Wagner M. General principles for the clinical use of the LCP. Injury. 2003;34 Suppl. 2:B31-42.

14. Wagner M, Frenk A, Frigg R. New concepts for bone fracture treatment and the locking compression plate. Surg Technol Int. 2004;12:271-7.

15. Rak V, Ira D, Masek M. Operative treatment of intra-articular calcaneal fractures with calcaneal plates and its complications. Indian J Orthop. 2009;43(3):271-80.

16. Hyer CF, Atway S, Berlet GC, Lee TH. Early weight bearing of calcaneal fractures fixated with locked plates: a radiographic review. Foot Ankle Spec. 2010;3(6):320-3.

17. Wang H, Zhang Q, Duan D, Yan L. The use of calcaneal anatomic plate in arthroscopically-assisted open reduction and internal fixation of intra-articular calcaneal fractures. J Huazhong Univ Sci Technol Med Sci. 2006;26(3):319-21.

18. Herlyn A, Brakelmann A, Herlyn PK, Gradl G, Mittlmeier T. Calcaneal fracture fixation using a new interlocking nail reduces complications compared to standard locking plates—preliminary results after 1.6 years. Injury. 2019;50(Suppl. 3):63-8.

19. Zhang G, Ding S, Ruan Z. Minimally invasive treatment of calcaneal fracture. J Int Med Res. 2019;47(8):3946-54.

20. Kim GB, Park JJ, Park CH. Intra-articular calcaneal fracture treatment with staged medial external fixation. Foot Ankle Int. 2022;43(8):1084-91.

21. Bába V, Kopp L. Calcaneal fractures: current trends and pitfalls. Rozhl Chir. 2021;100(8):369-75.

22. Kankare J. Operative treatment of displaced intra-articular fractures of the calcaneus using absorbable internal fixation: a prospective study of twenty-five fractures. J Orthop Trauma. 1998;12(6):413-9.

23. Rammelt S, Zwipp H. Fractures of the calcaneus: current treatment strategies. Acta Chir Orthop Traumatol Cech. 2014;81(3):177-96.

24. Wei N, Zhou Y, Chang W, Zhang Y, Chen W. Displaced intra-articular calcaneal fractures: classification and treatment. Orthopedics. 2017;40(6):e921-29.

25. Zhang J, Xiao B, Wu Z. Surgical treatment of calcaneal fractures with bioabsorbable screws. Int Orthop. 2011;35(4):529-33.

26. Min W, Munro M, Sanders R. Stabilization of displaced articular fragments in calcaneal fractures using bioabsorbable pin fixation: a technique guide. J Orthop Trauma. 2010;24(12):770-4.

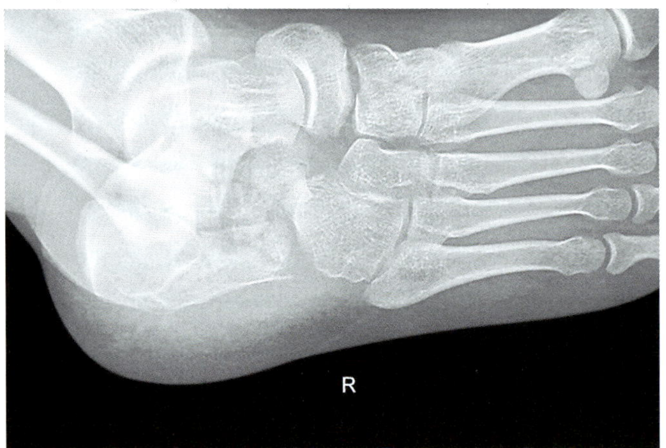

Fig. 3: Oblique radiograph of the midfoot showing disrupted lateral column, which is shortened and disrupted, and the fracture involves the calcaneocuboid joint while the medial column is seemingly normal.

series published predominantly recommend conservative treatment, and comparative studies and patient-rated outcome measures are missing **(Table 1)**. These fractures, being unusual, do not come to mind of the average orthopedic surgeon and are difficult to visualize in standard X-ray projections of the foot; therefore, they are often missed on initial radiographic inspection.

However, as has been mentioned in the literature, fractures of the anterior process of the calcaneus are often detected retrospectively on either magnetic resonance imaging (MRI) or computed tomography (CT) **(Figs. 4A to D)**.

■ PATHOANATOMY

The anterior process of the calcaneus has been described in the literature as a saddle-shaped bony protuberance

TABLE 1: A concise data review of all studies describing anterior end calcaneal fractures.

Study with year and journal	Number of cases	Mechanism of trauma	Management	Associated injuries/ conditions	Outcome	Complications
Dewar and Evans, 1968 JBJS (Br)[12]	5	Forced forefoot abduction	Three cases calcaneocuboid fusion ± fixation of navicular tuberosity if fractured two cases: Nonoperative management	Avulsion fracture of the navicular attached to the tibialis posterior	Patients who were managed nonoperatively: Pain and restricted ability to walk. Operatively managed cases: Free from symptoms and returned to full activity	Treatment by plaster immobilization alone has resulted in persistent disability
Hunt, 1970 JBJS (Br)[13]	1	Abduction injury	ORIF with K-wire	4th metatarsal fracture	*1-year follow-up:* Patient can walk bearing full weight with mild pain on uneven ground	NS
Langdon et al., 1994 JBJS (Br)[7]	26	Associated with DIACF	ORIF	DIACF	NS	NS
Trnka et al., 1998 Arch Orthop Trauma Surg[6]	1	Inversion and plantar flexion	Excision of fragment using sinus tarsi approach	NS	*12 months:* Relief of pain	Calcaneocuboid arthrosis
Ouellette et al., 2006 Skeletal Radiol[8]	14	Inversion injury with the foot in plantar flexion	Nonoperative	Talus ($n = 5$), navicular bone ($n = 3$), cuboid ($n = 2$), and calcaneal body ($n = 1$), anterior talofibular ligament (ATFL) tear ($n = 3$), and tears of the peroneus brevis ($n = 3$) and peroneus longus	NS	NS
Petrover et al., 2007 Skeletal Radiol[3]	15	Flexion, inversion injury and distraction of the bifurcate ligament leading to avulsion	NS	Calcaneonavicular coalition ($n = 9$) thickened ATFL ($n = 6$) thickened bifurcate ligament ($n = 9$)	NS	NS

Contd...

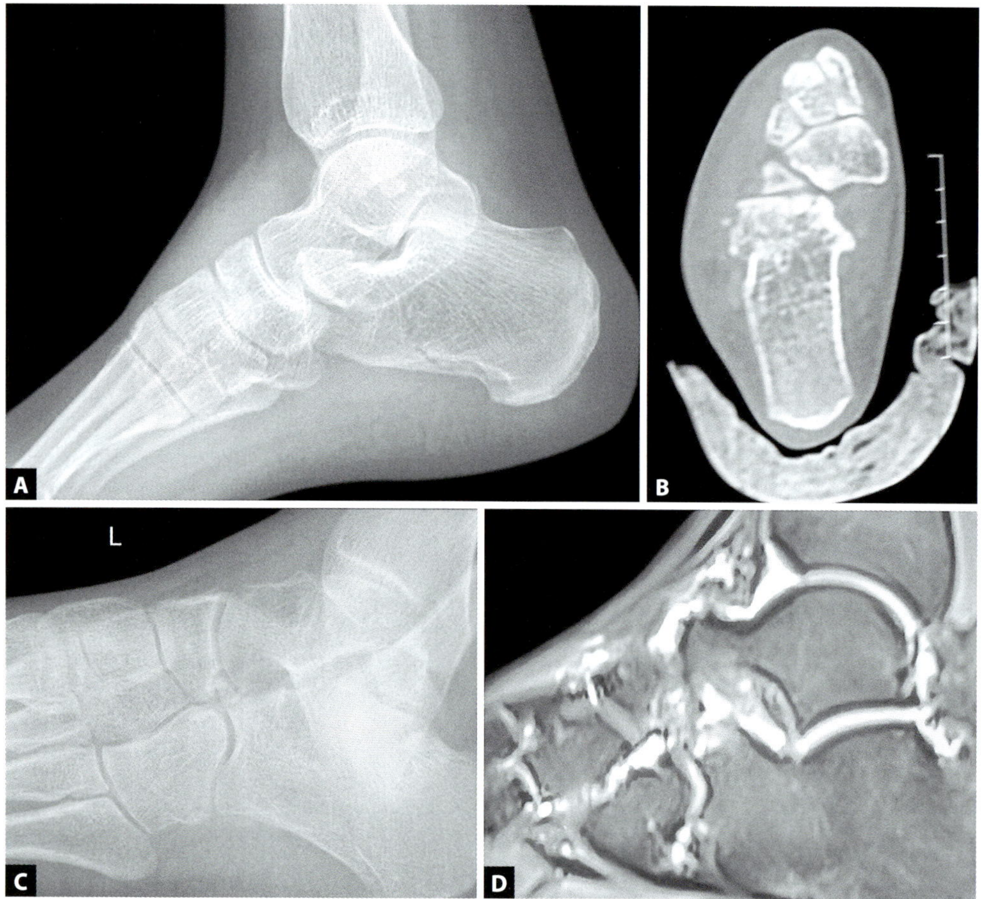

Figs. 4A to D: (A) Anterior end calcaneus fracture extending into the body; (B) Computed tomography (CT) shows actual extent of comminution, which extends into the calcaneus; (C) Oblique view of foot showing suspicious chip fracture of anterior end; (D) Magnetic resonance imaging (MRI) scan confirms fracture and adjacent bony edema.

beak of the cuboid. The superomedial corner of the articular surface makes a shelf-like projection anteromedially. This beak or rostrum of the os calcis overhangs the cuboid **(Fig. 5)**.

■ MECHANISM

The most frequent mechanism of fracture involving a part of the anterior end calcaneum is an inversion injury, with the foot in plantar flexion, leading to an avulsion of the bifurcate ligament. This may occur when participants are wearing high heels, which may explain the higher incidence of this injury in females. These patients may also have a calcaneonavicular coalition, long anterior calcaneal process, thickened anterior talofibular ligament, or thickened bifurcate ligament. Commonly, with a sudden twist, there is an immediate pain on the outer aspect of the midportion of the foot and discomfort on weight-bearing, which is later often in retrospect diagnosed as an "*anterior end calcaneal fracture.*" These are regularly missed on plain radiographs, and clinical differentiation from injury to lateral ankle ligaments is difficult. A fracture of the anterior process

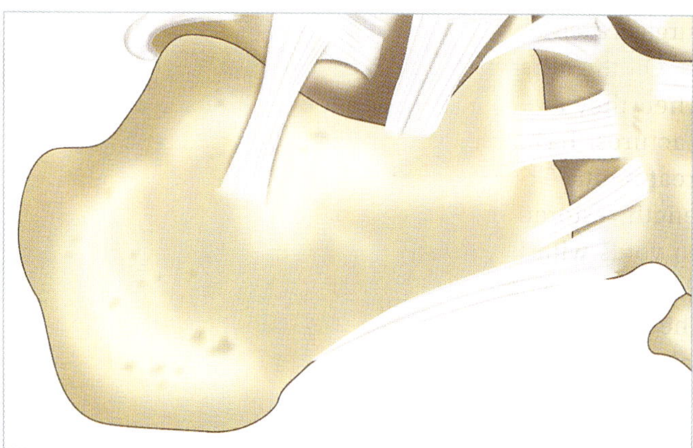

Fig. 5: Anatomic diagram of foot from lateral aspect showing ligamentous attachments.

of the calcaneus can also often coexist with a lateral ankle ligament injury. Patients may complain of lateral pain distal and anterior to the tip of the fibula.

- Compression injuries of the cuboidal articular surface of calcaneus, commonly due to abduction/eversion forces on the forefoot, are also well described. This occurs in

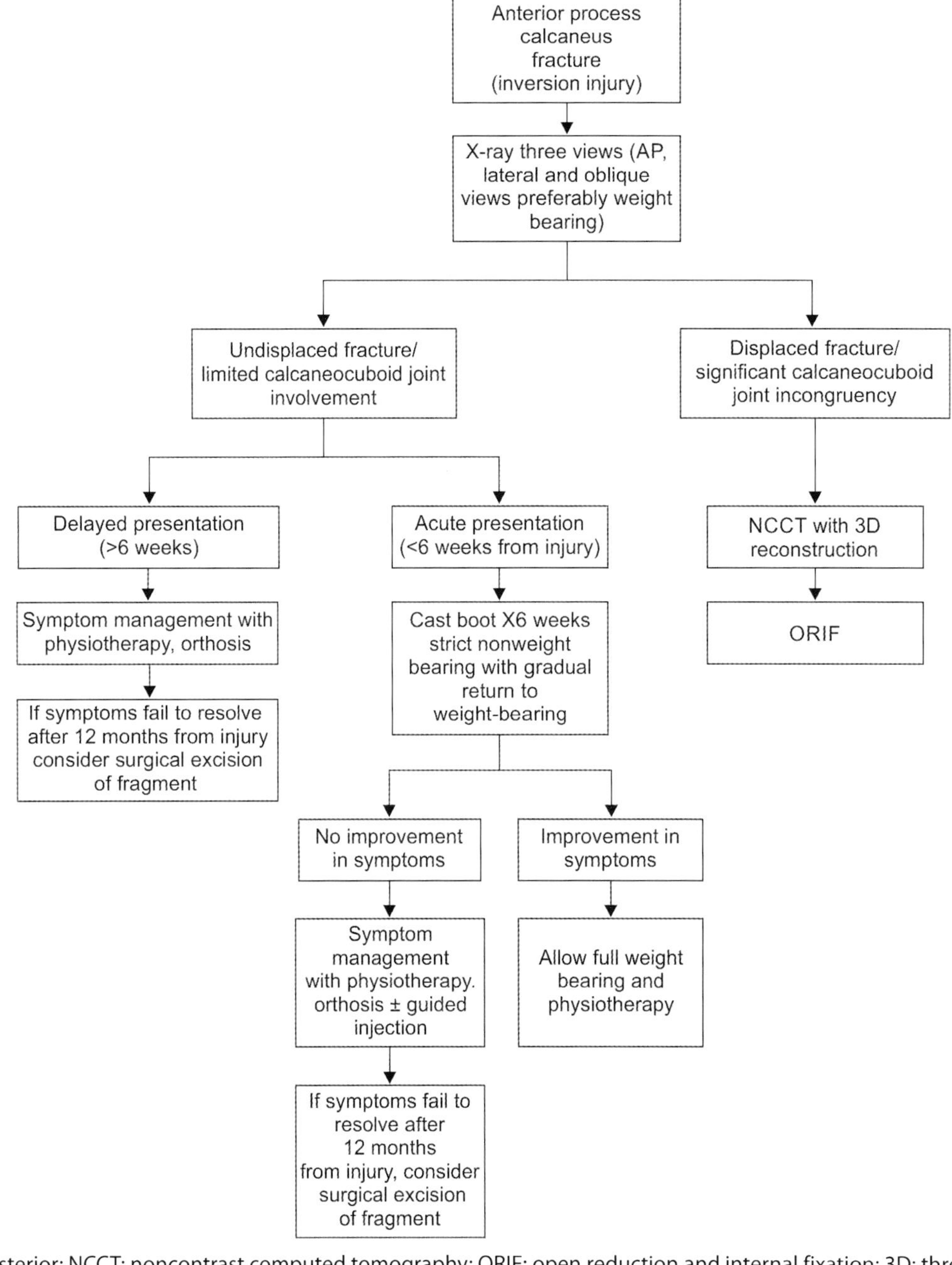

Flowchart 1: Treatment algorithm for management of anterior process calcaneal fractures seen in inversion injuries.

(AP: anteroposterior; NCCT: noncontrast computed tomography; ORIF: open reduction and internal fixation; 3D: three dimensional)

■ OUR RECOMMENDATIONS

- *Foot inversion injuries*: Most need nonoperative management in a cast or a boot with a period of nonweight-bearing for initial 4–6 weeks with gradual return to weight-bearing. If there is significant displacement of the articular surface of the anterior process of calcaneus involving the calcaneocuboid joint or involvement of over 40% of the articular surface, open reduction and internal fixation (ORIF) is indicated. A CT is needed prior to contemplation of surgery for better surgical planning.[10]

- *Foot eversion/abduction injuries*: Patients presenting with these high-velocity foot abduction injuries receive X-ray and CT scan with three-dimensional (3D) reconstruction to rule out associated injuries of the medial column or subtalar dislocation and to assess for reconstructability of the anterior process of calcaneus and involvement of the calcaneocuboid joint. Under fluoroscopic guidance, Joshi's external stabilization system (JESS) fixator or a spanning plate is used to regain length of the lateral column. Additionally, if the anterior process fracture is

We have found good-to-excellent American Orthopaedic Foot and Ankle Society (AOFAS) scores in our series at follow-ups over 2 years following surgery **(Fig. 7)**.

- *Anterior end fractures associated with DIACFs*: Management has been discussed in relevant section on DIACF management.

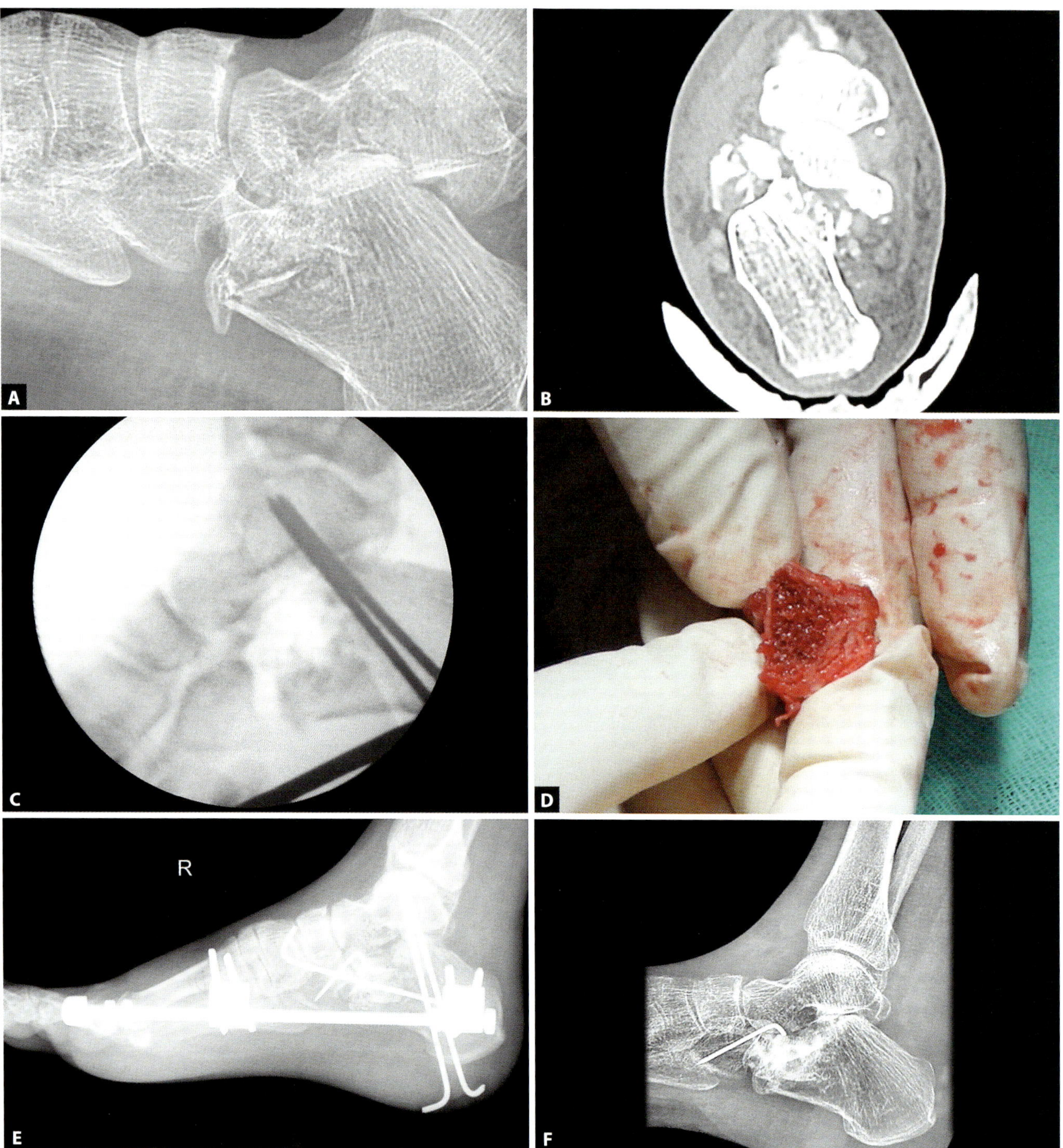

Figs. 7A to F: (A) Lateral view of foot showing comminuted anterior end fracture of calcaneus in a young school teacher; (B) CT scan shows the comminution and confirms the midfoot subluxation; (C and D) Intraoperative radiology showing reduction of the joints and temporary stabilization; tricortical iliac crest graft was added; (E) Postoperative x-rays with crossed K wires and fixater in situ; (F) Follow-up at 2 years showing graft incorporation and lateral column length maintained.

4. Pearce CJ, Zaw H, Calder JD. Stress fracture of the anterior process of the calcaneus associated with a calcaneonavicular coalition: a case report. Foot Ankle Int. 2011;32(1):85-8.

5. Hagino T, Tonotsuka H, Ochiai S, Hamada Y. Fracture of the anterior extremity of calcaneus together with calcaneocuboid joint dislocation. Arch Orthop Trauma Surg. 2009;129(12):1673-6.

6. Trnka H-J, Zettl R, Ritschl P. Fracture of the anterior superior process of the calcaneus: an often misdiagnosed fracture. Arch Orthop Trauma Surg. 1998;117(4-5):300-2.

7. Langdon IJ, Kerr PS, Atkins RM. Fractures of the calcaneum: the anterolateral fragment. J Bone Joint Surg Br. 1994;76(2):303-5.

8. Ouellette H, Salamipour H, Thomas BJ, Kassarjian A, Torriani M. Incidence and MR imaging features of fractures of the anterior process of calcaneus in a consecutive patient population with ankle and foot symptoms. Skeletal Radiol. 2006;35(11):833-7.

9. Taketomi S, Uchiyama E, Iwaso H. Stress fracture of the anterior process of the calcaneus: a case report. Foot Ankle Spec. 2013;6(5):389-92.

10. Dhillon M, Khurana A, Prabhakar S, Sharma S. Crush fractures of the anterior end of calcaneum. Indian J Orthop. 2018;52(3):244-52.

11. Dhinsa BS, Latif A, Walker R, Abbasian A, Back D, Singh S. Fractures of the anterior process of the calcaneum: a review and proposed treatment algorithm. Foot Ankle Surg. 2019;25:258-63.

12. Dewar FP, Evans DC. Occult fracture-subluxation of the midtarsal joint. J Bone Joint Surg Br. 1968;50:386-8.

13. Hunt DD. Compression fracture of the anterior articular surface of the calcaneus. J Bone Joint Surg Am. 1970;52:1637-42.

Initial evaluation includes foot and ankle X-rays. This injury is very difficult to accurately assess with standard X-ray. A noncontrast computed tomography (CT) scan is necessary to investigate the possibility of sustentaculum fractures and other associated injuries not readily identified on plain imaging. A well-padded short leg splint should be applied for immobilization and treatment of soft-tissue injuries. Rarely, swelling may be minimal, allowing immediate surgical intervention for displaced fractures. Nondisplaced fractures can be treated nonoperatively in a fracture boot or short leg cast with close clinical follow-up. Indications for operative fixation include loss of articular congruity of the medial facet and fracture fragment displacement. Fixation is also indicated if there is any clinical suspicion of entrapped tendon or neurologic structures. Finally, operative treatment typically allows early range of motion, improving long-term outcome.

Surgical Management

The approach to the medial calcaneus for intra-articular calcaneus fractures was initially described by McReynolds in 1958 and later modified by Burdeaux by addition of a percutaneous Steinmann pin into the calcaneal tuberosity to aid in fracture manipulation and to allow for a smaller incision.[14] The direct medial sustentacular approach, as described by Zwipp in 1994, moves the incision superiorly, and thereby avoids dissection of the neurovascular bundle.[15] This approach can be used alone for isolated sustentacular fractures or in conjunction with other lateral approaches for treatment of more complex calcaneal fractures **(Figs. 1A to G)**.

Operative treatment begins with the patient in a supine position, with a bump under the contralateral hip to provide access to the medial ankle. A 3–5 cm longitudinal skin incision is made, centered over the palpable sustentacular fragment, approximately 2 cm below the medial malleolus. The incision is kept posterior to the navicular tubercle. The deep fascia is divided in line with the skin incision. The posterior tibial tendon sheath is incised to allow for dorsal retraction of the posterior tibial and flexor digitorum longus tendons, while the FHL tendon is retracted plantarly. This allows for exposure of the medial calcaneal cortex. The sustentacular fracture line is identified and any debris or hematoma is cleared from the fracture. A K-wire can be used as a joystick within the sustentacular fragment to aid in manipulation and reduction. The middle facet of the subtalar joint is visualized to ensure accurate fracture reduction of the articular surface. The fragment is provisionally fixed with either multiple K-wires or a large Weber clamp, with one tine on the sustentaculum and the other on the lateral wall of the

calcaneus. Simple fracture patterns without comminution are stabilized with two lag screws, from the sustentaculum to the body of the calcaneus. Screw size varies due to the size of the fracture fragment and may be 2.4, 2.7, or 3.5 mm in diameter. The screws are placed in a posterior and inferior direction in order to remain extra-articular to the posterior calcaneal facet. Small, comminuted fractures may require the use of a mini-fragment plate and positional screws. A small rim plate may be used to support comminution of the articular surface. If the comminution extends down the medial side of the calcaneus, a T plate may be necessary to add buttress as well as raft the articulation of the middle facet. Rarely, the sustentaculum fracture is not reconstructable. Surgical excision is indicated in this scenario. Dissection is performed with care to protect the fibers of the superficial deltoid and prevent injury to the tendons and neurovascular bundle, which are in close proximity.

Initial postoperative care includes nonweight-bearing and immobilization. These injuries are often but one part of a more complex foot injury, and recovery may be prolonged as necessary. For an isolated injury, the patient's postoperative splint and sutures are removed at 2 weeks and a removable fracture boot is used. Early range-of-motion exercises are initiated at 2 weeks, with an emphasis on subtalar motion to reduce the risk of stiffness. If the patient shows radiographic and clinical signs of fracture union, they may begin to weight-bear at 6 weeks and transition out of the fracture boot as tolerated. Return to work or activities may begin as early as 12 weeks postoperatively.

Complications

Few complications of surgical fixation of sustentacular fractures have been reported. The most concerning complications arise with nonoperative treatment of displaced fractures including malunion and subtalar arthritis.[5,6] Varus hindfoot malunion can be avoided by restoring the height of the subtalar joint through visualizing the reduction of the sustentacular fragment and the corresponding articular surface of the middle subtalar facet.[16] Appropriate reduction of the middle facet also decreases the risk of subtalar arthrosis due to increased load on the posterior facet. Secondary subtalar arthrodesis has been performed in two patients for persistent post-traumatic arthritic pain and in one patient for progressive flatfoot deformity.[6,10,11]

Tendon irritation can occur with nonoperative or operative treatment. Impingement of the posterior tibial or flexor digitorum longus tendons on a malreduced fragment has been described.[17] Hardware can be removed after union if symptomatic. Neuropraxia or vascular injury is possible due to the proximity of the approach to the posterior tibial

AOFAS (American Orthopaedic Foot and Ankle Society) and mean SF-36 outcomes compared to patients with more complex injuries.[6] A recent case series of 10 patients also demonstrated improved AOFAS outcomes with isolated injuries compared to sustentacular fractures with associated talar neck or distal fibular fractures.[19] The authors' recommendations include open reduction and internal fixation of displaced sustentacular fractures or any nondisplaced fractures that have progressed to nonunion. Smaller incisions and specialized approaches have decreased the risk of postoperative complications, making surgical treatment a more favorable option than previously believed. Few wound complications have been described with more modern approaches and patient outcomes demonstrate improvement with operative fixation.[9,19]

■ MEDIAL PROCESS TUBEROSITY FRACTURES

Introduction

The medial process of the calcaneal tuberosity is an important anchor point for the medial longitudinal arch of the foot. As the bony origin of the plantar fascia, abductor hallucis, and flexor digitorum brevis, the medial process plays a key role in the maintenance of gait and foot biomechanics.[20]

A fracture to the medial process of the calcaneal tuberosity occurs after an impaction force to the heel with the hindfoot in an everted position.[21] The medial process fragment is further displaced by the pull exerted by the intact plantar fascia, resulting in anterior, plantar, and rotational displacement. All described cases in the current literature were a result of a fall from height.[21,22]

Indications for Surgery

Medial tuberosity fractures are most often treated operatively due to plantar fracture displacement. Left untreated, patients with these displaced fractures subsequently develop pain with weight-bearing and possible soft-tissue complications. Displaced fragments alter the weight-bearing surface of the calcaneus and can cause localized pressure points on the soft tissue, leading to painful callouses or ulcers.

Nonoperative Treatment

Nondisplaced fractures can be managed nonoperatively with close radiographic follow-up to monitor for fracture displacement (**Figs. 2A to D**). Nonoperative treatment consists of nonweight-bearing for 2–3 weeks in a removable fracture boot or short leg cast.[23] Patients often will have

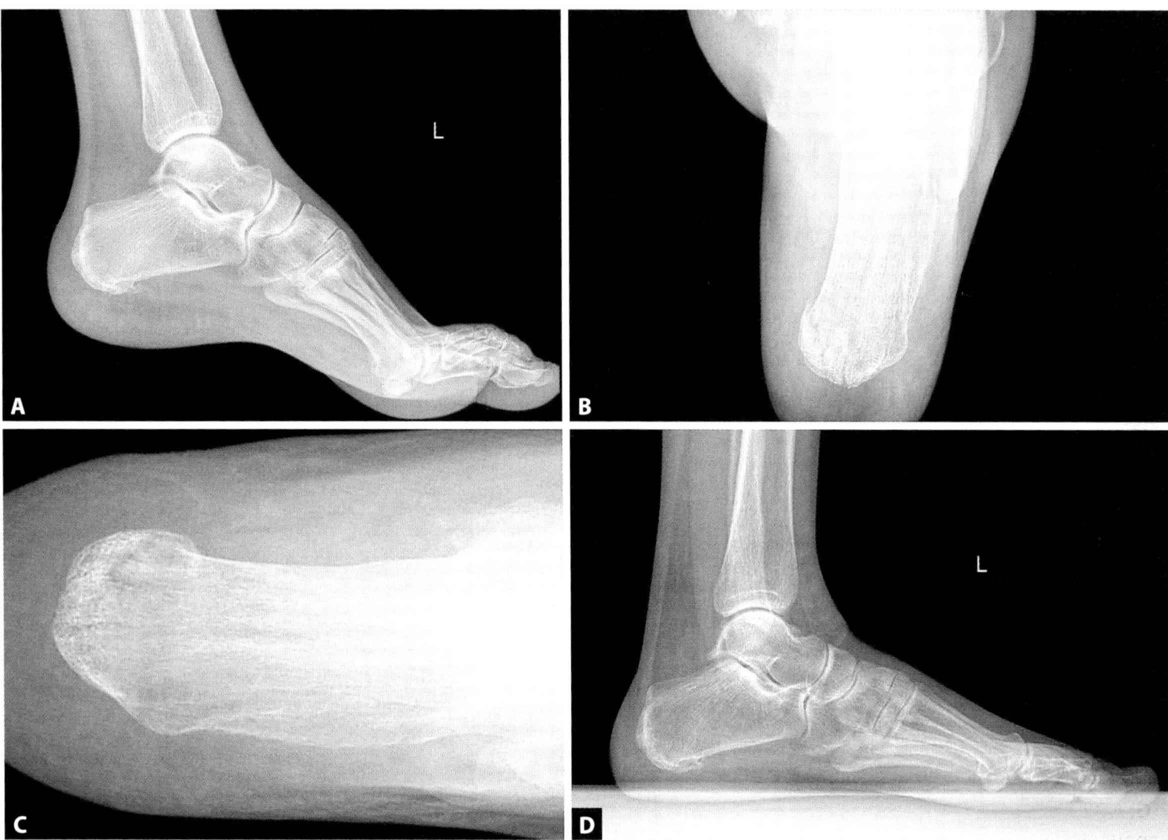

Figs. 2A to D: A 50 year old female fell from 2 steps off a ladder. (A and B) Lateral and axial x rays demonstrate a non displaced medial process fracture; (C and D) Lateral and axial x rays demonstrate the fracture is healed after 6 weeks of non weight bearing in a fracture boot.

Reduction of the fragment is surprisingly difficult. The fragment is usually displaced plantar and pulled distally and rotated by the soft-tissue attachments of the plantar fascia, abductor hallucis, and flexor digitorum brevis. Care must be taken during reduction to avoid creating comminution to the fragment. Provisional fixation is obtained with K-wires. Lag screws are placed into the medial process fragment for definitive fixation. Prominent hardware is avoided by countersinking screw heads located on the plantar aspect of the tuberosity.

Immediate postoperative care includes elevation and nonweight-bearing. Early range of motion exercises are encouraged. Immobilization in a fracture boot is necessary to avoid development of equinus. The patient may progress weight-bearing when clinical and radiographic evidence of bony union is present, typically seen at 6 weeks after surgery. Similar to patients treated nonoperatively, discomfort with barefoot weight-bearing on hard surfaces is common for several months after injury and the patient should be counseled on the importance of shoe wear.

Complications

Surgical complications such as malunion or nonunion are rare with appropriately reduced and fixed medial process fractures. Injury to the terminal branches of the medial plantar nerve can occur intraoperatively if care is not taken during dissection, but clinical consequences of this complication are low. Painful scarring of the incision can occur if placed too far onto the plantar surface of the heel.

Recommendations for Treatment

A prospective study of 19 displaced medial process tuberosity fractures compared nonoperative treatment to surgery using lag screws or mini-fragment plating.[21] Postoperative outcomes were compared, and the surgical group demonstrated improved time to weight-bearing and return to work while AOFAS ankle and hindfoot scores were comparable between groups.[21] There were no cases of wound complications, nonunion, or hardware failure. Long-term outcomes for isolated medial process fractures do not exist in the current literature. Therefore, definitive treatment guidelines are not available. The authors' recommendations for treatment of nondisplaced fractures include nonweight-bearing in a short leg cast with close monitoring. Displaced medial process fragments warrant open reduction and screw fixation to decrease the risk of malunion and mobility complications.

■ REFERENCES

1. Olexa TA, Ebraheim NA, Haman SP. The sustentaculum tali: anatomic, radiographic, and surgical considerations. Foot Ankle Int. 2000;21(5):400-3.

2. Wagner UA, Sangeorzan BJ, Harrington RM, Tencer AF. Contact characteristics of the subtalar joint: load distribution between the anterior and posterior facets. J Orthop Res. 1992;10(4):535-43.

3. Coughlin MJ, Mann RA (Eds). Surgery of the Foot and Ankle, 7th edition. St Louis: Mosby; 1999.

4. Rowe CR. Fractures of the os calcis: a long-term follow-up study of 146 patients. JAMA. 1963;184(12):920-3.

5. Della Rocca GJ, Nork SE, Barei DP, Taitsman LA, Benirschke SK. Fractures of the sustentaculum tali: injury characteristics and surgical technique for reduction. Foot Ankle Int. 2009;30(11):1037-41.

6. Dürr C, Zwipp H, Rammelt S. Fractures of the sustentaculum tali. Oper Orthop Traumatol. 2013;25(6):569-78.

7. Radley JM, Nicolaou DA. Bilateral isolated fractures of the sustentaculum tali: a case report. JBJS Case Connector. 2019;9(2):e0238.

8. Huri G, Atay AO, Leblebicioğlu GA, Doral MN. Fracture of the sustentaculum tali of the calcaneus in pediatric age: a case report. J Pediatr Orthop B. 2009;18(6):354-6.

9. Mu H, Xu X, Gang B. Isolated fractures of the sustentaculum tali: injury characteristics and surgical technique for reduction management. J Foot Ankle Surg Asia Pacific. 2014;1(2):48-51.

10. Marks RM, Antoniades S, Myerson MS. Injury to the sustentaculum tali. Foot. 1996;6(4):182-7.

11. Gatha M, Pedersen B, Buckley R. Fractures of the sustentaculum tali of the calcaneus: a case report. Foot Ankle Int. 2008;29(2):237-40.

12. Carr JB. Complications of calcaneus fractures entrapment of the flexor hallucis longus: report of two cases. J Orthop Trauma. 1990;4(2):166-8.

13. Komiya K, Terada N. Entrapment of the flexor hallucis longus tendon by direct impalement in the osseofibrous tunnel under the sustentaculum tali—an extremely rare complication of a calcaneal fracture: a case report. JBJS Case Connect. 2014;4(4):e100.

14. Burdeaux BD. Reduction of calcaneal fractures by the McReynolds medial approach technique and its experimental basis. Clin Orthop Relat Res. 1983;(177):87-103.

15. Zwipp H. Chirurgie des Fußes. Wien: Springer; 1994.

16. Rammelt S, Pitakveerakul A. Hindfoot injuries: how to avoid posttraumatic varus deformity? Foot Ankle Clin. 2019;24(2):325-45.

17. Myerson MS, Berger BI. Nonunion of a fracture of the sustentaculum tali causing a tarsal tunnel syndrome: a case report. Foot Ankle Int. 1995;16(11):740-2.

18. Sauer ST, Burdeaux BD, O'Connor DP, Oates JC. Calcaneus fractures: medial approach and indirect reduction. Tech Foot Ankle Surg. 2004;3(4):245-9.

19. Al-Ashhab ME, Elgazzar AS. Treatment for displaced sustentaculum tali fractures. Foot (Edinb). 2018;35:70-4.

20. Sarrafian SK. Anatomy of the Foot and Ankle: Descriptive, Topographic, Functional. Philadelphia: Lippincott; 1983.

21. Li B, Wu G-B, Yang Y-F. Conservative versus surgical treatment for displaced fracture of the medial process of the calcaneal tuberosity. J Orthop Surg (Hong Kong). 2016;24(2):163-6.

22. Squires B, Allen PE, Livingstone J, Atkins RM. Fractures of the tuberosity of the calcaneus. J Bone Joint Surg Br. 2001;83-B(1):55-61.

23. Browner BD (Ed). Skeletal Trauma: Basic Science, Management, and Reconstruction, 5th edition. Philadelphia, PA: Elsevier, Saunders; 2015.

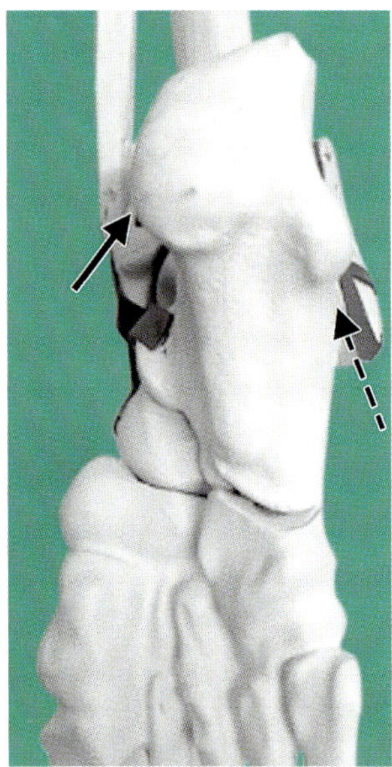

Fig. 2: Inferior surface of calcaneal tuberosity. The solid arrow points to the medial tubercle, whereas the dotted arrow points to the lateral tubercle.

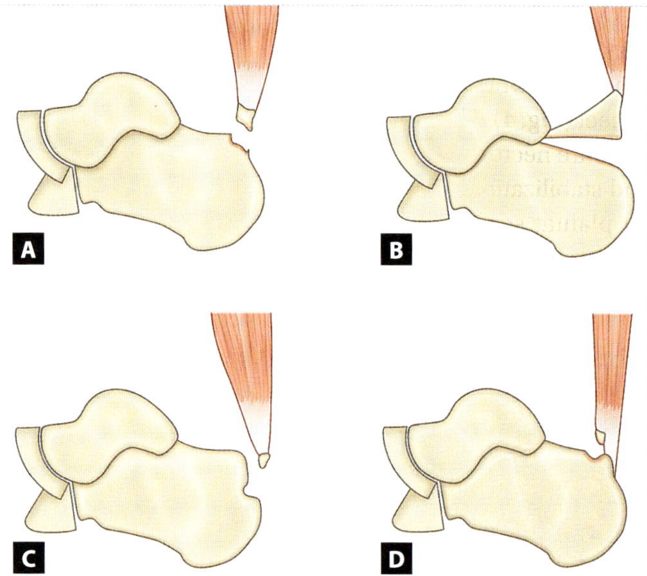

Figs. 3A to D: The modified Beavis classification of tuberosity avulsions: (A) Type 1; (B) Type 2; (C) Type 3; (4) Type 4.

PATHOMECHANISMS OF TUBEROSITY AVULSIONS

Avulsions of the calcaneal tuberosity can be traumatic or pathological. *Traumatic* avulsions can be caused by either indirect or direct mechanisms. Indirect mechanisms most commonly involve eccentric contraction of the gastrosoleus coupled with forced dorsiflexion. However, concentric contraction of the gastrosoleus in a fully flexed knee has also been reported to result in tuber avulsions. Direct mechanisms, such as road traffic accidents and gunshot injuries, generally result in *open* fractures.

Pathological avulsions occur in patients with neurogenic conditions such as peripheral neuropathy, diabetic foot, and Charcot's neuroarthropathy. Such avulsions occur with minimal trauma.

Whether traumatic or pathological, elderly are more susceptible to these injuries. This may be attributable to two important risk factors: A physiological decrease in the trabecular bone strength of the tuberosity and an increase in the intrinsic tightness of the gastrocnemius–soleus complex.[4]

EPIDEMIOLOGY

The burden of tuberosity avulsions has been reported variably in the literature. In a series of 180 calcaneus fractures, Essex-Lopresti[5] reported tuberosity fractures (including tuberosity avulsions, plantar fascia avulsions, and other fracture patterns) in 17.4% of the cases. In contrast, however, Schepers et al.[6] reported tuberosity fractures in 8% of a total

of 151 calcaneus fractures. Tuberosity avulsions were noted to account for 3% of all calcaneal fractures in this series.

CLASSIFICATION

Beavis et al.[7] have classified tuberosity avulsions into three types. *Type 1* avulsions, also known as *"sleeve avulsions"*, involve avulsion of a thin shell of the tuberosity along with the Achilles tendon. *Type 2* avulsions represent the classical *"beak"* avulsions and involve avulsion of a variable part of the tuberosity. *Type 3*, or *infrabursal*, avulsions involve avulsion of the middle third of the posterior tuberosity. Lee et al.[8] added another variant, *type 4* avulsions, which result from avulsion of only the deep (anterior) fibers of the Achilles tendon **(Figs. 3A to D)**.

The 2018 classification categorizes the calcaneus bone as "82". Extra-articular fractures of the calcaneus are classified as "82A", and extra-articular tuberosity avulsions are classified as "82A1".[9]

CLINICAL FEATURES AND PREOPERATIVE ASSESSMENT

It is important to elicit whether or not the patient had significant trauma; pathological avulsions can occur with minimal or no trauma. In such cases, a detailed history focusing on risk factors such as peripheral neuropathy, diabetes mellitus, smoking, tobacco consumption, and Charcot's disease must be elicited. The mechanism and time since injury must also be elicited.

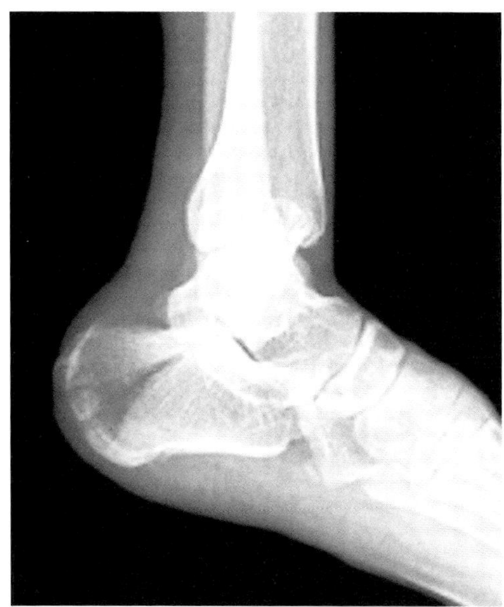

Fig. 6: Completely undisplaced tuberosity avulsions, such as the one seen in this radiograph, may be managed nonoperatively in the low-demand elderly patients with comorbidities.

tissues, especially in patients with peripheral neuropathy, a window can be cut into the cast to permit regular inspection. The cast is maintained till there is evidence of radiological healing.

■ OPERATIVE MANAGEMENT

The vast majority of displaced tuberosity avulsions are managed operatively. As mentioned earlier, emergent reduction and fixation is necessary to prevent pressure necrosis of the skin of the posterior heel. The goals of operative treatment are twofold. Foremost is anatomic reduction; nonanatomic reduction will lead shortening of the gastrocnemius–soleus lever arm and consequent impairment of plantarflexion. The other equally important goal is to ensure stable fixation, as fixation failures are common and can be disastrous.

Surgical Approaches

Minimally Invasive/Percutaneous Approach

The patient is placed in a prone position with a radiolucent bolster under the ankle. In this position, reduction is easily achieved by knee flexion, which neutralizes the pull of gastrocnemius, and by ankle plantarflexion, which neutralizes the pull of soleus. If need be, a K-wire or a Schanz pin may be used as a joystick to reduce the fragment anatomically. One or two large fracture reduction clamps are applied; stab skin incisions are used. We prefer to use two clamps if the fragment is large, as this gives better control and

compression. The proximal spike of each clamp engages the avulsed fragment on medial and lateral sides of the Achilles tendon, and the distal spike engages the plantar surface of the tuberosity. Sequential tightening results in anatomical reduction. Thereafter, cannulated screws can be used to maintain the reduction (**Figs. 7A to D**).

If the avulsed fragment is small or if reduction fails by closed means, a "mini-open" approach can be employed. This entails a 2–3 cm straight incision placed posterolaterally or posteromedially, directly over the avulsed fragment. Sharp dissection is used to expose the fragment. Any interposing fibrous tissue is cleared, and the fragment can be reduced by means of a K-wire or sutures. This approach can also be used if suture anchors or transosseous suture repair is contemplated.

Posterior Approach

If anatomic reduction cannot be achieved by percutaneous means, or if the presentation is delayed, an open posterior approach is warranted (**Figs. 8A to C**). Positioning for this approach is similar to the minimally invasive approach. An important pearl is to prepare and drape the uninjured leg; this helps to evaluate the tension on the gastrocnemius-soleus complex after repair and need for gastrocnemius recession intraoperatively.

A straight midline incision is used starting from the point of insertion of the Achilles tension and extending several centimeters proximally, as deemed necessary by the surgeon. Sharp dissection is used to expose the avulsed fragment, taking care to minimize soft-tissue stripping. The fragment can be turned proximally along with the Achilles tendon, and the crater visualized and cleared of any interposing tissues.

Fixation Modalities

The choice of fixation depends on the type of avulsion, size of the avulsed fragment, and quality of the host bone. The surgeon must not hesitate to supplement fixation if need be.

Cannulated Screw Fixation

6.5- or 7.0-mm cannulated screws can be used for Beavis type 2 avulsions. A minimum of two and preferably four screws should be used. Care must be taken to maximize the spread of the screws so as to obtain an optimal hold on the avulsed fragment. The Achilles tendon insertion must be respected and avoided during screw placement. We prefer to use 6.5 and 32 mm partially threaded cannulated screws; two screws are placed posteriorly and one or two screws anteriorly. Care is taken to place the screws perpendicular to the fracture line, which ensures compression. Whenever

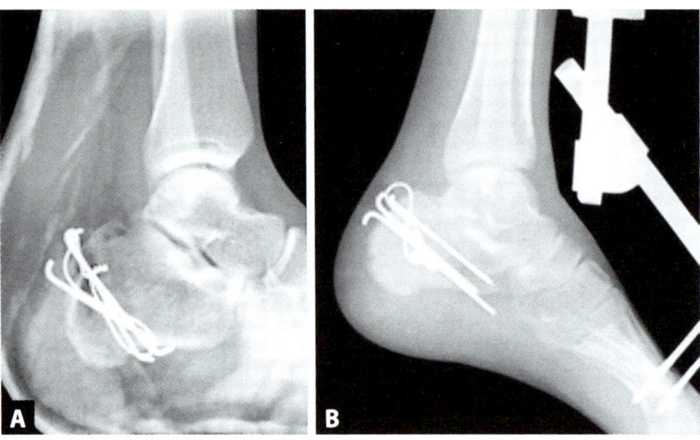

Figs. 9A and B: Tension-band wire fixation. (A) The technique by Squires et al. (B) A modification—proximally, the wire loop is passed around the Achilles tendon and distally through a screw placed in the lateral wall of calcaneus. An external fixator was also used as this was an open fracture.

feasible, the plantar cortex of the calcaneus must be engaged to improve pullout strength. Washers may be used in osteoporotic bones to prevent the screw head from sinking into the soft bone.

Tension-band Wiring

The technique of tension-band wiring for tuberosity avulsion was described by Squires et al.[10] Two K-wires are placed from the posterosuperior aspect of the tuberosity into the anteroinferior aspect of calcaneus. A tension band is around the ends of the wires over the lateral wall of calcaneus **(Figs. 9A and B)**. Alternatively, the tension band can be passed around the Achilles tendon and a screw placed in the lateral wall of calcaneus. The tension-band technique may also be used to supplement other forms of internal fixation.

Transosseous Suture Fixation

Banerjee et al.[4] have described a technique of transosseous repair that may be used for avulsions with small fragments (Beavis type 1 or 3) or to supplement other forms of internal fixation. A modified Krackow suture is passed through the Achilles tendon and the avulsed fragment. The free ends of the suture are then passed through two tunnels drilled in the body of the calcaneus and tied over the plantar aspect of calcaneus. Wakatsuki et al.[11] modified this technique by using a side-locking loop suture technique, which is believed to have a better pullout strength than the conventional Krackow sutures.

Fixation with Suture Anchors

Suture anchors may also be used to fix Beavis type 1 and 3 avulsions or to supplement other forms of fixation. Several suture-anchor configurations have been described. Common to all of these is the fact that anchors are used in pairs and are inserted into the body of the tuberosity. The free end of suture is then passed through the avulsed fragment and the Achilles tendon to achieve reduction and stabilization. Robb and Davies[12] used two 6.5 mm corkscrew anchors to achieve fixation, and the proximal ends of the sutures were passed through the avulsed fragment and the Achilles tendon using a Kessler technique. Lui[13] described a modification of this technique. Two limbs of each suture are tied over the avulsed fragment. The remaining limbs of one suture are weaved through the peripheral zone of the Achilles tendon, whereas the remaining limbs of the other suture are weaved through the central zone. This reduces overcrowding of the sutures.

Gastrocnemius Recession

Gastrocnemius recession may be indicated if there is tightness of the gastrocnemius–soleus complex. Intraoperatively, this is determined by placing both knees in equal flexion and comparing the amount of plantarflexion at the ankle with the uninjured side. Tightness is indicated by decreased plantarflexion of the ankle. Recession may also be indicated in late presentations when anatomical reduction of the fragment may be impossible owing to tightness of the gastrocnemius–soleus. We used the Strayer procedure[14] to perform the recession through a separate incision at aponeurosis of the gastrocnemius–soleus.

■ AFTERCARE

The ankle is placed in gravity equinus to protect fixation, which may be unnecessary if a concomitant gastrocnemius recession has been performed. A below-knee cast or splint is used with a window incorporated into the cast to enable wound check. Toe-touch weight bearing is permitted. There are no guidelines as to how long the equinus position should be maintained; a decision is, therefore, taken on a case-to-case basis. We prefer to maintain an equinus position till at least early evidence of healing is noted and longer if the bone is osteoporotic and cutout is anticipated. The cast or splint is discontinued only when there is evidence of sound radiological union; a CT scan may be sometimes indicated to assess union. Range-of-motion and strengthening exercises are initiated after complete healing **(Figs. 10A to D)**.

■ COMPLICATIONS

The two most-feared complications of tuberosity avulsions are skin breakdown and failure of fixation, respectively. Wound breakdown occurs due to pressure necrosis from the

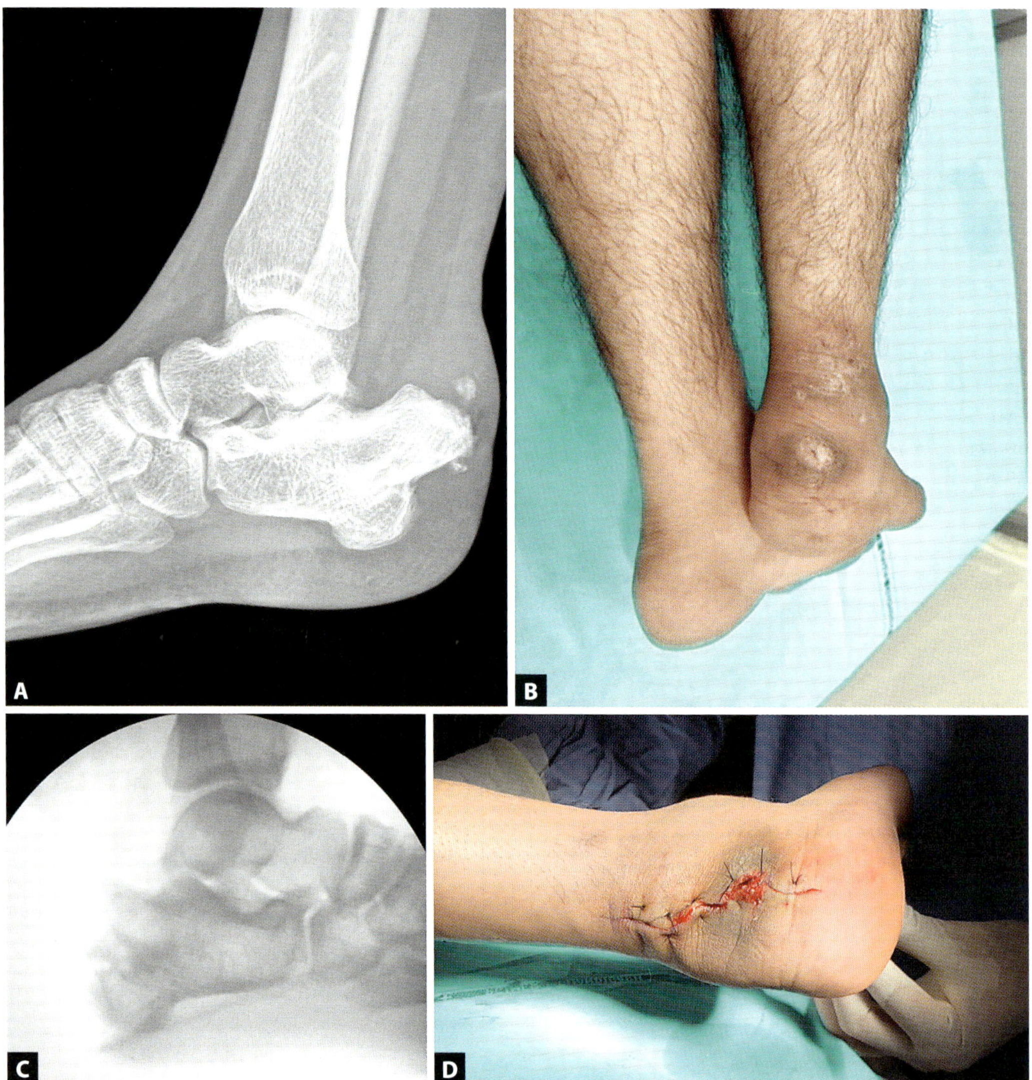

Figs. 11A to D: Neglected tuberosity avulsion, resulting in malunion and soft-tissue problems. (A) Lateral view of the ankle, demonstrating malunion of the tuberosity; (B) Wound breakdown is noted on the posterior aspect of the heel, corresponding to the prominence of the malunited tuberosity; (C) Intraoperative fluoroscopy image, demonstrating resection of the malunited tuberosity; (D) Loose closure could be achieved after resection of the tuberosity.

complications, especially soft-tissue complications, whereas those with <2 cm displacement had 30% probability of complications.

SUMMARY

Avulsion fractures of the calcaneal tuberosity are more common in the elderly and patients with peripheral neuropathy. They are associated with significant soft-tissue complications, and emergent reduction and fixation is therefore indicated. Inadequate fixation and immobilization, as well as poor bone quality, can lead to fixation failures. Hence, a close follow-up is necessary till union occurs, and outcomes are guarded at best.

REFERENCES

1. O'Brien M. The anatomy of the Achilles tendon. Foot Ankle Clin. 2005;10(2):225-38.
2. Keener BJ, Sizensky JA. The anatomy of the calcaneus and surrounding structures. Foot Ankle Clin. 2005;10(3):413-24.
3. Lohrer H, Arentz S, Nauck T, Dorn-Lange NV, Konerding MA. The Achilles tendon insertion is crescent-shaped: an in vitro anatomic investigation. Clin Orthop Relat Res. 2008;466(9):2230-7.
4. Banerjee R, Chao JC, Taylor R, Siddiqui A. Management of calcaneal tuberosity fractures. J Am Acad Orthop Surg. 2012;20(4):253-8.
5. Essex-Lopresti P. The mechanism, reduction technique, and results in fractures of the os calcis. Br J Surg. 1952;39(157):395-419.

Calcaneal Fracture Dislocation

Cristian Ortiz, Andrew Sands

"Great things are done by a series of small things brought together".

–Vincent Van Gogh

INTRODUCTION

Calcaneus fracture dislocations are uncommon but potentially devastating injuries if not treated in time. The term fracture dislocation is used when a bone fracture is associated with a dislocation of a surrounding joint. The calcaneus has three superior facets that articulate with the talus, forming the subtalar joint complex. The anterior surface of the calcaneus has a saddle-shaped joint that connects with the cuboid to form the calcaneocuboid joint, which is part of the midtarsal joint (Chopart joint). Any fracture of the calcaneus associated with the dislocation of the joints surrounding the bone should be called a calcaneus fracture dislocation. This can involve the subtalar or the Chopart joint. This type of injury has been described by several authors. Initially, Merle d'Aubigné and Wilmoth in 1936 and then Biga and Thomine in 1977 identified four cases that they termed fracture dislocations of the calcaneus. Case reports and series of at most 17 patients are currently described in the literature. A high-energy mechanism from an axial force applied to an inverted foot causes calcaneal fracture dislocation. The posterolateral calcaneal tuberosity fragment is displaced laterally, impacting the tip of the lateral malleoli. It frequently produces irregular distal fibular fracture with avulsion of the superior peroneal retinaculum and other adjacent soft tissue lesions. Calcaneus fracture dislocation can be misdiagnosed as isolated lateral malleolus fractures, resulting in catastrophic outcomes for the patients. The importance of correctly evaluating radiographs and computed tomography (CT) scans in the foot and ankle is fundamental to define the severity and evaluate associated occult injuries. If the injury is left dislocated or nonoperative treatment is decided, the outcome is poor, leading to chronic disability in most cases. Severe complications such as prompt post-traumatic subtalar joint arthritis, nonunion, and malunion are the results of missed injuries. Early fixation of fracture dislocation of the calcaneus is needed to avoid early evolving complications. Important prognostic factors are anatomical reduction of the subtalar joint and restoration of the normal structure of the calcaneus. Operative treatment options include closed reduction and percutaneous pin fixation, external fixation, open reduction with internal fixation, and arthrodesis. The approach recommended for this injury is a lateral approach modified by palmer; however, percutaneous and minimally invasive fixation has the potential advantages of restoring hindfoot alignment and articular congruity with less extensive soft-tissue dissection. Severe wound complications can occur in patients with comorbidities such as diabetic patients, elderly, or smokers. Minimally invasive or percutaneous techniques for reduction and internal fixation may be considered when there are risk factors. The importance of calcaneal fracture dislocation lies in prompt detection, evaluation of associated injuries, early reduction, and stabilization.[2]

ETIOLOGY

Most calcaneal fractures are produced by traumatic axial loading due to falls from height or motor vehicle accidents. More than 75% of all calcaneal fractures are intra-articular, and the posterior facet of the subtalar joint is involved in almost 90% of all intra-articular calcaneal fractures. The extent and direction of the collision force, foot position, and characteristics of the bone will determine the fracture pattern. The mechanism of calcaneal fracture dislocation is a vertical force combined with an inversion position of the hindfoot. The primary fracture line from oblique shear separates the calcaneus into an anteromedial fragment that maintains its normal relationship to the talus and a posterolateral fragment that is dislocated from the subtalar

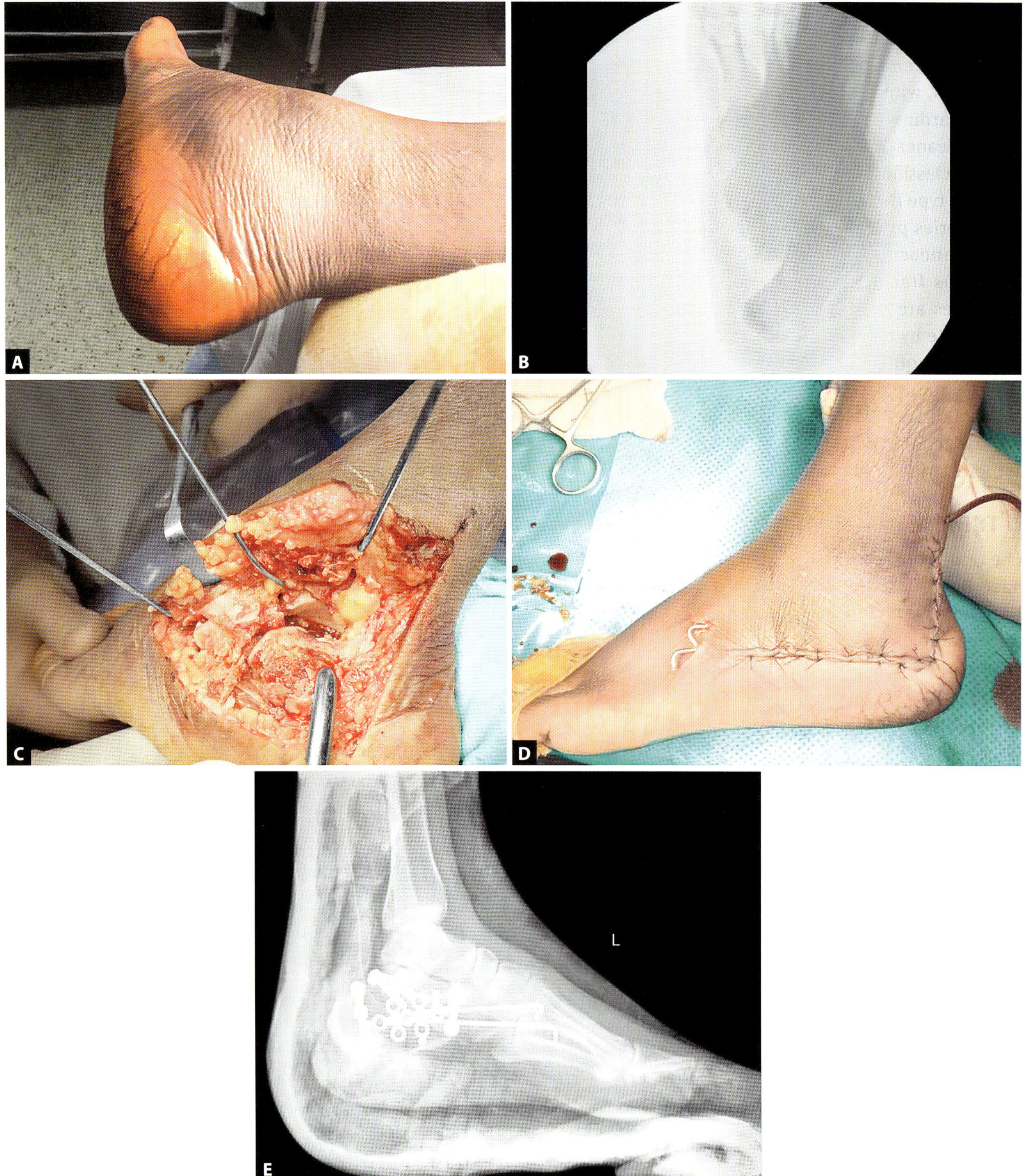

Figs. 1A to E: Case report of a calcaneal fracture dislocation pattern. (A) Swelling and deformity in the lateral region of the foot secondary to a calcaneus fracture dislocation; (B) Axial radiographic view demonstrating a calcaneus fracture dislocation pattern; (C) Extended lateral approach used for the reduction and fixation of the fracture dislocation pattern; (D) Immediate postoperative wound closure over drain with 3-0 nonabsorbable sutures placed using Allgower–Donati technique; (E) Final lateral radiographic view showing the postoperative result.

variety of associated injuries. These lesions are classified by subtype variants of the multiple classical calcaneus fractures classification system proposed in the literature. The Sanders classification evaluates the amount of displaced fracture

until week 12, when full bone callus formation is confirmed with CT scan. Propioceptive, standin leg balance (BOSU), and articular range of motion are increased progressively as tolerated until week 20. Continuation and progression of previous exercises associated with lower extremity closed chain strengthening until week 24. Progression to light jogging (treadmill) and returning to daily activities.

COMPLICATIONS

Calcaneal malunions regularly result from displaced fractures treated conservatively. It is unacceptable to leave calcaneus fracture dislocations conservatively. The main complications of nonoperative calcaneal fracture dislocation include symptomatic subtalar arthritis, varus or valgus malalignment, shortening and widening of the hindfoot, impingement and/or subluxation of the peroneal tendons, and sural or posterior tibial neuritis. Anatomical reconstruction of the calcaneal shape and especially of the joint surfaces may be problematic in missed calcaneal fracture dislocations, and primary subtalar arthrodesis is the ideal treatment. This procedure must be combined with reconstruction of heel height and width in order to achieve a plantigrade foot. Therefore, even in high-risk patients, some kind of reduction has to be made to avoid severe malunion. In the Stephens and Sanders classification for calcaneal malunions based on CT scan, calcaneus fracture dislocation will develop into a type III if left untreated. This type of pattern includes lateral wall exostosis, subtalar arthrosis, and malalignment of the calcaneal body, resulting in significant hindfoot varus or valgus angulation. The solution proposed by this type of pattern is lateral wall exostectomy, peroneal tenolysis, distractive subtalar arthrodesis, and a calcaneal osteotomy to correct hindfoot malalignment. Zwipp and Rammelt described five types of posttraumatic calcaneal malunions Type IV in their classification system is the subtalar joint incongruity associated with arthritis, hindfoot malalignment, loss of height and lateral translation of the tuberosity[6] Multiplanar corrective osteotomy through the former fracture line and distractive subtalar arthrodesis using bone block is the prefer treatment. The realignment involves a medial shift of the displaced lateral calcaneal body, fixation to the sustentacular fragment, restoration of the calcaneal height, and elimination of axial malalignment. Postoperative protocol differs from early reduction and fixation treatment in the restrictive weight bearing for 12 weeks. Progressive weight bearing is indicated according to bone callus formation seen in the CT scan.

CONCLUSION

Calcaneal fracture dislocations are rare injuries. Prompt diagnosis involves adequate physical examinations and correct imaging with basic set of calcaneal radiographs and CT scans. There are no classifications for this type of injury, and the studies reported in the literature are small series or isolated case reports. Independent of the type of calcaneal fracture dislocation, early reduction and fixation are essential for favorable outcomes and to avoid complications. Surgeons should be aware of this type of injury and other variants in order to prevent inappropriate treatment or misdiagnosis. The subtalar arthrodesis is the option of treatment when this injury is discovered late and used as a salvage procedure associated with a corrective osteotomy to correct calcaneus malunion.

REFERENCES

1. Rammelt S, Marx C, Swords G, Swords M. Recognition, treatment, and outcome of calcaneal fracture-dislocation. Foot Ankle Int. 2021;42(6):706-13.
2. Miller TJ, Kwon JY. The "joint-elevation" calcaneus fracture: a rare variant of the intra-articular calcaneus fracture-dislocation. Foot Ankle Spec. 2015;8(2):125-9.
3. Sanders R, Vaupel ZM, Erdogan M, Downes K. Operative treatment of displaced intraarticular calcaneal fractures: long-term (10–20 years) results in 108 fractures using a prognostic CT classification. J Orthop Trauma. 2014;28(10):551-63.
4. Schepers T, Backes M, Schep NW, Goslings JC, Luitse JS. Functional outcome following a locked fracture-dislocation of the calcaneus. Int Orthop. 2013;37(9):1833-8.
5. Rider CM, Olinger CR, Szatkowski JP, Richardson DR. "Locked lateral" calcaneal fracture-dislocation treated with primary subtalar fusion: a case report. JBJS Case Connect. 2020;10(1):e0467.
6. Rammelt S, Marx C. Managing severely malunited calcaneal fractures and fracture-dislocations. Foot Ankle Clin. 2020; 25(2):239-56.

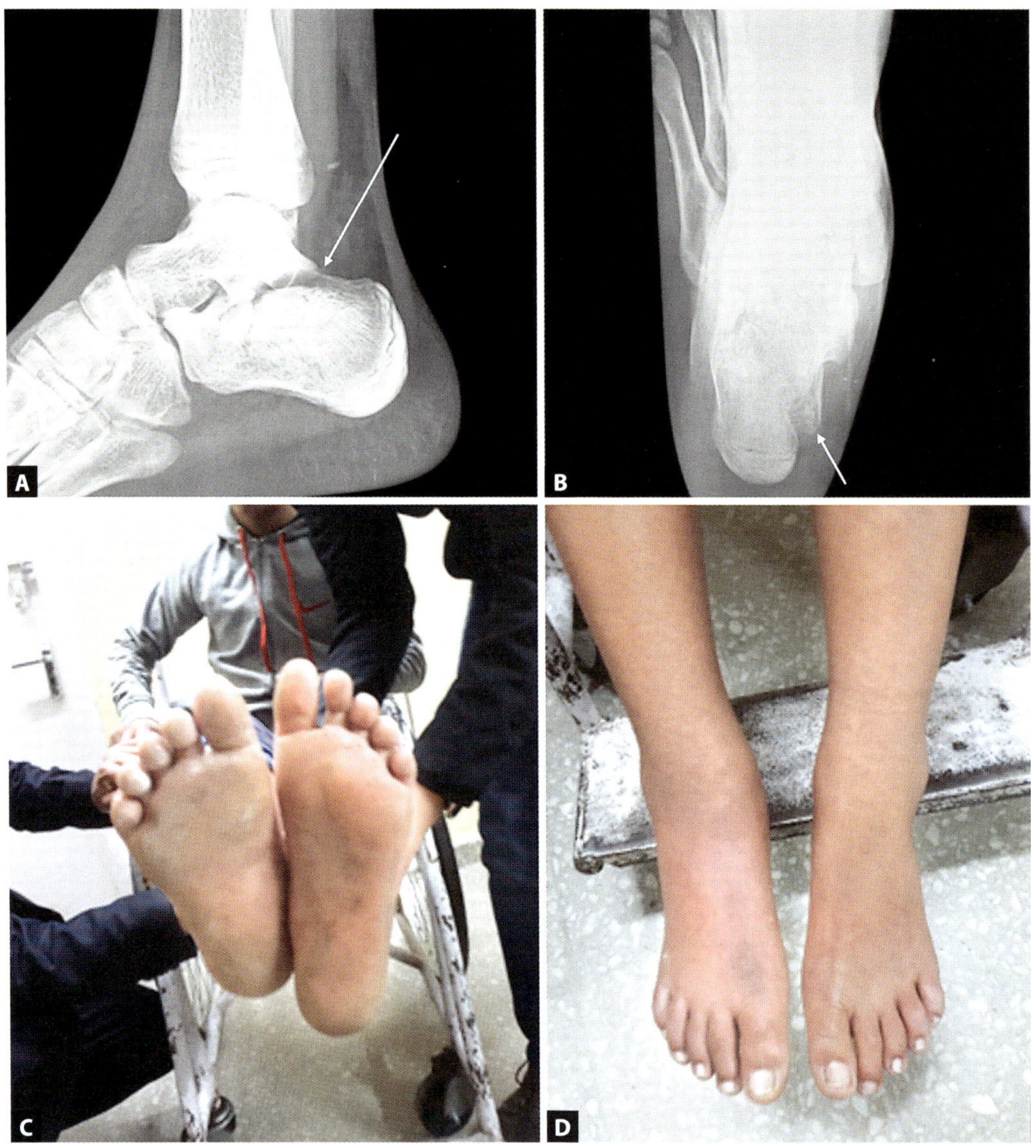

Figs. 1A to D: (A and B) Anteroposterior (AP) and axial views of a 15-year-old male with open physis who fell from a height; there is facet depression, heel varus, and lateral wall blowout, similar to that of an adult. (C and D) Clinical picture of the same child viewed from below and above; note the foot swelling and heel broadening.

lower extremities and the spine. Pain, swelling, and typical heel broadening **(Figs. 1A to D)** are seen in displaced fractures, although only pain and some soft-tissue swelling could be the only clinical presentation in undisplaced or minimally displaced fractures. The heel should be examined for swelling, blisters, or any open wounds. Open injuries are much less common in children than adults, both from our experience and from the available literature. Both feet should be examined because a tell-tale bruise may be seen in children presenting a few hours after injury. Unilateral injuries in older children may allow them to walk with a limp at presentation. Finally, a complete neurological and vascular evaluation is essential.

■ INVESTIGATIONS/RADIOGRAPHY

Pediatric calcaneus fractures have been commonly missed as radiographic abnormalities are often more subtle than in adults. The majority of the missed ones are extra-articular fractures. Radiography is the primary evaluation tool in calcaneus fractures, although it may not be the gold standard. For interpretation, one should be familiar with the ossification centers and accessory bones in the pediatric foot. Standard anteroposterior and lateral foot views are usually taken, but it is important to add an axial (Harris) view if the child is cooperative. The lateral view is the one that renders more information, and the clinician must evaluate the following:

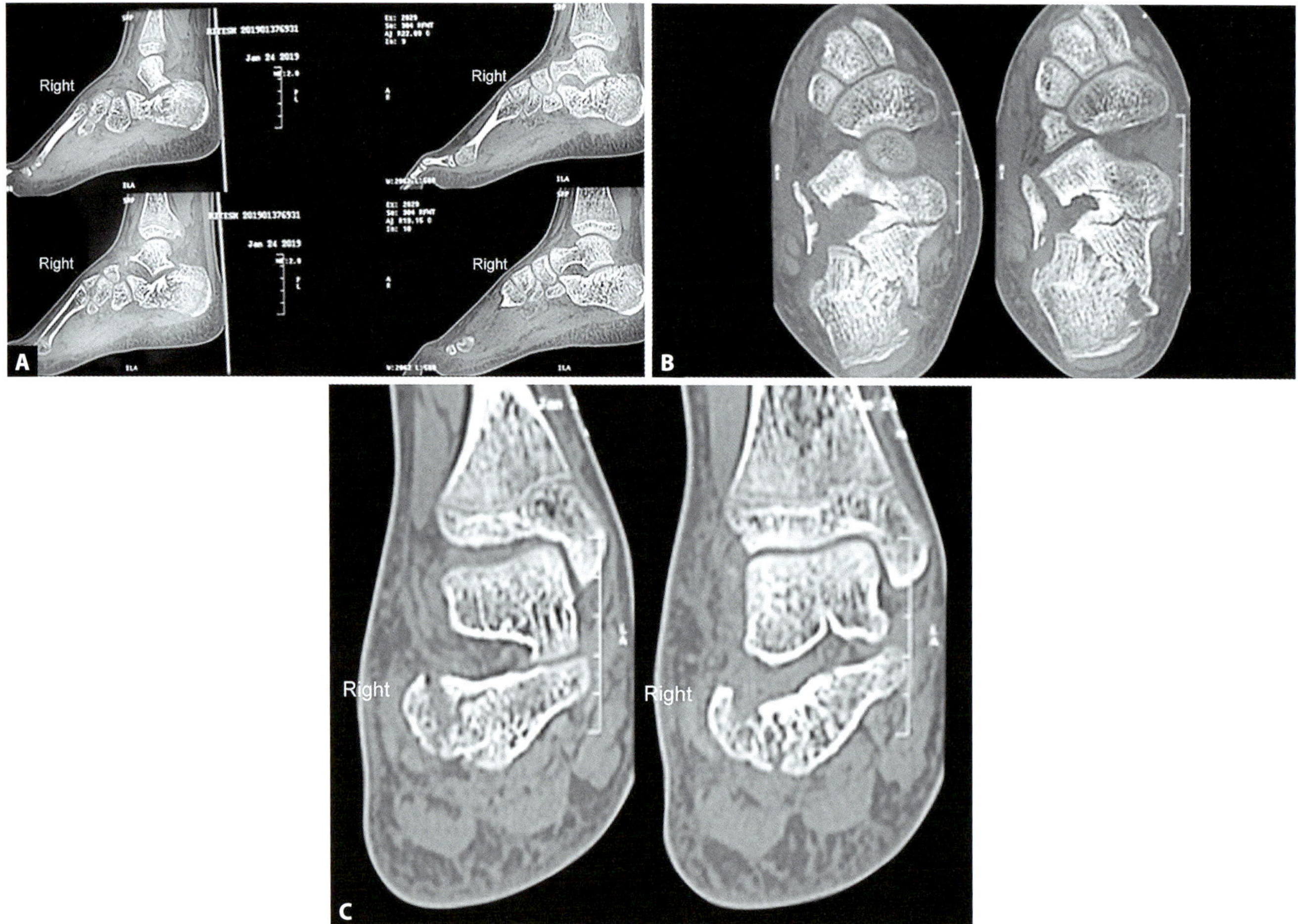

Figs. 3A to C: Computed tomography (CT) scan of a patient. (A) Sagittal sections showing tuberosity depression; (B) Axial cuts showing lateral wall and anterior end involvement; (C) Coronal cuts showing the extent of subtalar joint involvement and lateral wall blowout.

TABLE 1: Classification of pediatric calcaneus fractures.[4]			
Type 1	1A	Fracture of tuberosity/apophysis	Extra-articular
	1B	Fracture of sustentaculum tali	Extra-articular
	1C	Fracture of anterior process	Extra-articular
	1D	Distal inferolateral aspect	Extra-articular
	1E	Small avulsion off body	Extra-articular
Type 2	2A	Beak fracture	Extra-articular
	2B	Avulsion fracture of insertion of Achilles tendon	Extra-articular
Type 3		Linear fracture not involving subtalar joint	Extra-articular
Type 4		Linear fracture involving subtalar joint	Intra-articular
Type 5	5A	Tongue type	Intra-articular
	5B	Joint depression type	Intra-articular
Type 6		Significant bone loss of posterior aspect with loss of Achilles tendon insertion	Extra-articular

stabilization (similar to adults) to achieve predictable good outcomes.

The study by Petit et al.[13] suggested that surgical intervention is preferable while managing displaced intra-articular fractures as they were able to get a good surgical outcome in 14 displaced intra-articular fractures in 13 children. Brunet,[9] in a study on 17 children with 19 fractures with a mean review of 16.8 years after injury, concluded that only adolescents with displaced fractures require open management, and nonoperative management is sufficient for almost all children with pediatric os calcis fractures. But closer evaluation of their published cases reveals more; although follow-up showed "good results", there was the persistence of radiological abnormality (axial deformity) and loss of Böhler angle. This indicates that intra-articular remodeling is not as complete as expected. This contradicts Thomas' hypothesis that the articular surface of the talus remodels in a growing child to accommodate deformity of the calcaneus; hence, subtalar function is not affected much in children.[14] Although these patients at follow-up

Thus, the concept of chidren being seen as capable of tolerating even malreduction and articular step-off needs to be questioned as subtalar malalignment results in long-standing morbidity and joint degeneration in middle age and old age has been documented with adult unreduced injuries. Summers et al. believed that if there are no contraindications, displaced intra-articular calcaneus fractures should be managed by surgical intervention, irrespective of age.[17]

■ METHODS OF TREATMENT

Nonoperative Management

Most pediatric calcaneus extra-articular and intra-articular undisplaced/minimally displaced can be managed on the below-knee cast for 4–6 weeks. Najefi et al.[12] reported a guide for the management of pediatric calcaneal fractures.

The nonoperatively managed joint depression-type fractures had poor outcomes in 21% of patients. Nonetheless, it is notable that 79% had good outcomes after nonoperative treatment, with or without displacement. Poorer outcomes occurred in those patients treated with surgery in case of a displacement (Sanders classification 2, 3, or 4) **(Figs. 5A to D)**. Full recovery occurred in all undisplaced intra-articular fractures (Sanders 1) with surgical management and with good outcomes.

Operative Management

Most of the displaced intra-articular calcaneus fractures in adolescents can be treated using the minimally invasive surgery (MIS) technique **(Figs. 6 and 7)**. Surgical treatment open reduction and internal fixation (ORIF) is usually

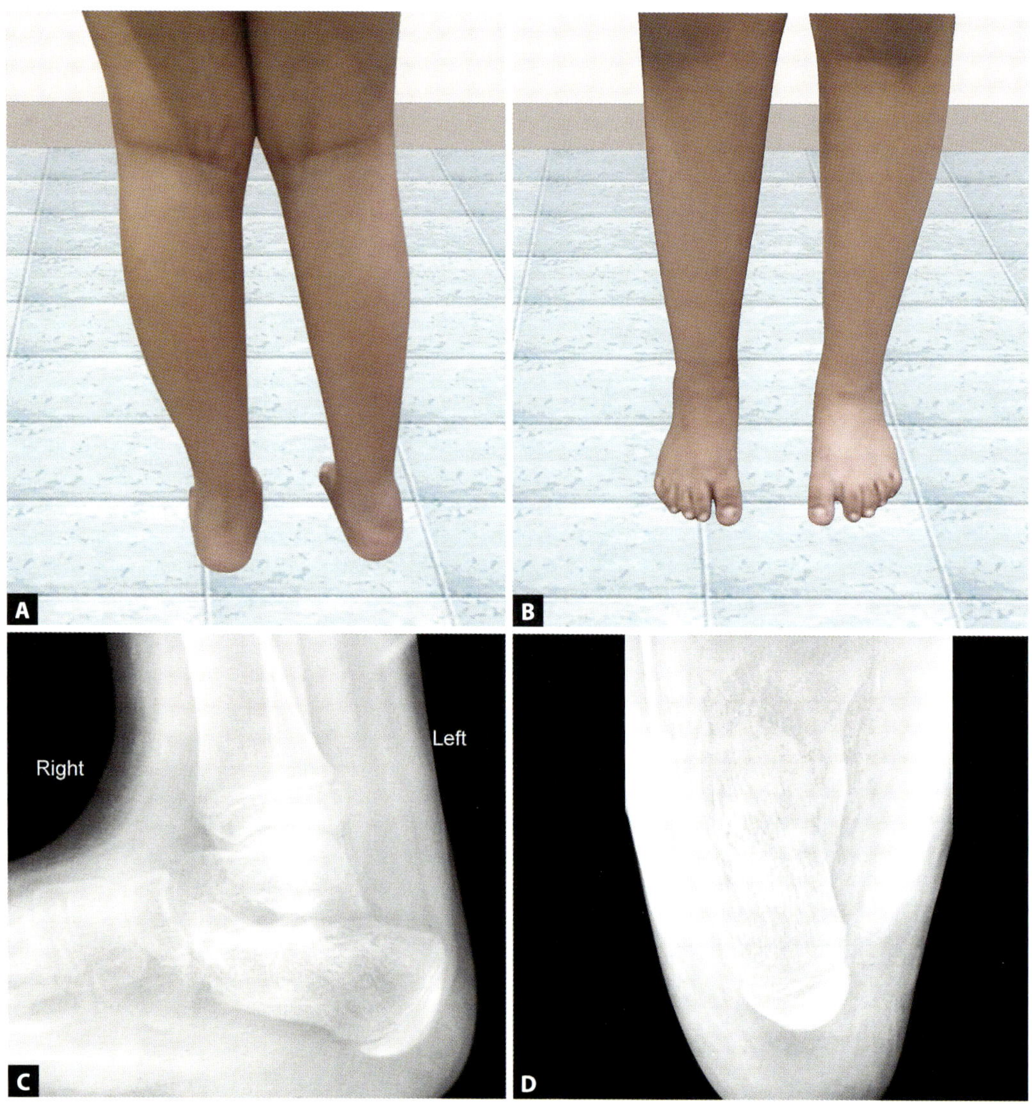

Figs. 5A to D: (A) 1-year follow-up after nonoperative treatment of case; (B) There is some heel broadening, heel valgus, and mild gait alteration; (C and D) Radiology shows significant change in Gissane and Böhler angles.

reserved for adolescents and older children with significant alteration of radiological angles and deformity **(Figs. 8A to G)**.

Complications

Compartment syndrome of the foot following the injury can occur. Skin blisters and necrosis may relate to the severity of the injury. Subtalar arthrosis can be a late complication following intra-articular fractures in adolescents, similar to adults.

To summarize that in younger children, most pediatric calcaneal fractures can be managed nonoperatively by 4–6 weeks of the below-knee cast. In older children (>10 years), the extra-articular and undisplaced intra-articular fractures

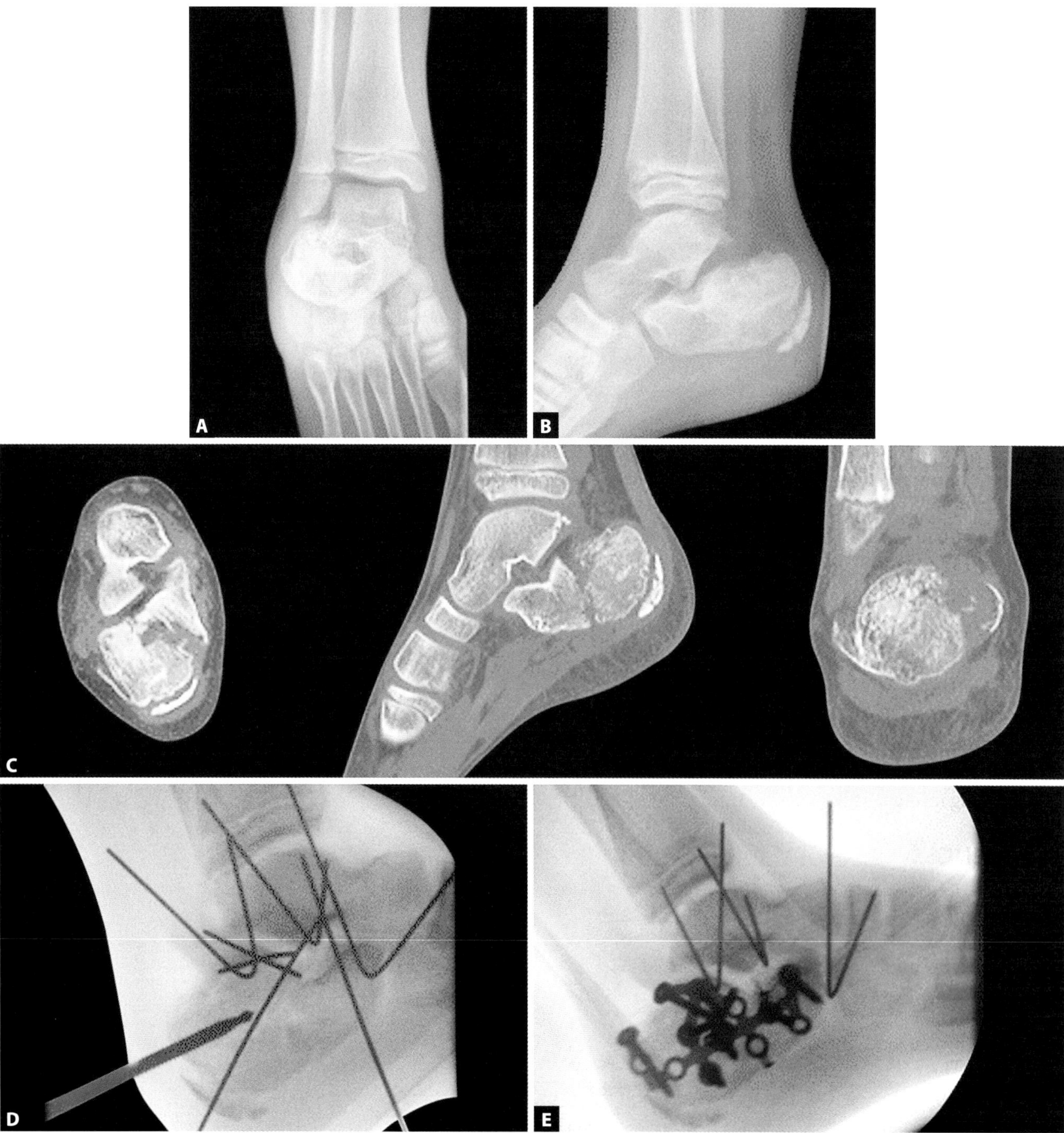

Figs. 8A to E

11. Beaty JH, Kasser JR. Rockwood and Wilkins' Fractures in Children. Philadelphia: Lippincott Williams & Wilkins; 2010.

12. Najefi AA, Najefy A, Vemulapalli K. Paediatric calcaneal fractures: a guide to management based on a review of the literature. Injury. 2020;51(7):1432-8.

13. Petit CJ, Lee BM, Kasser JR, Kocher MS. Operative treatment of intraarticular calcaneal fractures in the pediatric population. J Pediatr Orthop. 2007;27:856-62.

14. Thomas HM. Calcaneal fracture in childhood. Br J Surg. 1969;56(9):664-6.

15. Schneidmueller D, Dietz HG, Kraus R, Marzi I. Calcaneal fractures in childhood: a retrospective survey and literature review. Unfallchirurg. 2007;110:939-45.

16. Tong L, Li M, Li F, Xu J, Hu T. A minimally invasive (sinus tarsi) approach with percutaneous K-wires fixation for intra-articular calcaneal fractures in children. J Pediatr Orthop B. 2018;27(6):556-62.

17. Summers H, Ann Kramer P, Benirschke SK. Pediatric calcaneal fractures. Orthop Rev (Pavia). 2009;1(1):e9.

Op

...ant problems we have cannot be solved at the sa...

ne... a... a fracture in which a break
rec... c...mmunication of the fracture
om a ...ith the elements external
of th... skin.[1] The already difficult
erm in... calcaneal fractures is further
is a...o...en wound and compromised
the h...dfoot. Since intra-articular
tor...i...eduction with stable internal
...f good joint mobility and
...agement options arises
...n, and variable options
...may lead to suboptimal

...mmon as these form
...s.[2] Mitchell et al. noted
...'52 calcaneal fractures
...dy conducted at Royal
...gdom.[2] Randle et al.[3]
...es and discovered no
...es for open calcaneal
...d only find five articles
...t of open calcaneal
...t al.), we encountered
...s (22%) over a period
...f Medical Education
...hese open fractures
...staining road traffic
...this higher incidence
...tertiary care center,
...rauma cases are

refe...
frac...
leve...

...
not...
in a...
pub...
occu...
of o...
gun...

So...

The...
hin...
The...
the...
st...

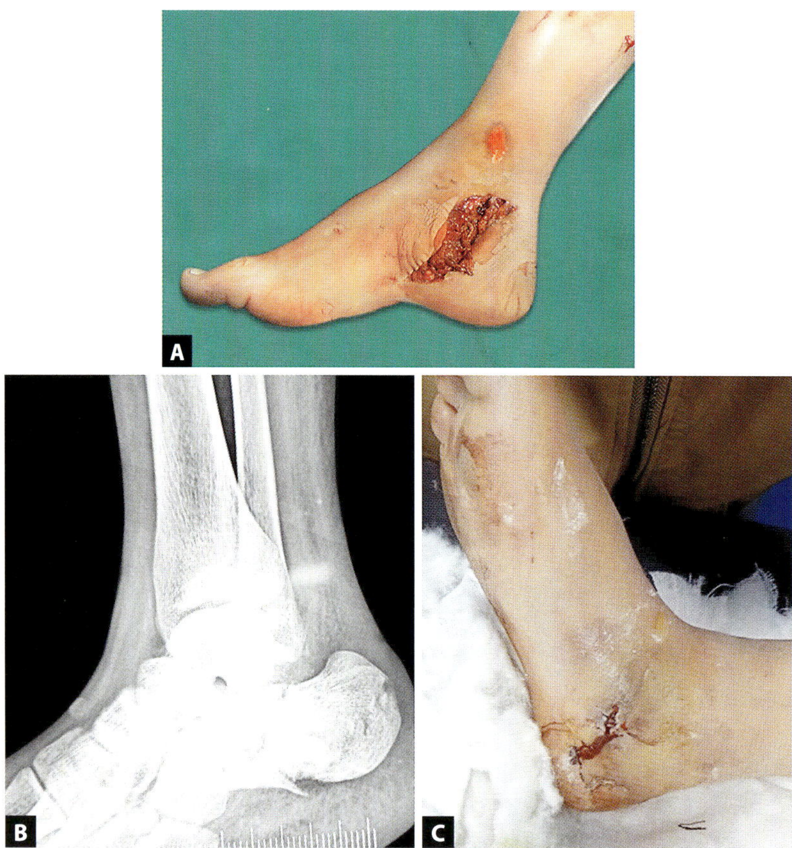

Figs. 2A to C: (A) Type II open fracture, with medial wound; (B and C) Type II open fracture, with medial wound. The radiological anatomy may not be too complex in some of these cases.

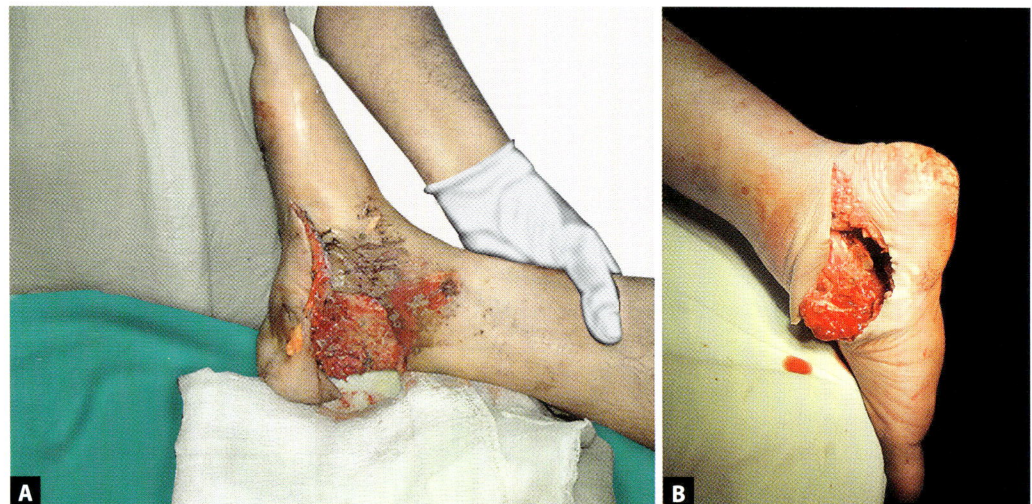

Figs. 3A and B: (A) Type III open fracture with medial wound and associated polytrauma; (B) Type III open fracture with large medial wound and complex fracture.

walking and running activities. Heel pad injury may result from crushing injury or avulsion from the plantar surface of the calcaneus. Injuries with exposed bone and tendons require timely coverage to promote a healing environment. Many traumatic wounds associated with open fractures may be approximated with primary or delayed closure. However, extensive soft tissue loss may require plastic surgery intervention in the form of soft-tissue transfer. The ultimate goal is to restore soft-tissue integrity in a timely fashion with durable, functional, and aesthetic coverage.

inserted superolateral to the Achilles tendon. The pin is inserted into the tongue fragment, which is manipulated to restore the posterior facet as described by Essex-Lopresti.[7] In cases where reduction is difficult to achieve, a fine wire fixator is applied to the tibia and calcaneum to achieve distraction, and in the process, restore Böhler's angle to as near its anatomical status as possible **(Fig. 4)**. The fine wire fixator works on the principle of ligamentotaxis. By ligamentotaxis, the reduction of displaced bone fragments is indirectly achieved through distraction on the ligaments

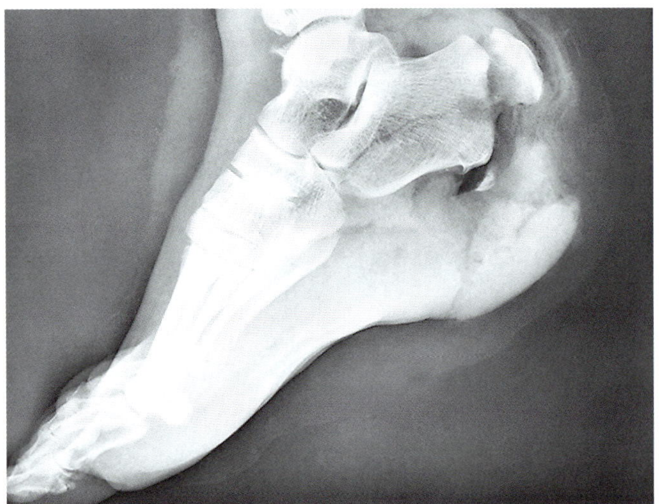

Fig. 4: An X-ray of avulsed tuberosity with open wound. This type of fracture can be treated by primary debridement and definitive fixation with screws.

attached to these fragments, which in turn restores the height of the posterior talocalcaneal joint and reduces the varus/valgus malalignment as well as the width of the calcaneal tuberosity. However, the lateral joint fragment usually remains depressed in joint depression–type fractures because the fracture lines run lateral to the interosseous ligament. This fragment needs to be directly lifted upward using Kirschner wire leveraging or a bone punch inserted plantarly via the primary fracture line to restore the joint congruence. Rarely, the fracture can be directly manipulated through the open wound.

There have been few published studies aimed at finding a universally acceptable protocol for open calcaneal fractures **(Table 1)**. In a retrospective study of 36 open calcaneal fractures (35 patients), Siebert et al.[8] reported outcomes following an array of surgical and nonsurgical treatment strategies.

Complications were seen in >60% of the injuries. Deep infection developed in 14 fractures (39%) and 5 affected extremities (14%) were amputated. Two amputations were performed during the primary hospital stay because of devitalized tissue, while three had to be carried out because of a bone infection and soft-tissue defect at a later point in time. When immediate fracture fixation was carried out, the complication rate was 100%. Only 16% of patients achieved good or excellent results. The authors emphasized that acute treatment should focus on the soft-tissue injury and that bone injury management must never compromise the soft tissues.

TABLE 1: Details of some published series of open calcaneal fractures.					
Author/year	**Number of cases**	**Types of wounds**	**Wound locations**	**Mechanism of injury**	**Outcomes**
Aldridge et al., 2004	19	5 type I, 8 type II, 1 type IIIA, 3 type IIIB, 2 type IIIC	17 medial, 1 posteromedial, 1 posterolateral	11 RTA, 5 fall from height, 1 gunshot wound, 1 lawn mower accident, 1 industrial crush injury	2 infections (1 needed below-knee amputation)
Mehta et al., 2010	14	4 type II, 10 type IIIA	All medial wounds	9 RTA, 1 crush	2 infections
Berry et al., 2004	30	5 type I, 12 type II, 9 type IIIA, 2 IIIB, 2 type IIIC	25 medial, 2 posterior, 3 plantar	18 RTA, 8 fall from height, 3 suicide attempts	2 below-knee amputations for type IIIC injury
Heier et al., 2003	43	9 type I, 8 type II, 12 type IIIA, 13 type IIIB, 1 type IIIC	19 medial, 5 lateral, 3 plantar, 2 posterior, 14 extensive	25 RTA, 2 parachute jumps, 3 boating accidents, 1 crush injury, 1 gunshot wound, 2 lawn mower accidents, 1 explosion	5 below-knee and 1 above-knee amputations, 11 primary subtalar or triple arthrodesis
Siebert et al., 1998	36 (all intra-articular fractures)	9 type I, 10 type II, 2 type IIIA, 13 type IIIB, 2 type IIIC	Not mentioned	13 fall from height, 11 RTA, 12 crush injuries	5 below-knee amputations, 4 ankle arthrodesis, 9 osteomyelitis, 1 partial calcanectomy

(RTA: road traffic accident)

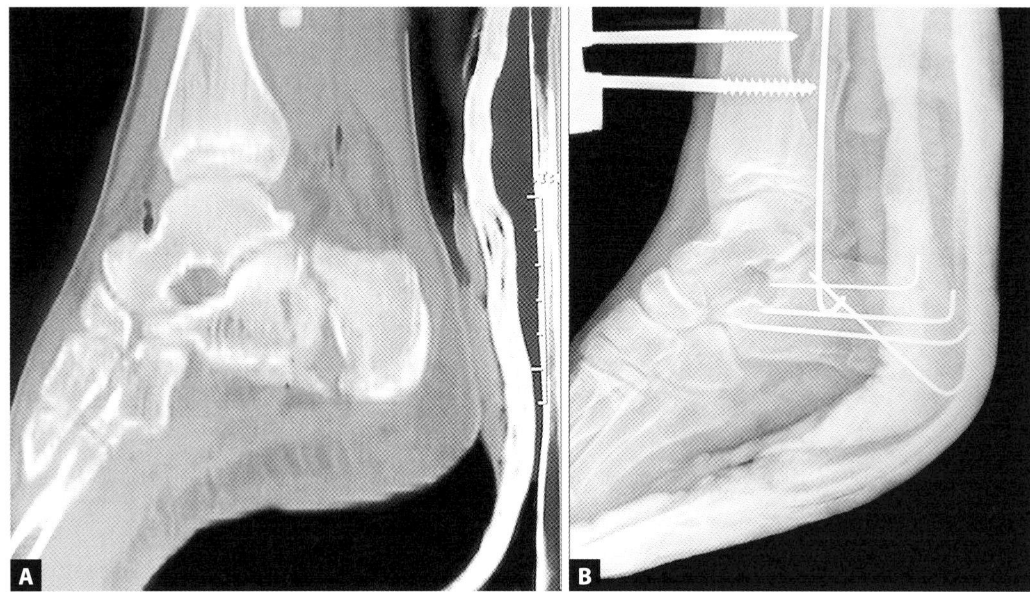

Figs. 6A and B: Open fracture treated with multiple K-wires. (A) Extra-articular open fracture with grade II open injury; (B) After debridement and stabilization with multiple K-wires and plaster of Paris (POP) splint.

the patients had a medial wound, which was taken up for debridement, irrigation, and percutaneous fixation within 8 hours of presentation. Definitive fixation was carried out on an average of 18 days after the initial presentation through an extensile lateral approach with plating.

A superficial infection developed in one patient and a deep infection in one patient and all the fractures went on to union. Mehta et al. concluded that a staged treatment strategy consisting of urgent debridement, provisional internal stabilization, and late definitive reconstruction offers a protocol that may reduce infections associated with open calcaneal fractures.

Some problems are unique to underdeveloped countries; patients with open injuries are often not seen early enough as facilities at peripheral centers are limited and referral is often late. Polytrauma and comorbidity may take precedence in management and calcaneal injuries are often given low priority. This may preclude the option of stable internal fixation as this is ideally done in the case that has been debrided early, stabilized in the best possible position, and then taken up for deferred internal fixation, which in our scenario is often a problem keeping in mind overworked trauma centers and limited operation theater times.

Recommendations for Treatment

Taking into account the various complications found in an open calcaneal fracture, the following treatment guidelines can be recommended for these complex injuries:

- Emergent irrigation and debridement, along with intravenous antibiotics and tetanus prophylaxis, are mandatory. Even in cases with delay, debridement is essential at whatever stage the patient presents.
- Provisional fracture stabilization may be undertaken with minimal risk of complications using minimally invasive techniques, such as inserting percutaneous K-wires or utilizing distractors and external fixators **(Figs. 6 and 7)**. Most centers still use a plaster of Paris (POP) slab, which has a limited role and will compromise subsequent fracture stabilization if wound healing is delayed.
- Grade I wounds, especially when on the medial side, can be taken up for early definitive treatment through a lateral approach. It is better to delay definitive fixation of grade II and grade III open calcaneal fractures with particular reference to wounds involving the lateral side to minimize the risk of disastrous outcomes, such as infection and wound slough.
- Some open fractures are badly crushed; the aim in these should be limb salvage, and this can be achieved by a combination of methods, principal among which is wound closure or coverage, and as much of foot alignment as possible. External fixation devices help in this scenario, as POP splints often hinder wound dressings and if loose, hang from the leg rather than support it. Delayed reconstruction often means the management of complications such as malunion, infection, and subtalar arthritis.
- There is a role for vacuum-assisted closure (VAC) as a primary support to enhance wound healing **(Figs. 8A to G)**.

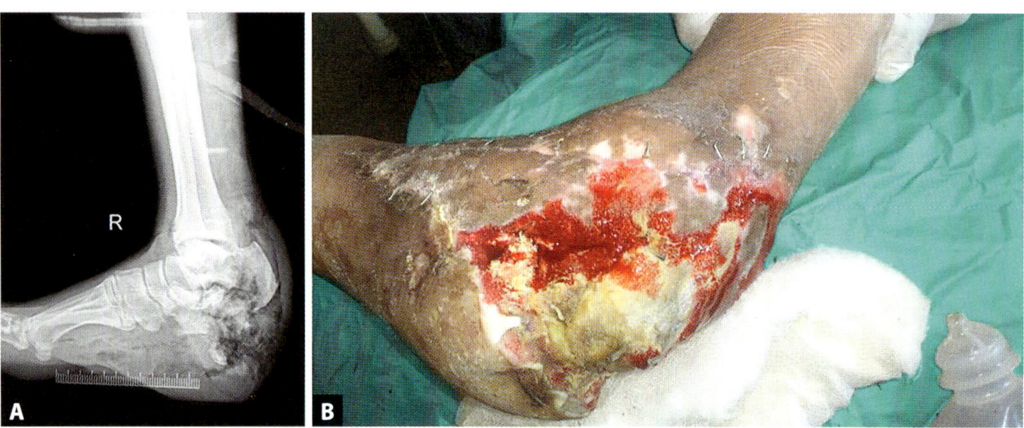

Figs. 9A and B: Severe crushing of calcaneus and heel pad with a large wound. Same case after repeated debridement and failed cross-leg flap. This case may be best helped by amputation and prosthesis fitting due to insensate heel and chronic infection.

The role of primary amputation is limited to the nonsalvageable limb, or with severe soft-tissue loss despite reconstruction attempts **(Figs. 9A and B)**.

■ REFERENCES

1. Sanders WR, Clare MP. Fractures of the calcaneus. In: Bucholz RW, Heckman JD, Court-Brown CM (Eds). Rockwood and Green's Fractures in Adults, 6th edition. Philadelphia: Lippincott Williams & Wilkins; 2006. pp. 2293-36.
2. Mitchell MJ, McKinley JC, Robinson CM. The epidemiology of calcaneal fractures. Foot (Edinb). 2009;19:197-200.
3. Randle JA, Kreder HJ, Stephen D, Williams J, Jaglal S, Hu R. Should calcaneal fractures be treated surgically? A meta-analysis. Clin Orthop Relat Res. 2000;(377):217-27.
4. Aldridge 3rd JM, Easley M, Nunley JA. Open calcaneal fractures: results of operative treatment. J Orthop Trauma. 2004;18:7-11.
5. Heier KA, Infante AF, Walling AK, Sanders RW. Open fractures of the calcaneus: soft-tissue injury determines outcome. J Bone Joint Surg Am. 2003;85-A:2276-82.
6. Gustilo RB, Anderson JT. Prevention of infection in the treatment of one thousand and twenty-five open fractures of long bones: retrospective and prospective analyses. J Bone Joint Surg Am. 1976;58:453-8.
7. Essex-Lopresti P. The mechanism, reduction technique, and results in fractures of the os calcis. Br J Surg. 1952;39: 395-419.
8. Siebert CH, Hansen M, Wolter D. Follow-up evaluation of open intra-articular fractures of the calcaneus. Arch Orthop Trauma Surg. 1998;117:442-7.
9. Lawrence SJ, Grau GF. Evaluation and treatment of open calcaneal fractures: a retrospective analysis. Orthopedics. 2003;26:621-6.
10. Berry GK, Stevens DG, Kreder HJ, McKee M, Schemitsch E, Stephen DJ. Open fractures of the calcaneus: a review of treatment and outcome. J Orthop Trauma. 2004;18:202-6.
11. Mehta S, Mirza AJ, Dunbar RP, Barei DP, Benirschke SK. A staged treatment plan for the management of type II and type IIIA open calcaneus fractures. J Orthop Trauma. 2010;24:142-7.

possible displacement of the joint. This classification presents moderate inter-rater reliability. It divides the body of the calcaneus into four columns, using the lines that are correlated with the most frequent fracture lines. This classification does not consider the other CT sections and CT reconstructions and may therefore fail to pick up other possible fracture lines nor does it take into account the degree of displacement of the fracture, the complexity of the fracture line, any osteochondral injuries, tendon entrapment, or the state of the soft tissues affected by the energy of the trauma. For this reason, we may encounter fractures that could be classified as grade II, which are nonetheless high-energy injuries with major displacement and affection of the cartilage and soft tissues.

Ball et al.[13] recently demonstrated that the viability of the joint cartilage declines after fractures of the calcaneus, which may cause post-traumatic degeneration of the latter in the mid- to long-term. According to Allmacher et al.,[14] the long-term result of treatment of fractures of the calcaneus is mainly conditioned by the degree of osteoarthritis of the subtalar joint since early elimination of this joint leads to major disorders of gait and of the neighboring joints. However, most patients aged over 15 years who undergo subtalar arthrodesis have not been found to have significant or symptomatic disorders. For this reason, the sacrifice of the subtalar joint is a reasonable price to pay in the long term to prevent problems in this joint which, though it could be reconstructed satisfactorily using an aggressive approach, often degenerates because of post-traumatic chondrolysis or undergoes spontaneous ankylosis.

In the view of Csizy et al.,[3] the prognostic factors which favor late subtalar arthrodesis in displaced fractures of the calcaneus are, in order of importance, a negative Böhler's angle, a patient who suffered the injury in the workplace, grade IV fracture, and conservative treatment.

Certain authors have also extended indications to Sanders type 3 and few Sanders type 2 injuries. Bloomer et al.[15] had 10 Sanders type 2, 36 Sanders type 3, and 32 Sanders type 4 in their series. Other aspects to consider are presence of severe comminution, loss of Böhler's angle, and presence of workmen's compensation.

Calcaneal fractures can occur in any accident but are much more common in the work environment or in road accidents. In this particular situation, the influence on the outcome of compensation claims may be significant, and the results of any treatment could be biased.

Thornes et al.[16] compared conservative and surgical treatment in 54 patients (33 surgical, 21 conservative), with a median follow-up of 40 months (range 14–78 months). With similar groups of fractures, similar comorbidities and energy of trauma were seen to be insignificant in the outcome in litigants ($p < 0.0001$). The problems related to the wearing of shoes were higher in the litigants. Low time was more than double that in nonlitigants (14.5 vs. 6 months, $p < 0.01$). The results were similar between the surgical and conservatively treated groups by comparing the functional scales, problems of footwear, and low time. The disputes are the major determinants of the evolution of disabling symptoms after the repair of fractures.

In the classic work of Buckley et al.,[9] 512 patients with intra-articular calcaneus fractures treated at different centers were evaluated. The 36-item short form survey (SF-36) between cases treated conservatively and those operated was 64.7 and 68.7, respectively ($p = 0, 13$) and visual analogical scale readings were 64.3 and 68.6 ($p = 0, 12$). However, patients who did not receive financial compensation and were operated upomhad greater satisfaction ($p = 0, 001$) with their outcomes. It seemed that functional results of conservative treatment were similar to those of surgical treatment. However, after further evaluation of data, after eliminating the patients who received financial compensation, the results were seen to be much better in patients receiving surgical treatment.

McCormack et al.[17] presented their results in evaluating the failure of the treatment in fractures of calcaneus and development of secondary subtalar arthritis. Out of 424 patients with displaced intra-articular calcaneus fracture, 44 required subtalar fusion between 1 and 4 years after the accident. Thirty-seven of these 44 patients (84%) initially had been treated conservatively. In the opinion of these authors, the main prognostic factor in determining the evolution of a displaced intra-articular fracture of calcaneus was the amount of energy dissipated in the bone at the time of injury. Males, heavy-duty workers, those with issues of financial compensation, smokers, and those fractures having a Böhler's angle of 0° or lesser were high-risk candidates who would probably end up with subtalar arthrodesis.

Keeping these arguments in mind, a trend is evolving in the management of a specific subset of calcaneal fractures, where aggressive primary intervention may reduce long-term disability and multiple surgeries. The authors' proposed indications for primary subtalar fusion along with calcaneal reconstruction in displaced intra-articular calcaneus fractures are listed in **Box 1**.

■ SURGICAL TECHNIQUE

The primary fusion can be done by the classical exposure, through a conventional extensile lateral approach, or by percutaneously fixing the calcaneus and adding bone graft by a minimal approach.

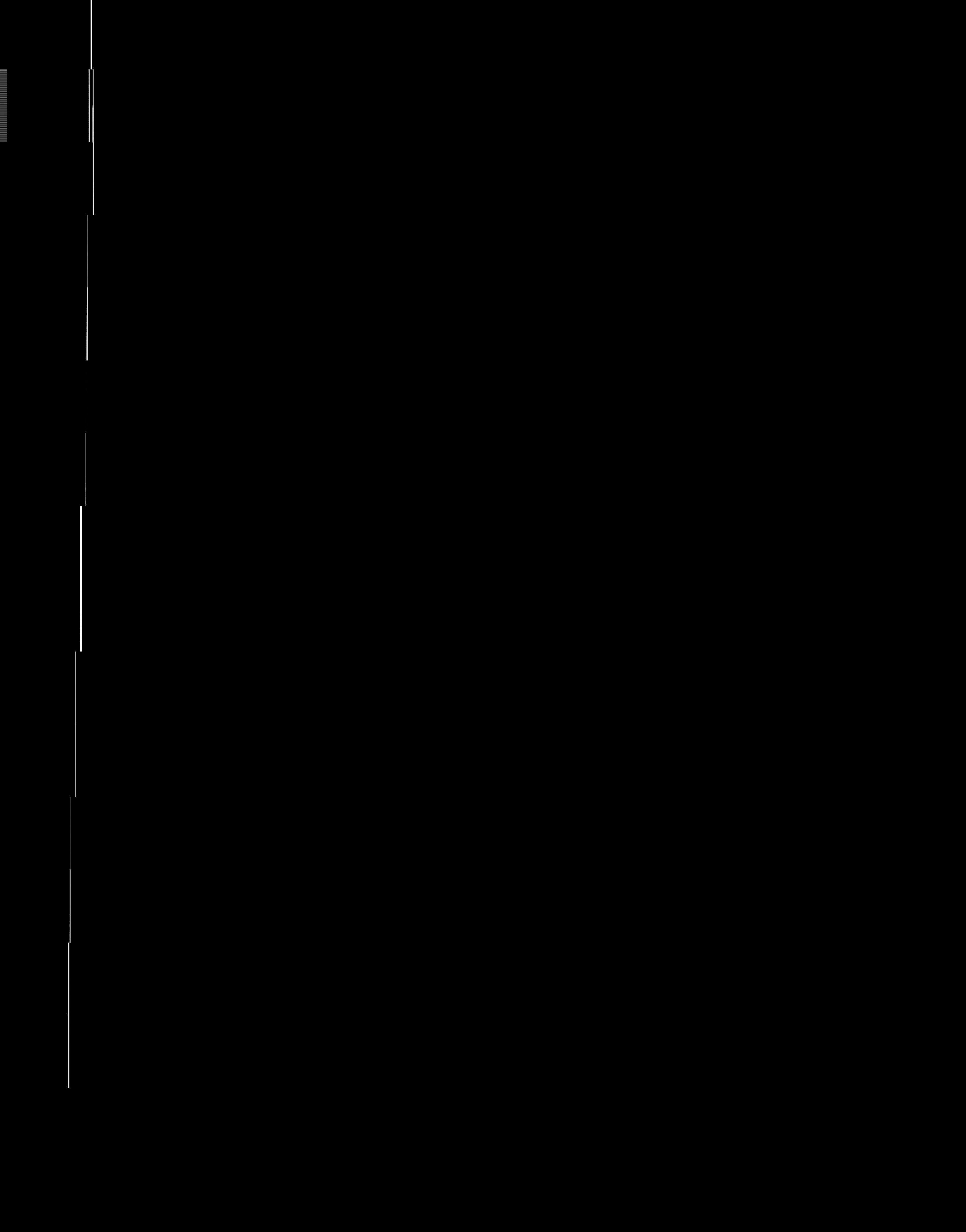

are made in reducing the other fragments. In fractures with significant elevation of the tuberosity and fracture of the inferior cortical wall, this maneuver can be time-consuming and unrewarding. After the reduction and its temporary maintenance with wires, we place back the removed lateral cortical bone and fix it with screws or a specific calcaneal plate. It is advisable to add stability to this osteosynthesis with 6.5 mm cancellous screws introduced from the heel through the subtalar joint and anchored into the body of the talus. We recommend two crossed, nonparallel screws to avoid the collapse of the calcaneal tuberosity **(Fig. 1D)**.

The authors also recommend the use of cannulated screws instead of the standard AO screws as positioning the guide wires and checking with image intensifiers allow correct screw position in the bone. This improves the reconstruction and ensures avoiding varus deformity and shortening of the os calcis.

Malik et al.[19] used minimally invasive surgery (MIS) approach with percutaneous subtalar joint screw fixation as a salvage in severe comminuted cases. In the MIS approach, a sinus tarsi approach can be used through which joint preparation, graft placement, and correction of alignment can be performed to achieve desired radiological parameters.

Postoperatively, the patient is placed in a below-knee posterior splint. Immobilization is continued for 6–12 weeks, depending on the stability of the internal fixation. Progressive weight-bearing is allowed after 8 weeks only in order to avoid calcaneal collapse which may accompany earlier weight-bearing ambulation.

■ VIRA® SYSTEM

The primary fusion as an option for the surgical treatment of fractures of the calcaneus has recently received a major boost with the development of the Vira® system.[20,21]

Technique and Treatment Protocol

The Vira® system (Biomet, Valencia, Spain) is a minimally invasive method for the reconstruction of severe calcaneal fractures with primary subtalar fusion. It comprises a small nail with two screws for fixation to the talus. The nail fixes the tuberosity of the calcaneus and is perforated by two cannulated screws (Tuberotalar), which enter through the heel and fixate the calcaneus to the talar body. The purpose of the locking nail is to simultaneously stabilize and reduce the calcaneal fracture and, at the same time, fix the subtalar joint.

The stainless steel nail is of a single diameter and length (10 × 38 mm) and has lateral wings to prevent the rotation. The holes have an angle of 20° to the axis of the nail for the two Tuberotalar screws. The screws have a core of 2.1 mm

and a double thread. They are available in seven sizes from 55 to 85 mm in length **(Fig. 2)**.

The Vira® guide is a complex and useful device to capture the calcaneal tuberosity, restore the axial alignment of the tuberosity, and regain the length and the height of the calcaneus. It makes it possible to perform a safe and accurate implantation and to achieve stability at both the displaced fracture and the subtalar joint via the nail and screw placement. The instrumentation comprises pincers with nails to capture the greater tuberosity of the calcaneus. The guide is made of titanium, with exception of the carbon fiber pincers to allow visibility on X-ray. This has a regulated support arch for the insertion of a reference wire in the head of the talus that carries out distraction. The insertion guide has a guidance system for the external wires and the Tuberotalar screws and a handle to hold and direct it **(Fig. 3)**.

The instruments are an important component of the system and they act as a guide that restores the morphology

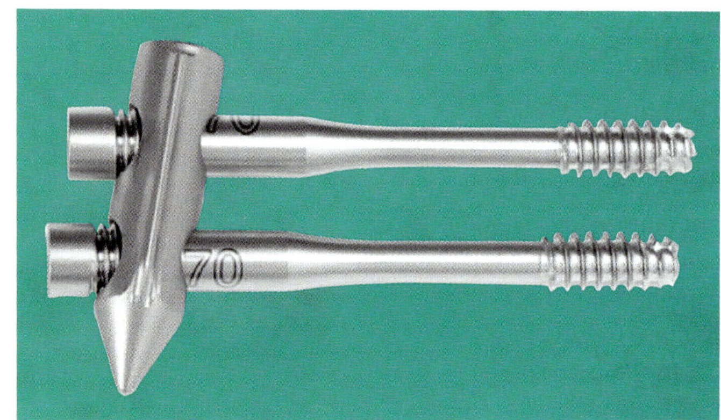

Fig. 2: Vira® system implant. Note the nail for the calcaneal tuberosity and the two Tuberotalar screws locking the nail and the talus body.

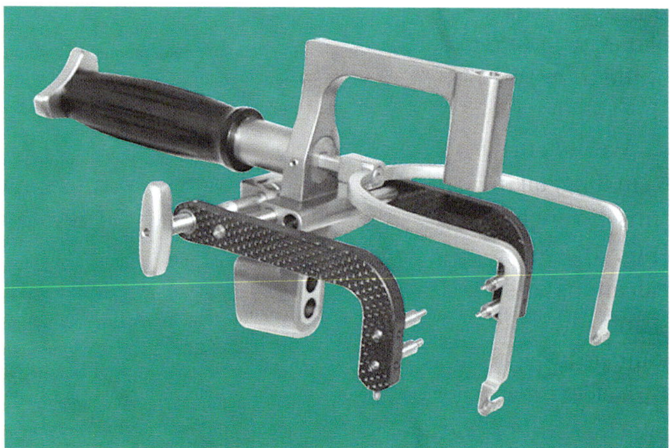

Fig. 3: Vira® system guide which allows the reconstruction of the calcaneus alignment and the insertion of the implant through a minimally invasive surgery.

The housing of the nail in the calcaneal tuberosity is burred using a 10 mm drill, taking care to protect the Achilles tendon **(Fig. 7B)**. When the drill is withdrawn, we must keep it running to extract the bone from the perforation in order to use this later as a graft for the subtalar arthrodesis. The drill should not be reversed. Once the site of the pin has been drilled and before the implant is positioned, the bone extracted during the perforation is placed in the subtalar joint. If there is severe sinking of the talus, the gap should be filled with autograft, allograft, or bone substitute as the surgeon considers fit.

With support from the guide, the nail is hammered into the channel that had previously been marked. The guide directs the nail to the inferior part of the tuberosity, where the plantar fascia is inserted. The nail must go in completely, up to the limit marked by the applicator. This ensures correct alignment of the orifices of the screws and the guide **(Fig. 7C)**. With the nail in place, it is possible to apply distraction, extension, and varus/valgus by moving the jig to the correct position **(Figs. 7D and E)**.

With the cannulas in position on the guide, we make a small (1 cm) incision with the scalpel, going as far as the bone. The guide wire is passed and the length of the screws is measured using the depth gauge. After the wire, we pass the cannulated 4.5 mm drill and then insert the screws **(Fig. 7F)**.

After inserting the implant, we suture the wounds in the standard way and apply a compressive bandage. It is not necessary to immobilize the ankle and foot as the system allows immediate partial support, depending on the surgeon's criteria and the patient's tolerance.

■ RESULTS OF PRIMARY FUSION

There are few published studies on primary fusion in calcaneal fractures, but those that exist are unanimous about the efficacy of this treatment and its good results. In an expected value decision analysis method of study by Eisenstein et al.,[23] they favored open reduction and internal fixation (ORIF) with primary subtalar arthrodesis (PSTA) over ORIF in terms of patient-reported outcomes, secondary fusion, and complications for the treatment of complex displaced intra-articular calcaneus fracture (DIACF).

Buch et al.[24] in a study of 14 patients reached 72.4 points in the outcome scales after 26 months of follow-up. Huefner et al.[25] averaged 88 points in patients evaluated at mean 4.9 years, and recently, Potenza et al.[6] published a series of six patients with a final outcome score of 85 points at 53 months.

In the retrospective series of 79 patients by Bloomer et al.,[15] 86% achieved fusion at a mean of 126.5 days and only 11 patients failed to achieve radiographic union. Nine of their 14 workers' compensation patients also returned to work within the period of observation. They concluded that PSTA has higher fusion rates and high rates of return to work.

The radiographic predictors for successful outcome after primary arthrodesis for comminuted fractures of calcaneus were evaluated by Holm et al.[26] They looked at talocalcaneal, calcaneal inclination, talo-first metatarsal, and Böhler's angles, and the height of the tibial plafond, width of the calcaneus, and the presence of a medial step-off on the injured and uninjured foot. They noticed statistically significant associations between greater postoperative function and increasing age, the quality of restoration of Böhler's angle, and the talocalcaneal angle.

Buckley et al.[27] in their randomized multicenter trial were unable to demonstrate a significant difference between treating Sanders type 4 fractures with either ORIF or ORIF + PSTA. They suggested careful evaluation of each case on a case-to-case basis and discussion with patient. In certain patients, ORIF + PSTA may be advantageous for both patients with Sanders type 4 fractures and the health care system as the fractures heal quicker. Furthermore, ORIF + PSTA may prevent the need for late secondary subtalar fusion, adding to increased costs and lost time from work.

The personal experience of the senior authors with this procedure using the minimally invasive Vira® system consists of more than 200 patients. This population has been evaluated prospectively and we can offer results of 169 cases with >1-year follow-up. This surgery was performed in severe calcaneus fractures (Sanders grade IV) or associated with bad prognostic comorbidities. All cases were treated in a work compensation health system. The evaluation was carried out by clinical, radiological, and biomechanical analyses.

The American Orthopaedic Foot and Ankle Society (AOFAS) score averaged 77.26 points at the end of follow-up. Forty-two cases (24.9%) obtained excellent results, 108 (63.9%) good, 12 (7.1%) mild, and 7 (4.1%) poor. The improvement in Böhler's angle after surgery was significant ($p = 0.05$), and this did not vary along the follow-up. Subtalar arthrodesis was achieved in all cases and only three cases needed additional bone grafting. Five major postsurgical complications were observed, and one deep infection in a case of open grade III fracture was encountered. The pedobarographic studies showed few but significant differences compared to the normal foot, mainly due to subtalar fusion. The restoration of plantar pressure achieved was considered satisfactory in most cases. A typical case is shown in **Figures 8A to D**.

From our experience, we can conclude that despite workplace injuries being a challenging population for any

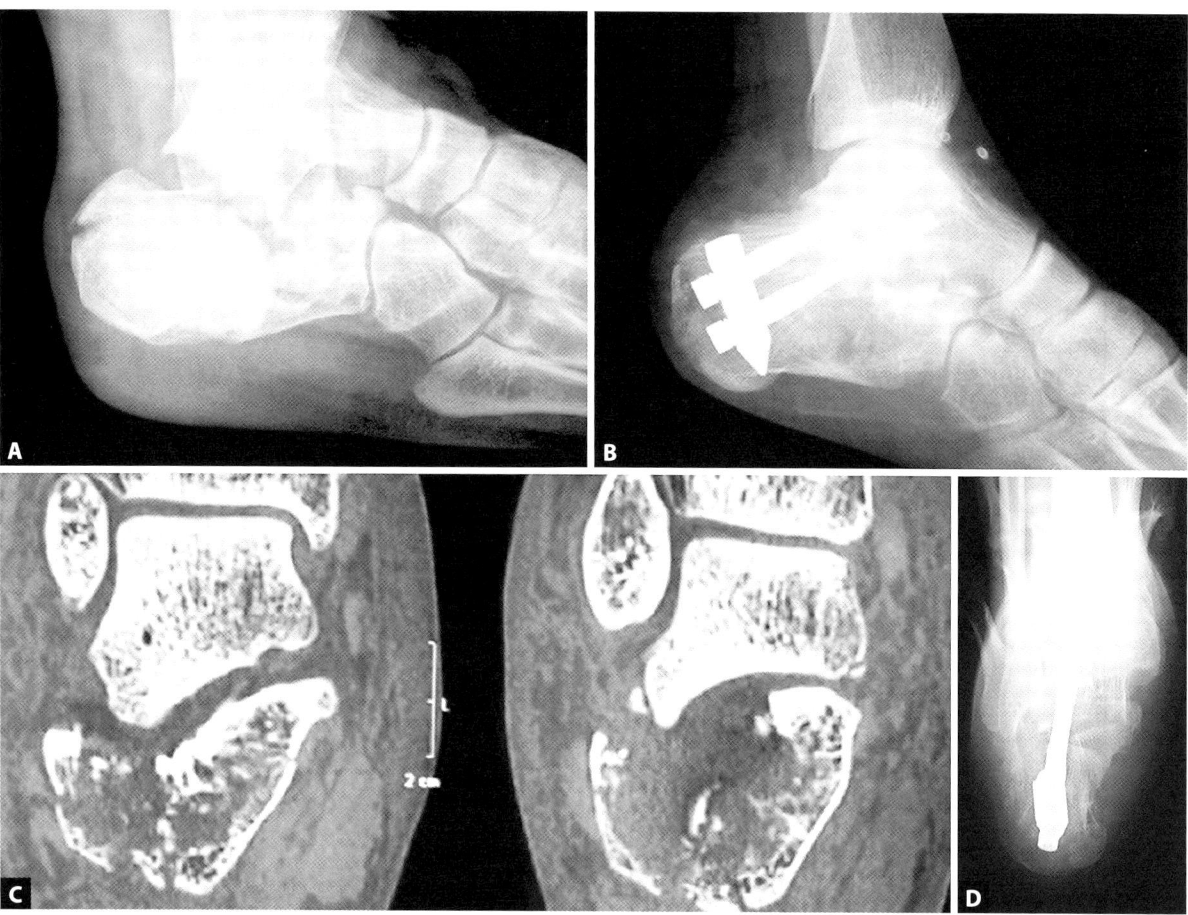

Figs. 8A to D: Case of a typical indication for treatment with Vira® system. Comminuted intra-articular fracture of the calcaneus grade IV of Sanders classification treated by minimally invasive reconstruction and primary subtalar fusion. (A) X-ray lateral view, (B) computed tomography (CT) scan showing the bone comminution of subtalar joint. (C) Postoperative X-ray lateral observe the good reconstruction of the shape of the calcaneus and Böhler's angle. The subtalar joint is refilled with bone yielded by the housing for the nail. (D) Axial X-ray postoperative view.

surgical technique, primary subtalar fusion with a minimally invasive method allows rapid recovery; this procedure should be judiciously used for a specified subset of patients where the potential for complications is significant.

The Vira® system is a new concept in calcaneal surgery which provides a definitive solution for these patients; it offers surgery with minimal invasion and has low complication rates combined with high clinical effectiveness.

Biomechanical Consequences of Subtalar Fusion After Calcaneus Fracture

Primary arthrodesis in the treatment of intra-articular fractures of the calcaneus involves the sacrifice of the subtalar joint, which has an important function in the foot. Nevertheless, the authors argue that this sacrifice may be advantageous for the patient under certain circumstances, especially if this intervention is performed using minimally invasive and safe procedures.

In 32 cases of primary subtalar fusion in patients treated with Vira® system, we performed a gait analysis 6 months after surgery (unpublished data). The biomechanical parameters of control group (contralateral healthy limb) and arthrodesis group (arthrodesis limb) were compared. The plantar pressure distribution was studied with the use of a pedobarographic platform (Emed, Novel, Germany). We collected data in barefoot static and dynamic position bilaterally. Patients were asked to walk back and forth at a self-selected velocity along the walkway to become familiar with the surroundings. In each condition, three trials were recorded and averaged for analysis. We evaluated the entire foot and divided it into six anatomical regions: Hindfoot, midfoot, forefoot (medial, middle, and lateral), and the hallux. The pressure (kPa) in each region of both feet was measured.

The kinetic parameters or ground reaction forces (GRF) were recorded using two, 90 × 60 cm, force platforms (Kistler,

of pressure in the sole of the feet involved is lower than the healthy foot, although this difference was not significant. The Vira® system reconstitutes the Achilles-calcaneal-planting, the adipose pad, and plantar fascia. However, we have observed in a kinetic study of ankle fusion that the support forces decrease[31] and are less on the healthy side. Thrust forces increase with the monopodal planting of the heel and foot and decrease during the impulse to take the foot off the ground. Differences in the anterolateral forces are significantly greater in the operated foot, and the time of the change of the forces is also of interest. These modifications are the consequence of a traumatic foot with a subtalar fusion which has difficulty in the rolling motion of the foot. Dubois et al.[32] noted that operated and healthy feet were different, and amplitude of joint ROM was lower for the arthrodesed foot side (16.5° vs. 21.5°); peak power generated for plantar flexion was lower at the end of the stance phase. Biomechanical studies comparing the operated foot and the healthy foot have not shown significant differences because the healthy foot to a large extent behaves similar to the operated foot. Dubois et al.[32] concluded that the gait pattern, after subtalar fusion, is globally symmetrical and has little functional impact on the knee and the hip.

■ REFERENCES

1. Essex-Lopresti P. The mechanism, reduction technique, and results in fractures of the os calcis. Br J Surg. 1952;39:395-419.
2. Lim EV, Leung JP. Complications of intraarticular calcaneal fractures. Clin Orthop Relat Res. 2001;391:7-16.
3. Csizy M, Buckley R, Tough S, Leighton R, Smith J, McCormack R, et al. Displaced intra-articular calcaneal fractures: variables predicting late subtalar fusion. J Orthop Trauma. 2003;17:106-12.
4. Dick IL. Primary fusion of the posterior subtalar joint in the treatment of fractures of the calcaneum. J Bone Joint Surg Br. 1953;35-B:375-80.
5. Hall MC, Pennal GF. Primary subtalar arthrodesis in the treatment of severe fractures of the calcaneum. J Bone Joint Surg Br. 1960;42-B:336-43.
6. Potenza V, Caterini R, Farsetti P, Bisicchia S, Ippolito E. Primary subtalar arthrodesis for the treatment of comminuted intra-articular calcaneal fractures. Injury. 2010;41:702-6.
7. Stulz E, Folscheveiller J, Naett R, et al. Traitement des fractures thalamiques du calcaneum para la reconstruction arthrodese. Lyon Chir. 1962;58:635-40.
8. Myerson MS. Primary subtalar arthrodesis for the treatment of comminuted fractures of the calcaneus. Orthop Clin North Am. 1995;26:215-27.
9. Buckley R, Tough S, McCormack R, Pate G, Leighton R, Petrie D, et al. Operative compared with nonoperative treatment of displaced intra-articular calcaneal fractures: a prospective, randomized, controlled multicenter trial. J Bone Joint Surg Am. 2002;84-A:1733-44.
10. Sanders R. Intraarticular fractures of the calcaneus: present state of the art. J Orthop Trauma. 1992;6:252-65.
11. Aktuglu K, Aydogan U. The functional outcome of displaced intra-articular calcaneal fractures: a comparison between isolated cases and polytrauma patients. Foot Ankle Int. 2002;23:314-8.
12. Lauder AJ, Inda DJ, Bott AM, Clare MP, Fitzgibbons TC, Mormino MA. Interobserver and intraobserver reliability of two classification systems for intra-articular calcaneal fractures. Foot Ankle Int. 2006;27:251-5.
13. Ball ST, Jadin K, Allen RT, Schwartz AK, Sah RL, Brage ME. Chondrocyte viability after intra-articular calcaneal fractures in humans. Foot Ankle Int. 2007;28:665-8.
14. Allmacher DH, Galles KS, Marsh JL. Intra-articular calcaneal fractures treated nonoperatively and followed sequentially for 2 decades. J Orthop Trauma. 2006;20:464-9.
15. Bloomer AK, McKnight RR, Johnson NR, Macknet DM, Wally MK, Yu Z, et al. Screws-only primary subtalar arthrodesis for calcaneus fractures. Foot Ankle Int. 2022;43(4):509-19.
16. Thornes BS, Collins AL, Timlin M, Corrigan J. Outcome of calcaneal fractures treated operatively and non-operatively. The effect of litigation on outcomes. Ir J Med Sci. 2002;171:155-7.
17. McCormack RG, Buckley RE, Leighton RK, Petrie DP, Galpin RD, Csizy M, et al. Displaced intra-articular calcaneal fractures: who fails treatment and needs subtalar fusion. Program and abstracts of the 16th annual meeting of Orthopaedic Trauma Association, San Antonio, Texas; 2000. pp. 12-4.
18. Benirschke SK, Sangeorzan BJ. Extensive intra-articular fractures of the foot. Clin Orthop. 1993;292:85-91.
19. Malik C, Najefi AA, Patel A, Vris A, Malagelada F, Parker L, et al. Percutaneous subtalar joint screw fixation of comminuted calcaneal fractures: a salvage procedure. Eur J Trauma Emerg Surg. 2022;48(5):4043-51.
20. López-Oliva F, Forriol F, Sánchez-Lorente T, Sanz YA. Treatment of severe fractures of the calcaneus by reconstruction arthrodesis using the Vira® system: prospective study of the first 37 cases with over 1 year follow-up. Injury. 2010;41(8):804-9.
21. López-Oliva F, Forriol F, Sánchez-Lorente T, Sanz YA. Vira® system—a minimally invasive technique for severe fractures of the calcaneus treatment with primary subtalar fusion: a preliminary report. Foot Ankle Surg. 2011;17(2):68-73.
22. Omoto H, Nakamura K. Method for manual reduction of displaced intra-articular fracture of the calcaneus: technique, indications and limitations. Foot Ankle Int. 2001;22:874-9.
23. Eisenstein ED, Kusnezov NA, Waterman BR, Orr JD, Blair JA. Open reduction and internal fixation (ORIF) versus ORIF and primary subtalar arthrodesis for complex displaced intraarticular calcaneus fractures: an expected value decision analysis. OTA Int. 2020;1(2):e005.
24. Buch BD, Myerson MS, Miller SD. Primary subtalar arthrodesis for the treatment of comminuted calcaneal fractures. Foot Ankle Int. 1996;172:61-70.
25. Huefner T, Thermann H, Geerling J, Pape HC, Pohlemann T. Primary subtalar arthrodesis of calcaneal fractures. Foot Ankle Int. 2001;22:9-14.

18

Interlocking Nailing for Calcaneal Fractures

Stefan Rammelt, Prasoon Kumar

"Creativity is seeing what others see and thinking what no one else ever thought".

–Albert Einstein

INTRODUCTION

Open reduction and internal fixation for displaced intra-articular calcaneus fractures has been a widely accepted surgery to achieve anatomical reduction with joint congruity and to put the calcaneal shape back into form, which is essential for favorable outcomes.[1-3] This regularly involves an extensile lateral exposure that carries the risk of postoperative wound complications such as wound gaping, skin necrosis, infection, and late scarring with resulting functional restrictions.[2-4] Minimally and less invasive techniques for reduction and fixation of displaced calcaneal fractures have been employed to minimize these complications, the most popular being the use of a sinus tarsi approach and its modifications and percutaneous methods.[5-9] When employing these methods, achieving an anatomic reduction of the calcaneal geometry and joint surfaces is essential for obtaining a favorable result.[10] Percutaneous fixation can be enhanced by the use of subtalar arthroscopy to ensure anatomic reduction of the posterior facet.[6,7] The sinus tarsi approach allows an adequate overview of the posterior facet of the subtalar joint with similar reduction rates to the extensile lateral approach.[8,9] Fixation methods with minimally invasive methods include percutaneous pinning and screw fixation as well as less invasive plate fixation and, more recently, intramedullary nailing.[5-11]

Interlocking nailing for treatment of a displaced intra-articular calcaneus fracture has been developed to provide accurate reduction and stable internal fixation with a limited exposure.[10,11] The idea was proposed way back in 1888 by Gussenbauer from Prague.[12] Nailing for calcaneal fractures and primary subtalar fusion have been used until the mid-20th century **(Figs. 1A and B)**. Recently, interlocking nails, such as CALCAnail® (FH Orthopedics SAS, Heimsbrunn, France) and C-NAIL (MEDIN, Nové Město na Moravě,

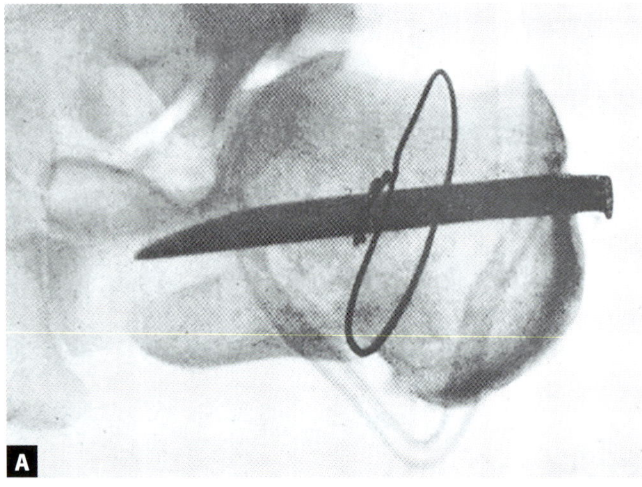
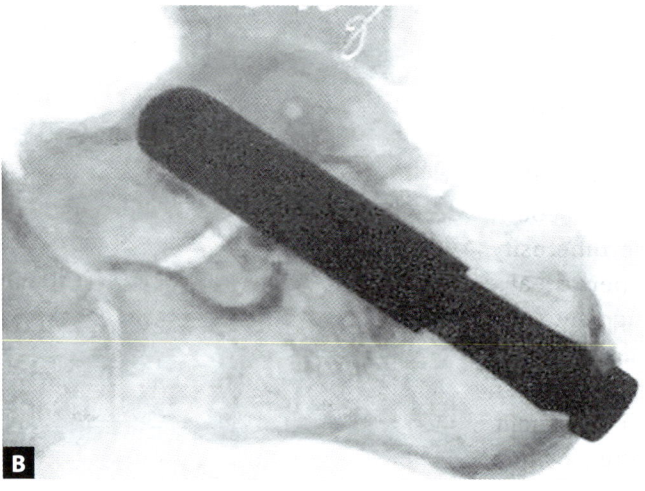

Figs. 1A and B: (A) Use of intramedullary nailing for the treatment of a calcaneal fracture in the classic textbook of Robert Danis (Danis R. Théorie et Pratique de l'Ostéosynthése. Paris: Masson; 1949); (B) Lorenz Böhler used a cylindric nail for minimally invasive subtalar fusion following calcaneal fractures (Böhler L. Die Technik der Knochenbruchbehandlung. 12./13. Auflage. Wien, München, Bern: Maudrich; 1953).

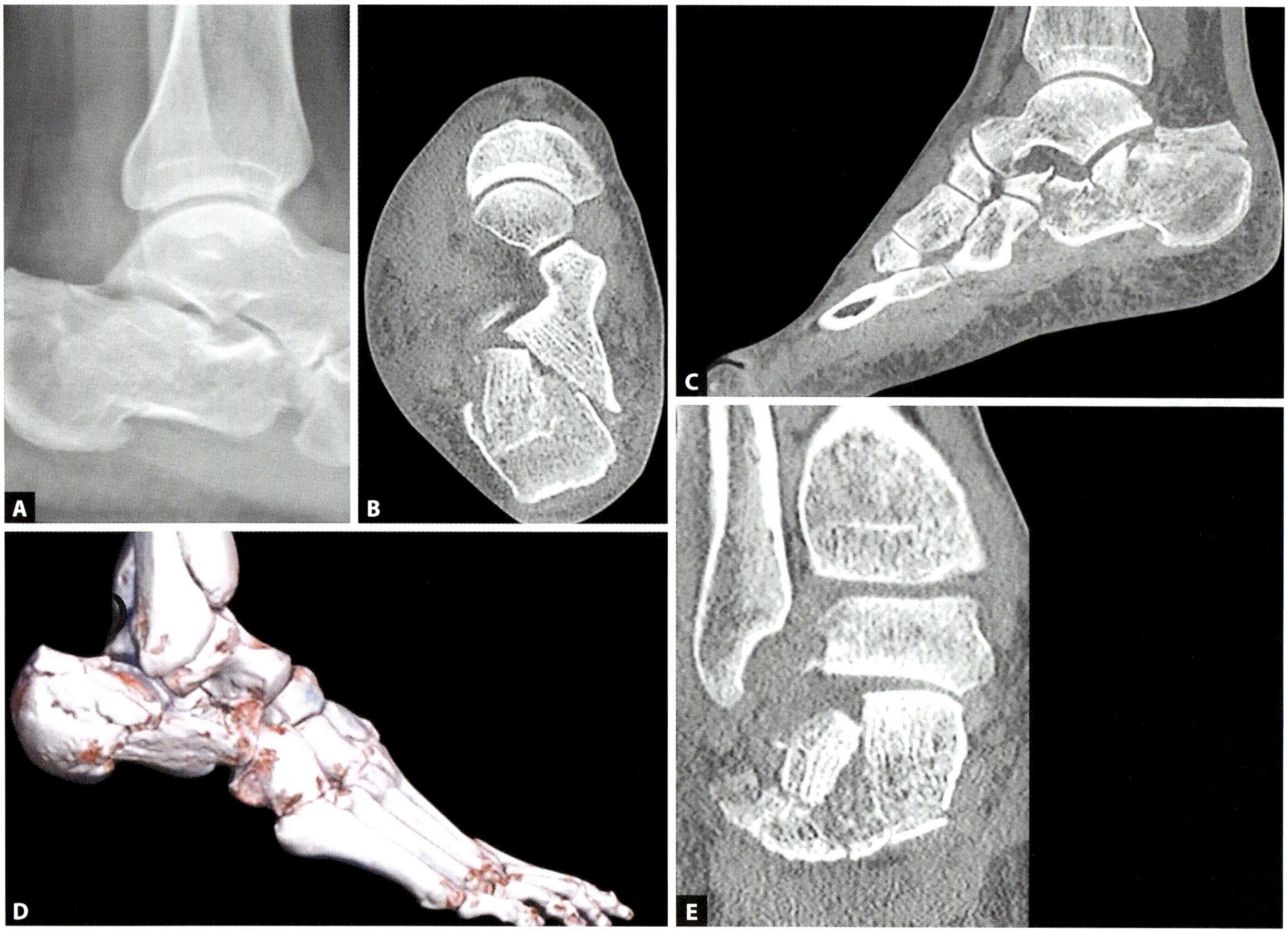

Figs. 4A to E: Preoperative imaging [plain radiographs, two-dimensional (2D) and three-dimensional (3D) computed tomography (CT) scanning] of a right calcaneal fracture Sanders type II in a 62-year-old male with mild osteopenia and no severe comorbidities.

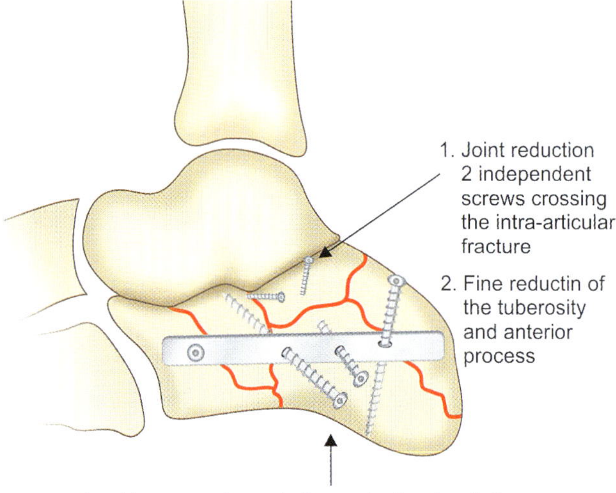

Fig. 5: Preoperative planning sketch by the surgeon.

After making the skin incision for insertion of the nail, a guidewire is advanced toward the center of the calcaneocuboid joint. The correct position of the guidewire along the calcaneal axis is verified fluoroscopically using a lateral and dorsoplantar ["anteroposterior (AP)"] view **(Fig. 7)**. After reaming over the K-wire with the 8 mm drill using a protection sleeve and stopping 5 mm short of the calcaneocuboid joint, the nail with the aiming device is introduced over the guidewire. The proximal 2.0 mm olive K-wire is forwarded into the sustentacular fragment close to the middle facet using the aiming device.

Note: Correct rotation of the nail is determined by the exact position of the sustentacular wire (and later screw). If the first K-wire does not hit the sustentaculum properly, the nail must be rotated accordingly with the aiming device.

A second olive K-wire is introduced through the aiming device. The K-wires are then gradually exchanged with screws. The locking cortical screws are guided by the same holes of that aiming device, which has three arms. The first screw is inserted into the sustentacular fragment, the second into the tuberosity, and the third screw into the anterior process fragment. Proper reduction and implant position are

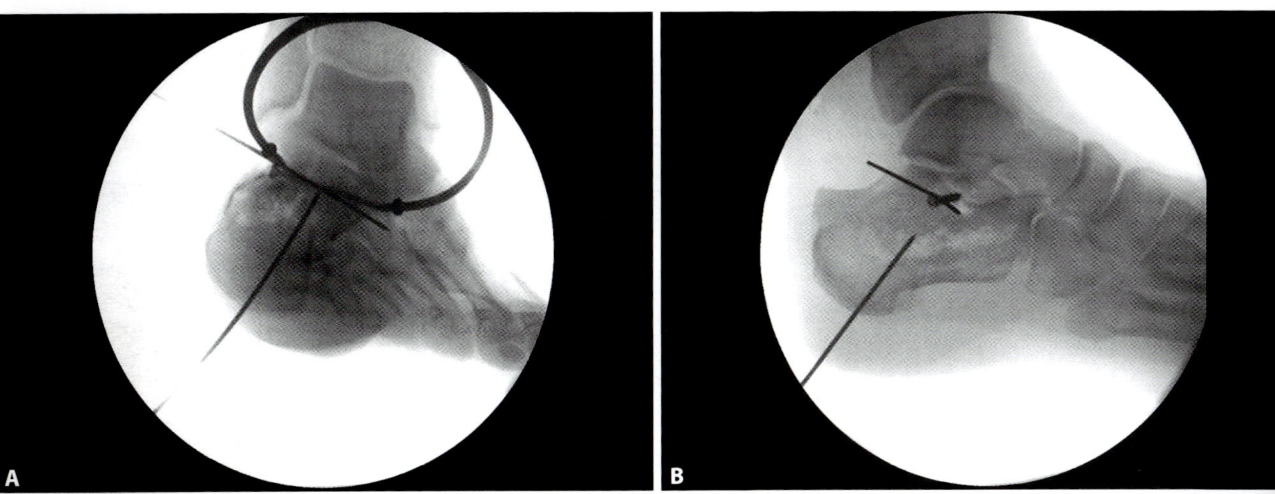

Figs. 6A and B: Intraoperative fluoroscopy after positioning of a large, pointed reduction clamp from the sustentaculum tali to the lateral wall and placement of the first screw confirming anatomic reduction of the posterior facet fragments.

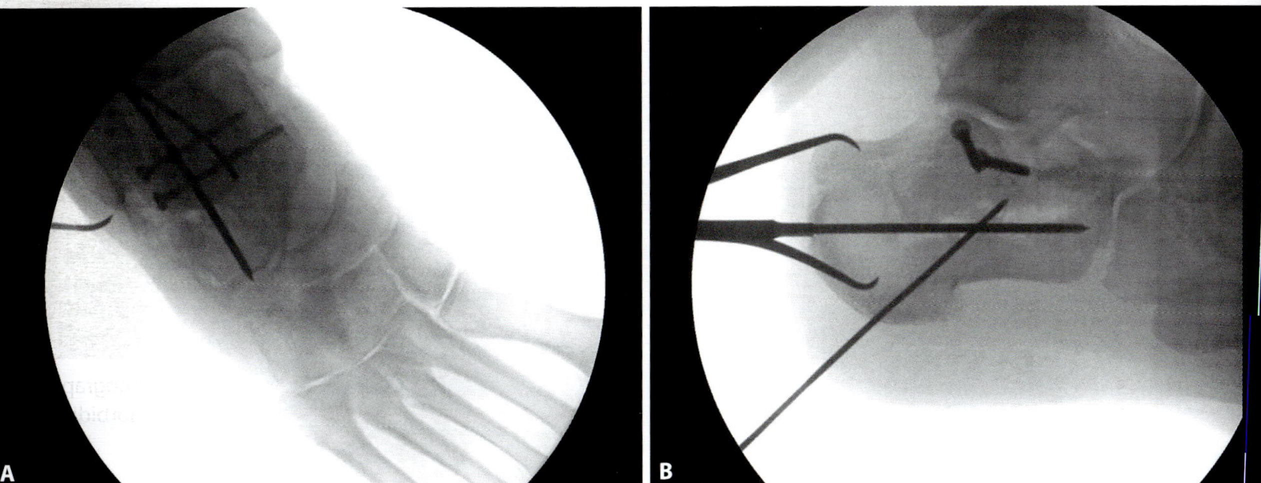

Figs. 7A and B: Fluoroscopy depicting ideal, central placement of the guidewire to create the nail track.

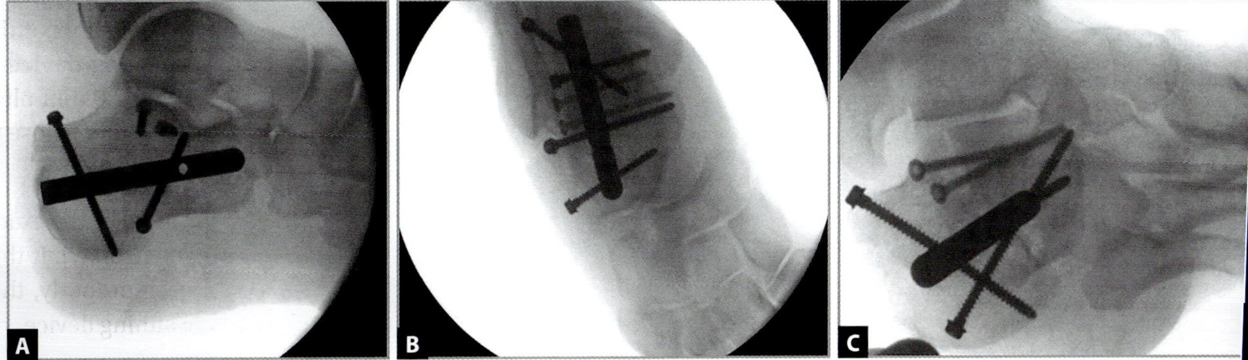

Figs. 8A to C: Fluoroscopy confirming ideal nail position and placement of the locking bolts in all three planes.

evaluated with a fluoroscopic lateral, 20° Broden, axial, and dorsoplantar views **(Fig. 8)**.

Postoperative rehabilitation: A short leg splint is used to immobilize the foot with the ankle in neutral for 3–5 days. Active and passive range of motion exercises begin on first postoperative day. The patient is mobilized with crutches and partial weight bearing of 20 kg in his own shoes for 6–8 weeks with physiotherapy to regain full range of motion and unassisted gait.

■ TECHNIQUE WITH CALCAnail[®11]

Design: It is a titanium nail with a diameter of 10 mm and at lengths of 45, 50, and 55 mm.

Indications and contraindications: These are similar to the C-NAIL.

Procedure: A working channel is created through the calcaneal tuberosity through which intrafocal reduction of displaced fragments is achieved. K-wires are introduced in the posterior tuberosity in the direction of the posterior surface of the talus (lateral view) and in the middle of the tuberosity (axial view). A Casper distractor is used with its two pins in the posterior calcaneal tuberosity and lateral process of talus. The distraction corrects the heel varus and opens up the talocalcaneal joint for articular reduction via the tract created over the first K-wire. Following this, the nail is inserted and fixed with two cannulated locking screws. In case percutaneous methods do not work, a sinus tarsi incision can be used for joint reduction under direct vision.

Postoperative rehabilitation: Similar protocols can be followed as those with the C-NAIL.

A special feature of the CALCAnail is that the same instrumentation can be used for subtalar arthrodesis if the surgeon decides so intraoperatively, depending upon the fracture and articular morphology. The implant available is of 12 mm in diameter, and the pins used for distraction can also hold a compressive device for facilitating contact at the proposed fusion site.

Interlocking nailing for calcaneal fractures utilizes a minimally invasive procedure, thus combining minimal soft-tissue dissection while maintaining a stable internal fixation. Avoiding the extensile lateral approach reduces postoperative wound-related issues, which have been a major concern with open reduction and lateral plate fixation. The peroneal tendons, lateral calcaneal artery, and sural nerve are protected, and scarring is minimized.[10,11,13]

■ BIOMECHANICAL DATA

Biomechanical studies have repeatedly shown the primary stability of these two nail designs to be at par and, in some cases, even superior to the currently used locking plates.[16-18] In a comparative biomechanical study on anatomical specimens, the C-NAIL showed significantly less dynamic failures and an insignificantly higher load to failure than the CALCAnail and a variable angle interlocking plate (Rimbus, Intercus GmbH, Rudolstadt, Germany), while there was no significant difference regarding stiffness, maintenance of Böhler's angle, or interfragmentary motion.[16]

■ RESULTS FROM THE LITERATURE

The results from the available clinical studies are summarized in **Table 1**. Interlocked nails have been shown to provide favorable outcomes, and computed tomography (CT)

TABLE 1: Studies reporting results of interlocking nailing for calcaneal fractures.

Authors	Journal	Number of feet	Nail used	Mean follow-up	Outcome	Conclusion
Simon et al.[11]	Int Orthop	63	CALCAnail®, FH	1 year	AOFAS: 85.9; good posterior facet reduction in 75%	Effective and reliable method with minimal complications
Zwipp et al.[13]	J Orthop Trauma	106	C-NAIL	12 months	AOFAS: 92.6; wound complications: 2.8%	Provides stable fixation with reduced soft tissue complications
Fascione et al.[14]	Foot Ankle Surg	15	CALCAnail®, FH	18 months	AOFAS: 85; excellent to good reduction in 93.5%	The nail provides good restoration of joint with good outcomes even in poor skin conditions
Fourgeaux et al.[15]	Int Orthop	26	CALCAnail®, FH	2.8 years	AOFAS: 79; excellent to good reduction in 81%	The surgery is efficient with a low rate of complications
Zeman et al.[19]	Acta Ortop Bras	19	C-NAIL	12 months	AOFAS: >80 in 13/19 and >70 in 17/19 cases	Suitable choice for Sanders II and III
Herlyn et al.[20]	Injury	20	CALCAnail®, FH	20 months	AOFAS: 71.6; complications in 5% (superficial infections)	The nail shows promising results with minimal risk of complications
Falis and Pyszel[21]	Ortop Traumatol Rehabil	18	CALCAnail®, FH	12 months	AOFAS: 82; no infectious complications	Minimally invasive procedure with low complications risk
Oliveira et al.[22]	Int J Orthop Sci	13	CALCAnail®, FH	16 months	AOFAS: 87.8; no skin complications in closed fracture; one infection in open type 2 case	Effective and reliable surgery for selected patients

(AOFAS: American Orthopaedic Foot and Ankle Society)

reconstructions in the follow-up periods have shown accuracy of reduction being maintained, with adequate increase in Böhler's angles, signifying that the nail provides a stable construct. The main indications for nailing are displaced Sanders type II and III fractures with documented favorable outcomes.[13] Selected Sanders type IV fractures may also be treated with interlocking nailing provided that anatomic reduction and stable fixation of the articular fragments can be achieved.[13,14] The authors, however, do caution against nailing in cases with severe comminution, as restoring the joint alignment becomes extremely difficult.[12] Primary or secondary fusion is another option for these severe fractures.[3,14] However, Sanders type IV fractures may also have favorable outcomes with few secondary fusions following anatomic reduction and stable fixation.[2]

Clinical comparative studies have also documented similar results in type II and III fractures. Zeman et al. compared the results of 217 Sanders type II and III calcaneal fractures treated with open reduction and internal fixation with locking compression plates with 19 calcaneal fractures treated with less invasive reduction and fixation with the C-NAIL. With comparable postoperative American Orthopaedic Foot and Ankle Society (AOFAS) scores (excellent to good score in close to 75% of cases in both groups) and reconstruction of Böhler's angle, the outcomes were similar with both techniques.[19] Herlyn et al., in their study, compared outcomes in 20 cases, each treated with a lateral locking plate or intramedullary nailing using the CALCAnail.[20] The duration of the surgeries was similar in both groups, but postoperative hospital stay and time away from work were less in the patients treated with intramedullary nailing. Although variables such as range of motion and usage of ambulatory aid favored the locking plates, the overall AOFAS scores did not show any significant difference at 20 months post surgery.[20]

The authors reported only one case of superficial infection following intramedullary nailing, while there was one case of deep infection requiring debridements, seven cases of impaired wound healing, and one case of hardware breakage in patients who underwent plating via an extensile approach resulting in complication rates of 5 versus 50% after nailing and plating, respectively.[20] The rate of implant removals was similar with four cases in both groups for reasons such as local pain, deep infection, arthrofibrosis, patient wish, and implant breakage.

■ COMPLICATIONS

While several authors report zero soft tissue-related complications with proper wound healing, optimal range of ankle movements and union **(Figs. 9 to 11)**,[14,21] others report superficial wound infections and deep infections, including osteomyelitis in 2–7%,[11,13,15,22] which compares favorably

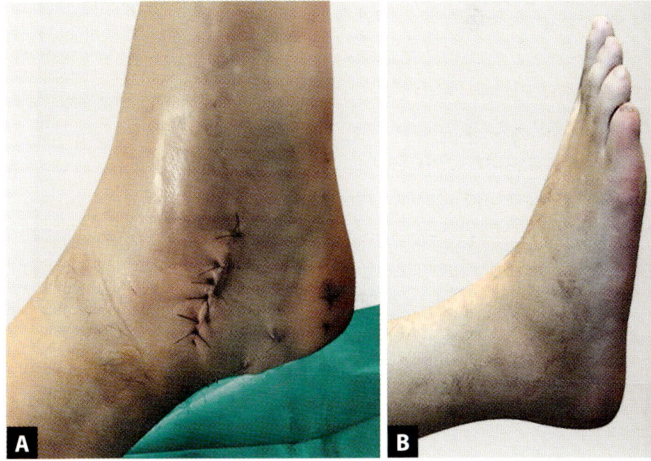

Figs. 9A and B: Wound healing over the sinus tarsi at (A) 2 days and (B) 6 weeks after fracture fixation.

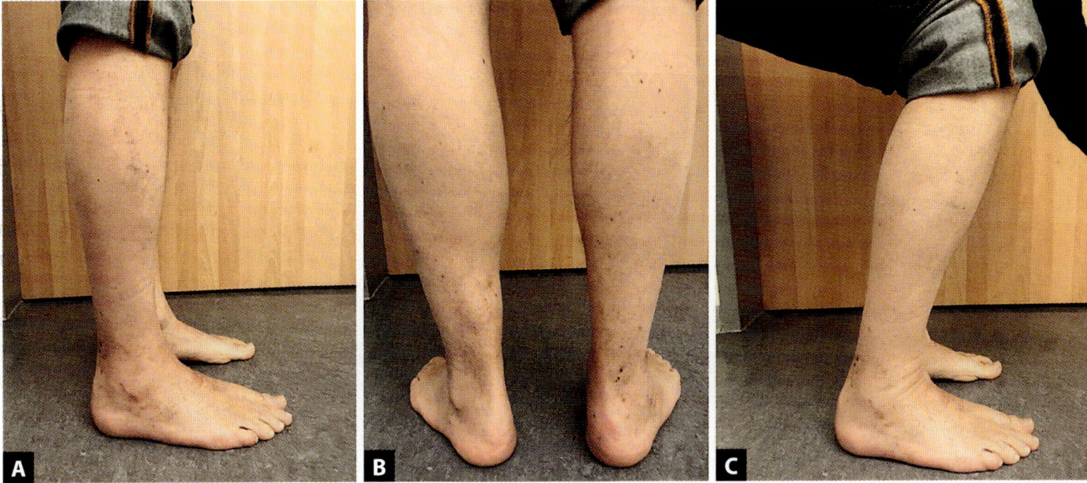

Figs. 10A to C: Full function of the ankle joint at 6 months' follow-up.

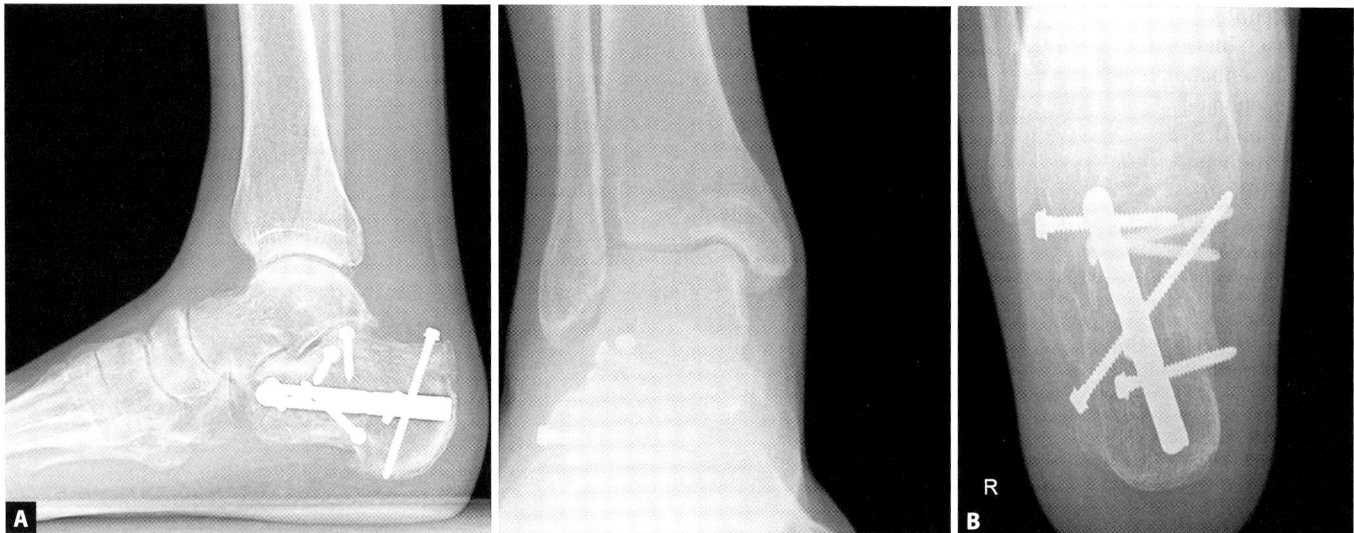

Figs. 11A and B: (A) Standing radiographs and axial view; (B) Complete union, anatomic alignment, and no signs of post-traumatic arthritis at 6 months' follow-up.

to open reduction and lateral plate fixation via extensile approaches[1-3] and is similar to reported rates with internal fixation other than intramedullary nailing using the same minimal-invasive (sinus tarsi) approach.[8-10,23,24]

Further, rarely reported complications include several cases of complex regional pain syndrome (CRPS), sural nerve entrapments that resolved spontaneously, arthrofibrosis, metal prominence at the heel or on the lateral aspect caused by the locking screws, requiring implant removal, and secondary subtalar fusions.[11,13,19,20]

Thus, the overall complication rates have been remarkably low.

SUMMARY

Less invasive reduction and stable internal fixation of displaced, intra-articular calcaneal fractures combine the benefits of minimally invasive surgery with superior biomechanical stability. However, to achieve good functional outcomes, anatomic reduction of the joint surfaces and the physiological shape of the calcaneus are indispensable.[25] While there are some encouraging data from clinical studies using two different nail designs, no high-level evidence is available.

REFERENCES

1. Makki D, Alnajjar HM, Walkay S, Ramkumar U, Watson AJ, Allen PW. Osteosynthesis of displaced intra-articular fractures of the calcaneum: a long-term review of 47 cases. J Bone Joint Surg Br. 2010;92(5):693-700.
2. Rammelt S, Zwipp H, Schneiders W, Dürr C. Severity of injury predicts subsequent function in surgically treated displaced intraarticular calcaneal fractures. Clin Orthop Relat Res. 2013;471(9):2885-98.
3. Sanders R, Vaupel ZM, Erdogan M, Downes K. Operative treatment of displaced intraarticular calcaneal fractures: long-term (10–20 years) results in 108 fractures using a prognostic CT classification. J Orthop Trauma. 2014;28:551-63.
4. Abidi NA, Dhawan S, Gruen GS, Vogt MT, Conti SF. Wound-healing risk factors after open reduction and internal fixation of calcaneal fractures. Foot Ankle Int. 1998;19:856-61.
5. Prabhakar S, Dhillon MS, Khurana A, John R. The "open-envelope" approach: a limited open approach for calcaneal fracture fixation. Indian J Orthop. 2018;52(3):231-8.
6. Rammelt S, Amlang M, Barthel S, Gavlik JM, Zwipp H. Percutaneous treatment of less severe intraarticular calcaneal fractures. Clin Orthop Relat Res. 2010;468:983-90.
7. Yeap EJ, Rao J, Pan CH, Soelar SA, Younger ASE. Is arthroscopic assisted percutaneous screw fixation as good as open reduction and internal fixation for the treatment of displaced intra-articular calcaneal fractures? Foot Ankle Surg. 2016;22(3):164-9.
8. Nosewicz T, Knupp M, Barg A, Maas M, Bolliger L, Goslings JC, et al. Mini-open sinus tarsi approach with percutaneous screw fixation of displaced calcaneal fractures: a prospective computed tomography-based study. Foot Ankle Int. 2012;33(11):925-33.
9. Schepers T, Backes M, Dingemans SA, de Jong VM, Luitse JSK. Similar anatomical reduction and lower complication rates with the sinus tarsi approach compared with the extended lateral approach in displaced intra-articular calcaneal fractures. J Orthop Trauma. 2017;31(6):293-8.
10. Rammelt S, Sangeorzan BJ, Swords MP. Calcaneal fractures; should we or should we not operate? Indian J Orthop. 2018;52:220-30.
11. Simon P, Goldzak M, Eschler A, Mittlmeier T. Reduction and internal fixation of displaced intra-articular calcaneal

fractures with a locking nail: a prospective study of sixty-nine cases. Int Orthop. 2015;39(10):2061-7.

12. Gussenbauer C. Ueber die behandlung der rissfracturen des fersenbeines. Prag Med Wochenschr. 1888;13:8.

13. Zwipp H, Paša L, Žilka L, Amlang M, Rammelt S, Pompach M. Introduction of a new locking nail for treatment of intraarticular calcaneal fractures. J Orthop Trauma. 2016;30(3):e88-92.

14. Fascione F, Di Mauro M, Guelfi M, Malagelada F, Pantalone A, Salini V. Surgical treatment of displaced intraarticular calcaneal fractures by a minimally invasive technique using a locking nail: a preliminary study. Foot Ankle Surg. 2019;25(5):679-83.

15. Fourgeaux A, Estens J, Fabre T, Laffenetre O, Lucas Y Hernandez J. Three-dimensional computed tomography analysis and functional results of calcaneal fractures treated by an intramedullary nail. Int Orthop. 2019;43(12):2839-47.

16. Reinhardt S, Martin H, Ulmar B, Döbele S, Zwipp H, Rammelt S, et al. Interlocking nailing versus interlocking plating in intra-articular calcaneal fractures: a biomechanical study. Foot Ankle Int. 2016;37(8):891-7.

17. Ni M, Wong DWC, Niu W, Wang Y, Mei J, Zhang M. Biomechanical comparison of modified CALCAnail system with plating fixation in intra-articular calcaneal fracture: a finite element analysis. Med Eng Phys. 2019;70:55-61.

18. Goldzak M, Simon P, Mittlmeier T, Chaussemier M, Chiergatti R. Primary stability of an intramedullary calcaneal nail and an angular stable calcaneal plate in a biomechanical testing model of intraarticular calcaneal fracture. Injury. 2014;45(Suppl. 1):S49-53.

19. Zeman J, Zeman P, Matejka T, Belatka J, Matejka J. Comparison of LCP and intramedullary nail osteosynthesis in calcaneal fractures. Acta Ortop Bras. 2019;27(6):288-93.

20. Herlyn A, Brakelmann A, Herlyn PK, Gradl G, Mittlmeier T. Calcaneal fracture fixation using a new interlocking nail reduces complications compared to standard locking plates; preliminary results after 1.6 years. Injury. 2019; 50(Suppl. 3):63-8.

21. Falis M, Pyszel K. Treatment of displaced intra-articular calcaneal fractures by intramedullary nail: preliminary report. Ortop Traumatol Rehabil. 2016;18(2):141-7.

22. Oliveira M, Grazina R, Ventura M, Cerqueira R, Lemos C. Calcaneal fractures treatment with locking nail: is it an option? Int J Orthop Sci. 2019;5(2):903-6.

23. Rammelt S, Zwipp H. Fractures of the calcaneus: current treatment strategies. Acta Chir Orthop Traumatol Cech. 2014;81(3):177-96.

24. Weber M, Lehmann O, Sägesser D, Krause F. Limited open reduction and internal fixation of displaced intra-articular fractures of the calcaneum. J Bone Joint Surg Br. 2008;90(12):1608-16.

25. Amlang M, Zwipp H, Pompach M, Rammelt S. Interlocking nail fixation for the treatment of displaced intra-articular calcaneal fractures. JBJS Essent Surg Tech. 2017;7(4):e33.

Role of Bone Graft and Bone Substitutes

Herman Singh Johal, Richard E Buckley, KV Menon, HK Verma, Rajesh Kumar Rajnish

"Statistics are no substitute for judgment".

–Henry Clay

"Substitute 'damn' every time you're inclined to write 'very;' your editor will delete it and the writing will be just as it should be".

–Mark Twain

■ INTRODUCTION

Almost every aspect of intra-articular calcaneal fracture management has been riddled with controversy over the years, and the decision to use bone graft or substitute during the operative treatment of these devastating injuries is no different.[1-9] As originally described by Böhler in 1931, the goals of treating these injuries are to attain anatomic reduction of the subtalar joint, restore calcaneal morphology, apply stable fixation, and allow for early range of motion.[10] The pendulum for treating these injuries has swung between conservative and surgical management, with the most recent shift being toward operative restoration of calcaneal height and anatomic reduction of the subtalar articular surface.[2,6,7,9,11-24] As with any articular fracture, depressed articular fragments crush the weak subchondral bone underlying the posterior facet, leaving a mean central defect of 11 cc following surgical reduction.[9,20,25-27] If internal fixation is not adequately stable, studies show that the presence of this bone void may predispose the calcaneus to collapse, resulting in loss of both the posterior facet reduction and calcaneal height.[5,7,9,28,29] This may contribute to the overall poor outcomes associated with these injuries,[18,30] as long-term issues such as pain, post-traumatic arthritis, and limitation of motion may occur if the joint surface collapses into the resulting defect.[19,21,24,27] Such bone voids are common sequelae of periarticular traumatic injuries, and various materials have successfully been used to augment fixation, improve fracture stability, and maintain reduction in other weight-bearing areas such as the wrist, femoral neck, tibial plateau, and tibial plafond.[6,27,31-37] However, each of these anatomic regions has different biological and biomechanical

needs, and it must be kept in mind that the validation of any bone graft or substitute in one anatomical location may not be indicative of its performance in another.[31,38]

Biomechanically, several features of displaced intra-articular calcaneal fractures are important to understand when considering the need to augment fixation with a bone graft or substitute. In the intact calcaneus, an area of low bone density exists under the anterior portion of the posterior facet. This is said to be a "force-neutral triangle", as the intact load-carrying trabecular bow disperses forces away from this weak cancellous bone **(Figs. 1A to D)**.[5,6,25,39-42] Typically, during displaced intra-articular calcaneal fractures, the calcaneal arc is disrupted, and the neutral triangle is transformed into an area that endures high compressive forces.[42] If the elevated articular surface is not adequately maintained with fixation methods, additional support may be provided by filling the "neutral triangle" with a bone graft or substitute that is able to withstand these high compressive forces.[6,9,25,43,44] Large bone voids may be present due to missing or impacted bone beneath the posterior facet, particularly in high-energy fractures or in patients with poor bone density.[6,45] In these situations, an additional void-filling buttress may contribute to maintaining reduction **(Figs. 2A to C)**. Despite these intuitive advantages, there has been mixed support for the use of bone graft or substitute in displaced intra-articular calcaneus fractures.

Studies have shown a spectrum of results, with some authors advocating for the use of various materials to augment fixation and maintain articular reduction.[1,5,9,11,25,28,29,42,43,45-48] Others argue that the regenerative capacity of the highly vascular cancellous bone of the calcaneus is enough

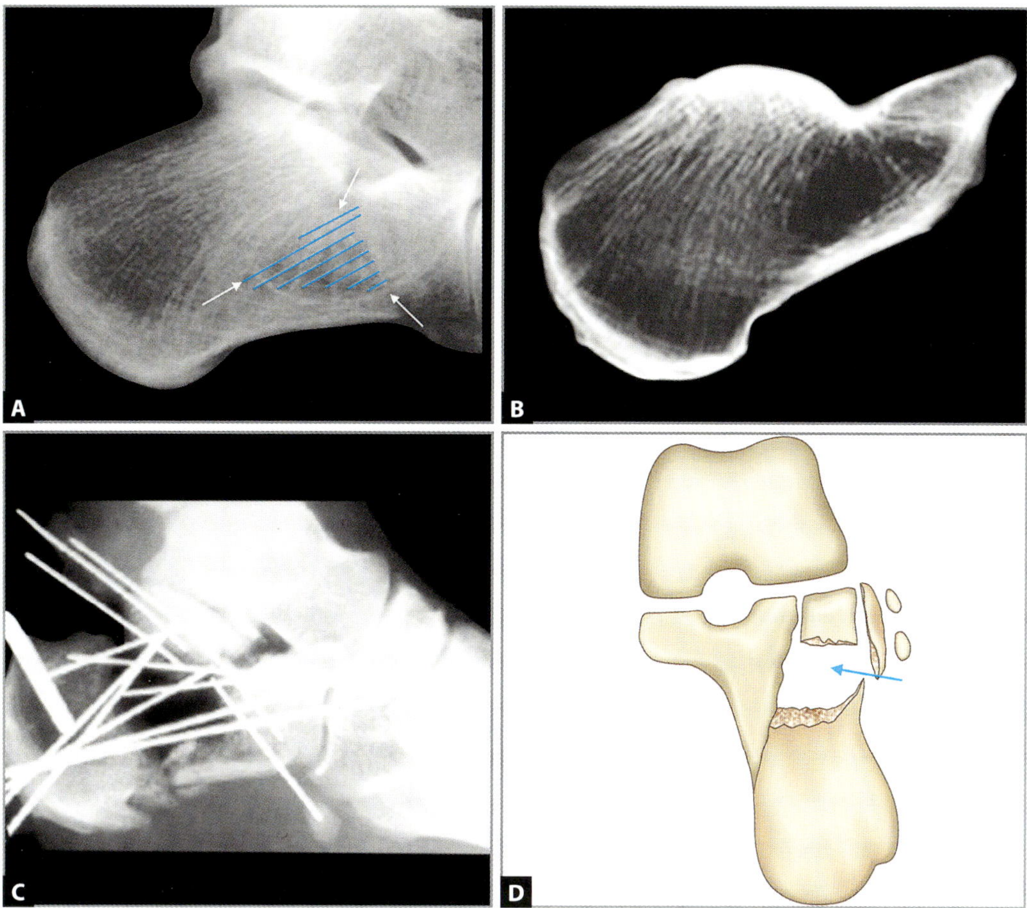

Figs. 1A to D: (A and B) Lateral radiographs of an intact calcaneus, with an area of low-density bone in the "neutral triangle" (blue in part A) underlying the posterior facet. Note the lack of trabeculae within this space in part (B). (C) Intraoperative radiograph showing the large void that is visible once the posterior facet is disimpacted from the underlying crushed cancellous bone and reduced in-line with the articular surface. (D) An illustration showing the defect present following articular surface reduction (blue arrow) in the coronal plane.
Sources: (A) and (B) Adapted from Schildhauer et al., (2000)[5] and Elsner et al. (2005)[42]; (C) Adapted from Banerjee et al. (2019)[44]; (D) Adapted from Palmer (1948).[1]

to fill the void over time,[49-52] and there is no need for augmentation if adequately stable internal fixation is achieved.[2,11,16,19,53-55] Methods of internal fixation in the literature have included lag screws, K-wires, and a one-third tubular plate, specialized calcaneal Y and H plates, and locking plates.[1,2,5,7,9,11,12,16,19,25,28,29,42,43,45-48,53-55] These constructs span a range of stability and can be implemented based on fracture type, surgeon familiarity, and available resources. However, limited stability with any form of internal fixation is achieved as the size of the cancellous bone void beneath the articular surface becomes larger.[25,45] Historically, bone grafts have included both autograft and allograft, each with its own advantages and disadvantages.[56] More recently, there has been an explosion of bone substitute products made available, eliminating the need to deal with the negative aspects of bone grafting such as donor site morbidity and risk of disease transmission.[42,45,48] These biological and synthetic options each have unique traits and variable suitability for

use in the management of calcaneal fractures.[38] Orthopedic surgeons must have an understanding of the defect to be grafted and choose a material that is able to address the need to fill the void, provide structural support, and resorb at an appropriate time.

BONE GRAFT AND SUBSTITUTE CHARACTERISTICS

In order to select an appropriate option to fill the calcaneal bone void left behind following articular surface reduction, orthopedic surgeons must be familiar with the properties inherent to bone grafts and substitutes. These characteristics include osteoconduction, osteointegration, osteoinduction, and osteogenesis.[38,48] Only the historic "gold standard" of autograft has all four of these properties, with all other options possessing one or typically two of these traits. Knowledge of these properties is critical as a specific fracture may require an option that maximizes only some of them.

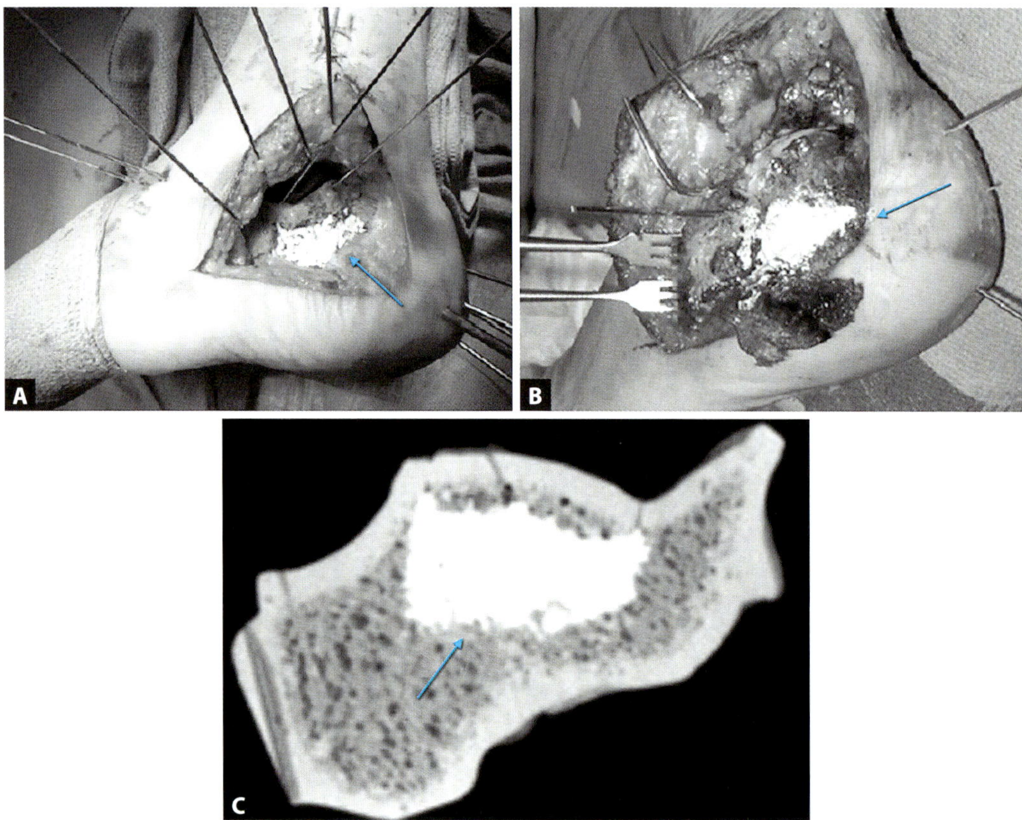

Figs. 2A to C: (A and B) Intraoperative placement of an injectable calcium phosphate cement (blue arrows) into the calcaneal bone void; (C) Anatomic cross-sectional specimen of human calcaneus filled with calcium phosphate bone cement (blue arrows) following articular surface reduction.
Sources: (A and B) Adapted from Banerjee et al. (2019)[44]; (C) Adapted from Elsner et al. (2005).[42]

Osteoconduction is the most common trait among the bone grafts and substitutes used in calcaneal fracture surgery.[31] It refers to the property of a three-dimensional matrix to act as scaffolding and support the attachment of bone-forming cells for subsequent bone formation.[31,48,57,58] The configuration of the material will dictate the orientation of ingrowth for new bone and blood vessels.[31,38,57] Capillaries, perivascular tissue, and osteoprogenitor cells migrate into the bone graft or substitute, and the newly formed bone is produced within the porous matrix.[31] The interconnectivity and pore size of this matrix are important factors in determining the overall osteoconductive nature of a substance, with the optimal pore size for bone ingrowth being between 150 and 500 μm.[31,59] Bone grafts and substitutes that are simply osteoconductive are indicated for filling voids, and aid in maintaining structural stability alongside some form of internal fixation.[31]

With the development of new bone substitutes and composite materials, osteoinduction is becoming a more prevalent trait in the landscape of options. It refers to graft materials which contain factors that induce the mitogenesis of undifferentiated mesenchymal stem cells from the surrounding tissue. These then progress down a bone-forming lineage, beginning with osteoprogenitor cells which then differentiate into osteoblasts.[38,60] This is most commonly seen with the integration of bone morphogenic proteins (BMPs) or bone marrow aspirate (BMA) with substitute materials possessing other properties. This can be differentiated from osteointegration, which simply refers to the surface bonding that occurs between the host bone and grafting material occurring at the periphery of the bone graft or substitute material.[38]

Finally, the relatively newly described trait of osteogenesis is one held by few of the available options, including autograft bone and bone marrow.[48] It can be defined as the generation of bone from bone-forming cells, with the critical component of viable osteoprogenitor cells being required as part of the graft.[48] These osteoprogenitor cells can proliferate and differentiate into osteoblasts and eventually osteocytes. Cancellous bone has a larger surface area than cortical bone and thus has a greater bone-forming potential.[57] Both osteogenic and osteoinductive grafts increase the rate at which bone voids are filled with native cancellous bone.

When choosing one material over another, the orthopedic surgeon needs to ensure that the mechanical and biological needs of the fracture are met by the option chosen.[61] If used in the management of calcaneal fractures, grafts or substitutes should be safe, osteoconductive, osteointegrative, and, if possible, osteoinductive as well.[62]

■ BONE GRAFT AND SUBSTITUTE OPTIONS

Options that have been used in the past to fill calcaneal fracture voids include biologic materials such as autogenous or allograft bone, synthetic materials such as cements and ceramics, and composites of both biologic and synthetic substances **(Table 1)**.[30,62] Cancellous autograft has been the historic standard used in orthopedic trauma surgery as it is easily obtainable. However, in calcaneal fractures, evidence has failed to show that it possesses the mechanical ability to resist collapse following weight-bearing.[44] More recently, a variety of allograft options have become more readily available through bone banks. Although these avoid many of the complications associated with harvesting and using autogenous bone, allograft still has limited mechanical resistance and poses infectious risks.[44,48] The development of synthetic and composite options attempts to provide a mechanically acceptable alternative to autografts that minimizes costs and complications.[31,63] These materials must be osteoconductive and have a resorption rate that accompanies the bone formation process while contributing mechanical strength.[63] The extent of bone substitute remodeling is influenced by a variety of factors, including the severity of fracture, time of weight-bearing, and stability of

TABLE 1: Bone graft and substitute characteristics.

Bone graft/ substitute	Implant	Osteogenic	Osteoinductive	Osteoconductive	Compressive strength	Resorption	Non- immunogenicity
Biologic							
Autograft							
	Cancellous (iliac crest)	+++	++	+++	No	+++	+++
Allograft							
	Fresh	No	+/–	++	No	+	+
	Frozen	No	+/–	++	No	No	++
	Freeze-dried	No	+/–	+	No	No	++
	Demineralized bone matrix (DBM)	No	+/–	+	No	No	+++
Synthetic							
Ceramics/ cements							
	Polymethyl methacrylate (PMMA)	No	No	No	++	No	++
	Hydroxyapatite (HA)	No	No	++	+/–	++	+++
	Calcium sulfate	No	No	++	No	+++	+++
	Calcium phosphate	No	No	+++	++	+	+++
Composite							
Bone marrow							
	Bone marrow aspirate (BMA) + synthetic	++	++	Varies by synthetic substitute		++	+++
Protein							
	Bone morphogenic protein (BMP) + synthetic	No	+++	Varies by synthetic substitute		No	+++

+++ = Excellent, ++ = Good, + = Fair, +/– = Poor, No = None

fixation.[61] Substitute and composite materials are becoming tailored and optimized for use in specific fracture situations, such as in the calcaneus.[61] Despite this proliferation of options, few studies exist that compare one type of bone graft or substitute to another or even to none at all, with a majority of options relying on anecdotal evidence, mechanical studies, or case series.

■ NO GRAFT OR SUBSTITUTE

The concept of filling calcaneal fracture bone voids dates back to the 1920s,[64,65] when fixation methods were less rigid, and autograft was used as a mechanical augment for stability. Since that time, fixation methods have improved, and there have been many authors arguing against the need for bone grafts or substitutes as part of the surgical management of these injuries. They state that rigid internal fixation alone will adequately prevent articular surface collapse, and that the use of grafts or substitutes may even block articular reduction as it could extrude into the subtalar joint.[2,12,16,19,53-55] Most of these studies are limited to small case series, the largest of which was an observational study of 120 displaced intra-articular calcaneal fractures.[2] Treatment across the studies involved open reduction with provisional K-wire fixation, followed by definitive fixation with lag screws and either a specialized calcaneal plate or contoured plate, without the use of any bone graft or substitute.[2,12,16,19] Patients were kept nonweight-bearing for as little as 6 weeks[16] but typically for a minimum of 10 weeks.[2,12,16,19] None of the studies described the size of the void remaining following reduction or any data regarding initial, postoperative, or final Böhler's angles. In a series of 12 operatively treated calcanei treated without the use of a graft, O'Farrell et al. stated that reconstituted cancellous bone was radiographically evident within the void at 4–8 weeks.[12] All of the studies indicated that none of the surgically treated fractures collapsed up to 2 years following surgery, and functional outcomes were excellent; however, there were no groups used for comparison.[2,12,16,19] Overall, little more than descriptive case series exist to support the use of no bone graft or substitute for all calcaneal fractures. With the evolution of fixation techniques, a rigid construct may be able to prevent collapse on its own; however, there is limited evidence in situations where a sizable bone void exists, or a rigid construct is otherwise unattainable.

■ BONE GRAFTS (BIOLOGIC)

Autograft

Autograft bone has long been used in orthopedic surgery to fill bone defects secondary to trauma. It provides an osteoconductive scaffold, osteoinductive growth factors, and osteogenic cells; however, most of the cellular elements and osteogenic potential are lost during harvest and transplantation.[38,66] The iliac crest is the most commonly chosen donor site and provides an adequate quantity of good-quality cancellous graft.[38] Despite being readily available, iliac crest autograft involves an additional surgical procedure and is commonly associated with donor site morbidity, with complication rates ranging from 6 to 39%.[20,31,57,67] Complications include hematomas, seromas, blood loss, injury to the lateral femoral cutaneous or cluneal nerves, superficial infections, cosmetic defects, hernia formation, infection, blood loss, cosmetic defects, iliac fracture, and chronic donor site pain.[38,57,67-70]

The use of cancellous autograft in calcaneal fracture surgery was initially described by a group of French surgeons when they were dissatisfied with the stability of fixation techniques being used at the time.[64,65] Its use was further popularized by Palmer as he explained that filling the bony defect with autograft following elevation of the articular fragment would avoid valgus collapse following weight-bearing.[1] Palmer described the void as being "about the size of one's thumb" **(Fig. 1D)**, for which he would tamp in a slightly larger piece of iliac crest autograft. Results were favorable at 2 years; however, there was no detailed description of outcomes beyond noting earlier mobilization, decreased pain, and increased mobility in 22 of 23 cases.[1] Issues with the ability of autograft bone to resist calcaneal collapse were highlighted by Longino and Buckley as they conducted a matched comparison within a larger randomized cohort study of calcaneal fracture management.[28] The authors prospectively matched 20 displaced intra-articular calcaneal fractures treated with open reduction internal fixation (ORIF) plus autograft with 20 similar fractures receiving ORIF alone based on age, sex, occupational workload, fracture classification, preoperative Böhler's angle, and fixation type. At final 2-year follow-up, Böhler's angles for those fractures treated with ORIF plus autograft compared with those fractures treated with ORIF alone measured 26 and 27°, respectively. Overall, ORIF supplemented with cancellous autograft provided no objective functional benefit and did not prevent calcaneal height collapse compared to ORIF alone.[28] This study, in combination with inherent donor site morbidity, renders autograft an inferior option in calcaneal fracture surgery when a void filler or ORIF augmentation is required.

Allograft/Demineralized Bone Matrix

The use of allograft bone emerged as a bone void filler in orthopedic trauma surgery to limit the donor-site morbidity associated with autologous grafts. However, its use requires a complex bone banking system, and processing typically eliminates any osteogenic and osteoinductive potential of the resultant graft.[38,57] The remaining osteoconductive capability and mechanical strength of the graft are dictated by the method of processing, with demineralized bone matrix (DBM) and fresh, frozen, and freeze-dried allograft, each varying in these properties. Furthermore, there may be lower union rates and problems with histocompatibility and disease transmission, despite vigorous sterilization techniques.[20,27,38,48,71]

Host immunogenic response decreases with increased tissue processing.[38,48] Fresh allograft is a historic entity that is rarely used in orthopedic trauma surgery due to the associated immune response and high potential for disease transmission.[38,48,57] Frozen or freeze-dried allograft possesses reduced immunogenicity; however, osteoinductive capability is also limited by processing.[38,48,57] The shelf life of fresh-frozen bone is 1 year when stored at –20°C and 5 years if stored at –70°C. Freeze-drying involves the removal of water from the tissue and subsequent vacuum packing, which allows for storage at room temperature and an indefinite shelf life.[48,57] The DBM has become more commonplace and involves treating allograft with a mild acid to extract and remove the mineral content of the graft. A collagenous structure is left behind and serves as an osteoconductive scaffold for new bone formation but provides little mechanical support on its own due to the loss of bone minerals.[38,48] The osteoinductive molecules are theoretically preserved; however, they have not been shown to exhibit any osteoinductive activity in humans.[48]

With regards to sterilization, bone banks are required to perform serological testing for human immunodeficiency virus-1 (HIV-1), HIV-2, and hepatitis C virus (HCV) antibody.[48] Depending on health legislation, some may also be required to test for human T-cell lymphotropic virus (HTLV) I and II antibodies, cytomegalovirus, and syphilis.[48] Terminal sterilization of allograft materials following harvest and processing is commonly done using gamma irradiation or ethylene oxide.[48] Gamma radiation has been shown to have a greater negative effect on the mechanical strength of allograft, whereas treatment with ethylene oxide may further affect osteoinductive potential.[48] With this complex preparation, the transmission rate of HIV is estimated to be 1 in 1.6 million; however, other contaminants still pose a problem as the use of allograft in calcaneal fractures has been linked to higher wound infection rates and breakdowns in several studies.[38,71,72] In a study of 49 patients, investigating the treatment of displaced intra-articular calcaneal fractures with primary reduction and external fixation followed by delayed definitive internal fixation, Baumgaertel and Gotzen

suggest that allograft may be associated with increased infection rates.[72] As indicated by positive wound cultures, those patients who received allograft had a 13% higher infection rate compared to those patients treated without graft.[72] The combination of costly, complex preparation, and storage alongside increased infection leads to allograft being an unfavorable choice in the management of calcaneal fractures.

■ SYNTHETIC BONE SUBSTITUTES

Synthetic bone substitutes have become an attractive option to fill cancellous bone voids in orthopedic trauma surgery. Overall, they avoid the donor site morbidity associated with autograft as well as the infection transmission risk associated with allograft materials.[27,61,73] With advances in technology and biological understanding, the number of bone substitute materials has rapidly grown. They are able to address the biological and structural needs of most periarticular defects by being osteoconductive and osteointegrative.[38,61] Although many of these products are used for similar indications, they vary in their chemical composition, structural strength, and resorption rates.[31] Mechanically, bone substitutes should provide similar strength to the cancellous calcaneal bone, which it is replacing to strike a balance that prevents stress shielding and provides resistance to collapse under cyclical axial loading.[38]

Each of the synthetic substitute materials has differing combinations of properties and, as a result, differing inter-actions with the surrounding bone following implantation. Porosity, osteoconductivity, biocompatibility, sterility, cost, ease of use, and ability to contour are all key features considered during the development of substitute materials.[20,38,61,73] The substitute material should not expose the host to inflammatory reactions, toxic, carcinogenic, or infectious risks.[20] Particularly, in the subtalar bone void, osteoconduction and mechanical stability outweigh the need for osteointegration to allow for early support of the articular surface following reduction. However, the goal of timely substitute material resorption via osteoclastic activity can only be achieved following rapid integration into the surrounding host bone, and thus osteointegration is still a necessity.[8,38,57,74] Ideally, the rate of substitute resorption and bone formation should be balanced to avoid premature collapse at the fracture site.[25] The major limitations of any substitute material typically revolve around their handling, ease of use, and maintaining the material in the desired location without extrusion into surrounding tissues and joints.[31] Additionally, there is concern that if a bone substitute is well incorporated, any subsequent infection may result in the destruction and removal of large quantities of normal bone.[31]

Polymethyl methacrylate (PMMA) cement and various ceramic/cement preparations, including coralline hydroxyapatite (HA), calcium phosphate, and calcium sulfate, have all been used in calcaneal surgery to varying degrees of success.[31,61] Evidence is, however, limited, coming mostly from biomechanical, animal, and case series data. Several randomized controlled trials do exist, but none directly compare one synthetic material to another. This places increased importance on interpreting the little clinical data available and understanding the properties of each material that may be beneficial for calcaneal fractures.

Polymethyl Methacrylate Cement

The concept of synthetic materials for use in orthopedic trauma surgery began with PMMA in the 1960s; however, its use did not gain widespread acceptance due to its biomechanical properties.[9,25,32] PMMA certainly provides mechanical support, but it is neither osteoconductive nor resorbable; therefore, it does not allow for incorporation or biological remodeling with native bone.[9,25,32] Bone healing is further inhibited by soft-tissue damage as PMMA sets via an exothermic reaction.[9,25,32] Only one report of two elderly patients has examined PMMA use in calcaneal fractures.[75] Despite these patients achieving cortical bone healing and early weight-bearing postoperatively, the long-term consequences of having PMMA in the calcaneus are unknown. This concern is especially relevant in the extension of its use to younger patients.

Ceramic Cements

Calcium-based ceramic materials are highly crystalline structures that consist of metallic and nonmetallic elements held together by ionic and covalent bonds.[48,56] These bonds are produced via sintering and result in HA, calcium phosphate, and calcium sulfate compounds. They are able to provide immediate structural support and porous osteoconductive scaffolding for new bone growth. However, ceramics typically possess no osteogenic or osteoinductive properties on their own, resulting in slow or incomplete resorption and replacement.[20,38,56] As a group, ceramics have been shown to be biocompatible and safe for human use.[55] Tricalcium phosphate has been extensively used in dentistry and orthopedic surgery since the 1980s. It has a chemical composition similar to that of amorphous bone precursors and is resorbed within months to years once bone grows onto the scaffold. HA has been investigated and used for over 30 years and has a chemical composition closer to that of bone mineral compared to calcium phosphate; however, it is much slower to resorb.[20,38]

Hydroxyapatite

Hydroxyapatite is a naturally found material obtained from sea coral. Certain sea coral species form an exoskeleton of calcium phosphate coralline, and this is similar to human cancellous bone.[31,38] It may be harvested directly from Goniopora sea coral or manufactured by subjecting natural coralline to high pressures and temperatures, with both methods producing a material with a pore size in the range that accommodates rapid normal bone ingrowth.[31,38] HA has a high compressive strength but a low tensile strength which makes it brittle overall.[38] Within orthopedic trauma, it has been used as a void filler in treating tibial plateau fractures, producing results comparable to tibial fractures in which autograft was used.[38] Resorption is extremely slow overall; however, rates do vary slightly by calcium and phosphate composition. At the extreme, some preparations have been shown to be radiographically visible beyond 10 years.[31] The use of natural coralline HA to treat calcaneal fractures requires careful handling of material as infection rates between 38% and 75% have been reported in French clinical studies.[76,77] The authors suggested that the high mechanical load sustained by the calcaneus contributed to the rapid resorption of the coralline HA implant, subsequent loosening, and infiltration with serous fluid. In their histological study, Huber et al. assessed the incorporation of a newer, fully synthetic, injectable HA nanocrystalline paste for various fractures.[78] Six adult fractures were assessed, including one calcaneal fracture where a calcaneal plate was augmented with 5 cc of HA to fill the bone void. Biopsy specimens were obtained 13 months postimplantation and showed good incorporation, no inflammatory reaction, osteofibrosis, or osteonecrosis.[78] The same group of authors reported a small case series of 24 intra-articular calcaneal fractures treated operatively with a stable calcaneal honeycomb plate, augmented with a nanocrystalline HA substitute if the bone void was >4 cc. Böhler's angle was adequately maintained at 27.7° 1-year postoperative, which was a slight, but not significant, drop from the immediate postoperative value of 31.5°. As synthetic HA bone substitutes continue to be perfected, they may serve as an acceptable option to fill bone voids >4 cc in calcaneal fractures; however, natural coralline HA options should be avoided.

Calcium Sulfate

Calcium sulfate is an osteoconductive substitute material, most commonly used in pellet form, but also available as a powder that may be mixed to form an injectable paste.[31] It provides a compressive strength similar to that of cancellous bone; however, it is too quickly resorbed in 4–12 weeks to support osteoconductive bone formation within the bone voids typically found in calcaneal fractures.[31] A single prospective cohort compared 33 calcaneal fractures treated with vancomycin-impregnated calcium sulfate plus ORIF to 11 calcaneal fractures treated with ORIF alone.[26] The defects filled ranged from 5 to 10 cc, and those treated with calcium sulfate were shown to have a significantly lower time to union and the incidence of infection compared to those treated with ORIF alone. However, this study reported no information on the maintenance of calcaneal height or functional outcomes and is further limited by small sample size and lack of randomized or blinded allocation. Calcium sulfate may be safe for use as an antibiotic delivery system in calcaneal osteomyelitic defects or for fractures at high risk for infection. However, its overall efficacy in maintaining articular reduction and augmenting fixation in a majority of calcaneal fractures remains to be shown.

Calcium Phosphate

Calcium phosphate has emerged as a favorable option for use in periarticular fractures.[79,80] Essentially, calcium phosphate is an osteoconductive substance that can be manufactured as cement to fill cancellous bone defects and improve articular stability. A variety of preparations are available and usually involves the mixing of two or more types of dissolvable calcium phosphate. This yields a saturated solution with a desired final composition that has a crystal structure similar to that of normal bone.[19,80,81] A variety of formulations are available, but each shares the same baseline characteristics.[31,48] The amorphous crystalline structure of calcium phosphates results in greater resorption and biocompatibility than HA, which favors overall bone

formation.[31,42,61] They also have the advantage of slower incorporation compared to calcium sulfate materials. This allows for sufficient structural support while bone formation and resorption occur in a balanced manner. According to animal models, calcium phosphate undergoes complete osteoclastic resorption over 26–86 weeks, followed by the invasion of small blood vessels that become surrounded by circumferential bone lamellae **(Figs. 3A and B)**.[31,48,80,82] The porosity of the hardened calcium phosphate cement facilitates bone colonization and vascular infiltration in both central and peripheral areas of the implant.[38,73] On their own, most calcium phosphate preparations lack osteoinductive and osteogenic properties and have an initial compressive strength similar to that of cancellous bone but a tensile strength that is considerably lower.[25,38,48,81] The average compressive strength of fully cured calcium phosphate varies from product to product according to the particle diameter.[74] Some formulations are able to resist loads of 10–15 MPa, while others have been shown to withstand loads up to 55 MPa but undergo slower resorption in vivo.[25,34,61,79,81,83] Compressive resistance is an asset within the neutral triangle following disruption of the calcaneal arc, and those calcium phosphates able to withstand higher axial loads possess a biomechanical advantage.[31,42] Human and animal histological studies show active resorption and biocompatibility of calcium phosphate without any evidence of immunogenic reaction.[80,82,83] Its use as a bone void filler in orthopedic tumor surgery was supported in a review by Galois et al., whose series included two benign calcaneal tumors.[79] Several clinical studies have indicated that it is superior to autogenous bone graft in providing

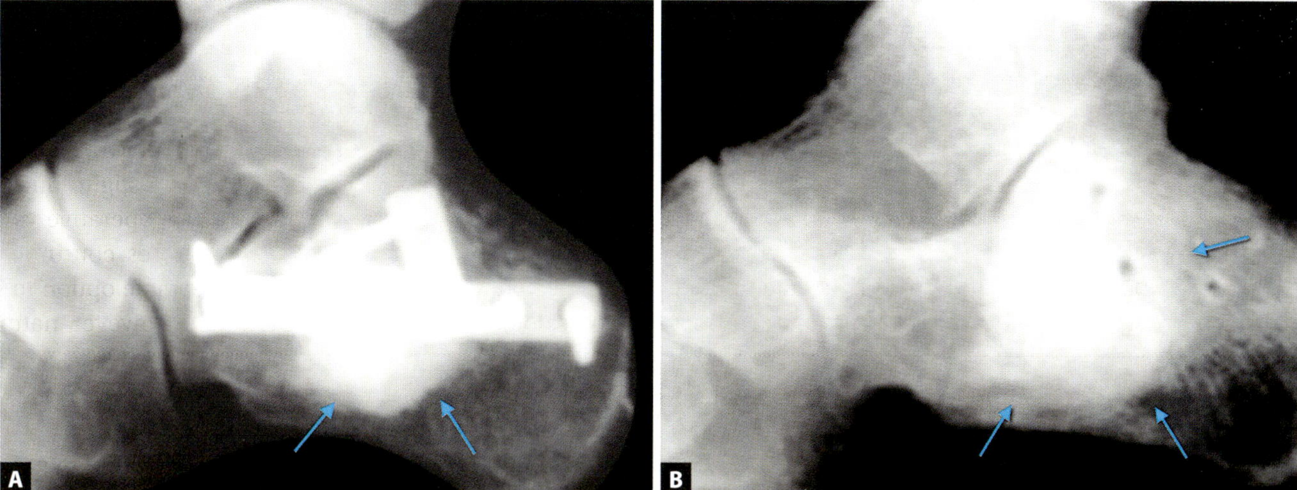

Figs. 3A and B: (A) Immediate postoperative radiograph of a calcaneal fracture managed with open reduction internal fixation (ORIF) and a calcaneal phosphate cement; (B) 18-month postoperative radiograph of the same patient following ORIF removal. Note that only slight resorption of the calcium phosphate cement has occurred as indicated by the decreased density and slight rounding at the peripheral edges. Blue arrows point to minimal resorption of bone substitute.
Source: Adapted from Schildhauer et al. (2000).[5]

stability and maintaining reduction in multiple areas of orthopedic trauma, including the distal radius, proximal humerus, proximal femur, and tibial plateau.[25,27,32-37,84] In a meta-analysis of 14 studies investigating the use of calcium phosphate in the management of periarticular injuries, Bajammal et al. showed that patients treated with calcium phosphate had similar rates of fracture healing and no increase of infection across all fractures treated regardless of the control group. Fractures augmented with calcium phosphate were shown to have a 68% lower risk of losing reduction compared to those managed with autograft alone, and a 56% decreased risk of pain at the fracture site compared to controls managed with no graft at all.[27]

Promising results in other areas of fracture surgery do not necessarily translate to the use of calcium phosphate in the management of calcaneal fractures; however, they do form a basis for further investigation. Studies in calcaneal fractures have typically assessed bioresorbable preparations that are typically mixed intraoperatively and injected or shaped to fill the irregularly shaped defects. Following implantation, the cement mixture hardens, in situ, at room temperature in an isothermic or endothermic reaction, which protects the surrounding tissue from thermal damage and allows for increased surgical working time.[20,25,80,81] Within 10 minutes of mixing, the substitute is able to provide initial compressive strength for the posterior facet and augment any additional internal fixation.[6,9,29,38,48,80] One formulation of calcium phosphate cement with a higher compressive strength was used in a cadaveric study where simulated Sanders IIB intra-articular calcaneal fractures were treated with ORIF plus bone graft or ORIF plus calcium phosphate cement.[29] They concluded that calcaneal stability and compressive strength are increased when ORIF is augmented with the high compressive strength cement. This same formulation was used by Csizy et al. as they emphasized the need to treat large bone voids with bone substitutes through the description of a case involving a pathologic intra-articular calcaneal fracture in a patient with a large, benign calcaneal bone cyst **(Figs. 4A to D)**.[45] The void measured 20 cc, and an injectable calcium phosphate substitute was used to fill the void and augment the limited K-wire fixation that could be obtained. Radiographic follow-up at 12 weeks postoperative did not indicate any calcaneal collapse, and 2-year functional outcomes were favorable.[45] Two small case series show that augmentation of fixation with high compressive strength calcium phosphate bone cement is able to allow for earlier weight-bearing following operative treatment of calcaneal fractures.[5,7] They found that the bone substitute supplementation was able to resist collapse with patients weight-bearing at 6 weeks as well as 3 weeks postoperative. Two European case series studies have investigated the use

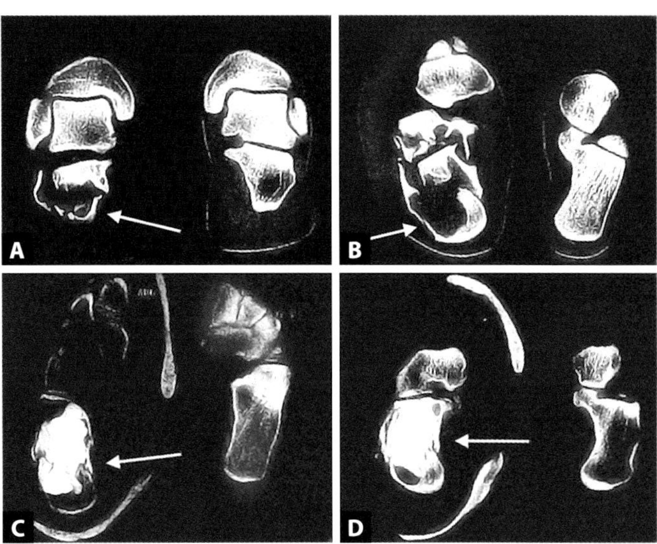

Figs. 4A to D: Preoperative (A) axial and (B) coronal computed tomography (CT) images of a pathologic intra-articular calcaneal fracture associated with a large benign bone cyst measuring 20 cc (white arrows). Postoperative (B) axial and (D) coronal CT images of the same patient following filling of the defect with a calcium phosphate bone cement (white arrows).
Source: Adapted from Csizy et al. (2001).[45]

of another formulation of calcium phosphate bone cement with a lower compressive resistance in trauma surgery and articular calcaneal fractures.[20,61] Calcaneal bone defects were filled with 1–9 cc of bone substitute to augment internal fixation and were followed for 1 year radiographically. The studies showed that resorbable calcium phosphate substitute is a safe alternative to autogenous bone graft for filling bone voids and augmenting fixation in the calcaneus. The bone substitute was biocompatible and resorbed within 6 months of implantation; however, these studies did not assess postoperative radiographic maintenance of reduction. The same formulation was investigated in a recent randomized controlled trial comparing the treatment of intra-articular calcaneal fractures ORIF plus an injectable calcium phosphate cement to treatment with ORIF alone.[9] A total of 52 fractures were randomized, and fixation consisted of K-wires, lag screws, and a one-third tubular plate **(Figs. 5A and B)**. At 1 year, there was some degree of collapse in both treatment groups; however, those fractures that were augmented with bone substitute lost less calcaneal height than those that were treated with ORIF alone. The difference between the groups may have been even more pronounced had a calcium phosphate preparation with a higher compressive resistance been used. The biological and mechanical properties of calcium phosphate cement bone substitutes have emerged as a favorable choice when filling medium- or larger-sized calcaneal bone voids present following articular reduction. However, anecdotally, it is the

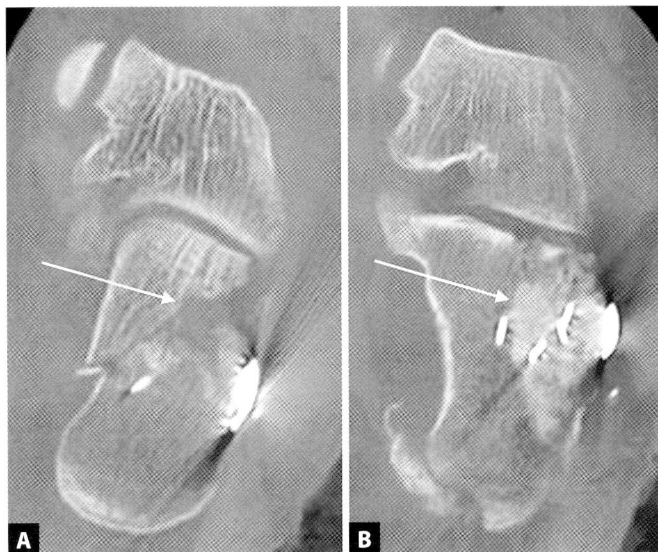

Figs. 5A and B: Postoperative coronal computed tomography (CT) scan illustrating a calcaneal fracture managed with (A) open reduction internal fixation (ORIF) alone and (B) ORIF augmented with an injectable calcium phosphate paste. Note that the white arrows indicated the bone void and calcium phosphate paste in (A) and (B), Respectively.
Source: Adapted from Johal et al. (2009).[9]

personal experience of these authors that some of the more recent injectable calcium phosphate cement preparations may be associated with continued serous wound drainage. This may be due to the initial viscosity of the formulations or possibly a mild inflammatory response. Regardless, caution must still be exercised in the use of calcium phosphate bone substitute to ensure that it is implemented only when indicated by the size of the bone void or need to augment fixation to prevent collapse following weight-bearing.

◼ COMPOSITE BONE SUBSTITUTES

There is yet to be any single bone graft or substitute that possesses all of the characteristics that would make the ideal filler for calcaneal fracture voids. Despite the fact that several of the above synthetic options possess adequate osteoconductive and osteointegrative ability,[48] they lack the osteogenic or osteoinductive potential that would accelerate bone healing and hasten the restoration of skeletal integrity. Composite grafts combine the scaffolding properties of synthetics, such as calcium phosphate, with biologic elements to stimulate cell migration, proliferation, differentiation, and, eventually, osteogenesis.[38,48] Ceramic cements are favored as carrier materials for osteoinductive agents such as BMP and BMA, and the synthetic chosen will dictate the overall osteoconductive nature of the composite graft.[57] The highly porous structure of ceramic cements provides a greater surface area for the vascular and bony

ingrowth that is induced.[38] In addition to osteoinductivity, BMA also contributes osteogenic potential as it contains mesenchymal precursor cells.[48] BMA may be obtained locally or from the iliac crest; however, more potent BMA cells may be developed through careful precursor selection, centrifugation, or clonal expansion.[57]

The compressive strength of composite grafts is also largely decided by the synthetic that is used as the carrier; however, the addition of polyelectrolytes or bovine serum albumin (BSA) may further enhance this characteristic. In a mechanical and X-ray diffraction study, Mickiewicz et al. tested several combinations of a calcium phosphate paste incorporated with either polyelectrolytes or BSA.[81] The BSA and polyelectrolyte calcium phosphate–polymer composites were respectably able to withstand compressive loads six and two times that of pure calcium phosphate. X-ray diffraction suggested that the addition of the polyelectrolyte or BSA possibly leads to a denser, more interdigitated microstructure, thus forming a more cohesive composite.[81]

Overall, the development of composite graft materials continues to move forward. As new combinations are developed, a material to address the specific needs of calcaneal fractures will eventually emerge, making composite grafts a promising option for the future.

Indian Experience with Ceramic Bone Graft Substitutes

The Bio-Medical Technology (BMT) wing of SCTIMST (Sree Chitra Thirunal Institute for Medical Sciences and Technology), Trivandrum, India, has been the pioneer in biomaterials research in India. Their first study on indigenously developed HA was published[85] in 1996 and, subsequently, the sol–gel derived bioactive glass (BG) (calcium phosphosilicate).[86] Both products were extensively tested in the laboratory before systematic animal and human trials.[87,88] Both cancellous bone augmentation and cortical replacement studies have been published using these materials.[89-91] As discussed in the preceding sections, optimizing the mechanical properties of ceramic against the biological properties (osteoinduction, osteoconduction, and eventual) is crucial for each particular clinical application. For cancellous bone augmentation needing mechanical support, the preferred combination has been reported to be 80% HA and 20% BG with 70% pore volume and pore size of 150–200 μm.[92] While the center has made extensive studies on ceramic matrix supplemented with autologous bone marrow-derived stem cells and growth factors, these were largely for cortical bone defects and not cancellous augmentation.[93]

The rationale for using bone grafts or substitutes in calcaneal fractures is perhaps intuitive with little evidence

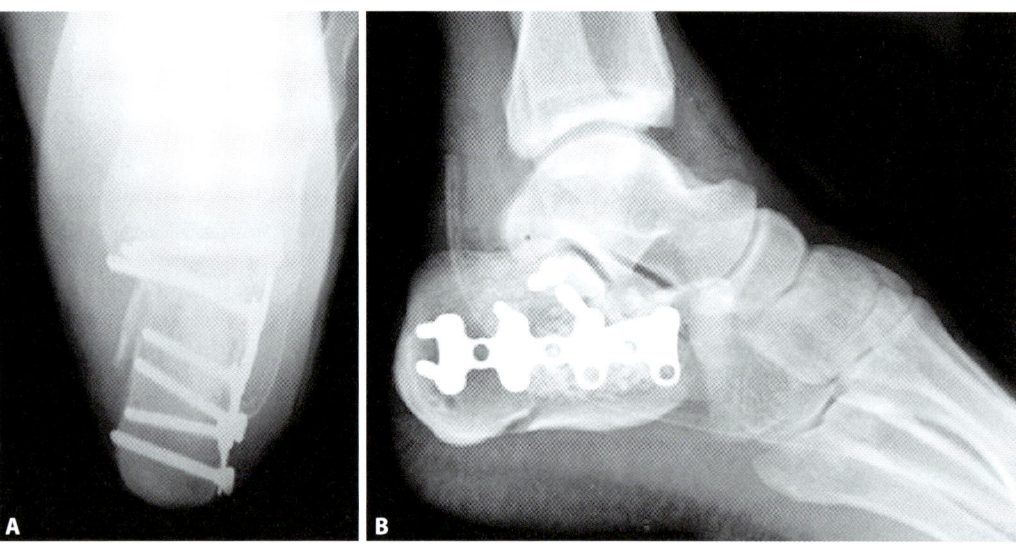

Figs. 6A and B: (A) Axial and (B) lateral roentgenogram of the calcaneal fracture immediately after ceramic augmentation and fixation.

as pointed out in the preceding sections. The biomechanical rationale is self-evident. The posterior subtalar joint, which consistently gets depressed during the trauma (in intra-articular fractures), is elevated during the surgery and fixed in place. The articular elevation does leave a large void in the subchondral region that predisposes to late collapse of the subtalar articular fragment. The "neutral triangle" is a trabeculae-free area directly under the thalamic region of the bone that is particularly vulnerable when axial loads are applied. The hypothesis is that during the healing process, patients are typically advised to "not weight bear", and therefore, the restitution (remodeling) of the compression trabeculae would take much longer than the tensile trabeculae that are subjected to muscular, tendinous, and ligamentous pulls even during rest. Since axial load-bearing seems to be the primary function of the os calcis, the load-bearing compression trabeculae are of paramount importance; yet they heal and remodel much later than is desired. All these arguments support the idea of augmentation of the depressed subtalar articular surface with a bone graft or graft substitute. In the foregoing discussion, it is already established that autograft is the gold standard, but significant donor site morbidity and the additional surgical time encourage the search for effective substitutes.[94]

Several cancellous bone augmentation studies were undertaken using the Chitra composite (HA:BG 80:20) involving the tibial plateau, vertebrae, and calcaneum.[89,90] Under strict ethics committee approval, the ceramic was used to augment subtalar articular fractures in six patients who had standard open reduction and internal fixation through the lateral approach. They were allowed immediate nonweight-bearing ambulation and partial weight-bearing

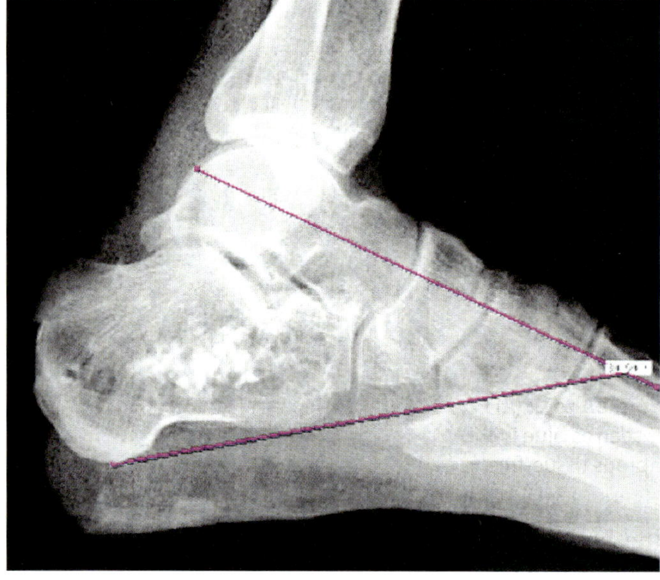

Fig. 7: Lateral X-ray of the calcaneus after removal of implant. Please note excellent restoration of anatomy and incomplete resorption of synthetic graft substitute.

at 6 weeks. Full weight-bearing was started at 3 months **(Figs. 6A and B)**. All the patients had uneventful healing of the surgical wounds and pain-free movements for 1 year. No clinical scoring system was used for outcome analysis though all cases were followed up radiologically for a year. One of the patients who reported for implant removal had histological sampling (with informed consent) of the ceramic bone interphase. The histological pictures correlate well with the radiological images—the HA component of the ceramic is incompletely resorbed at 1 year **(Fig. 7)**. The newly formed bone shows excellent osteonal bone formation with well-formed Haversian systems and the interphase between

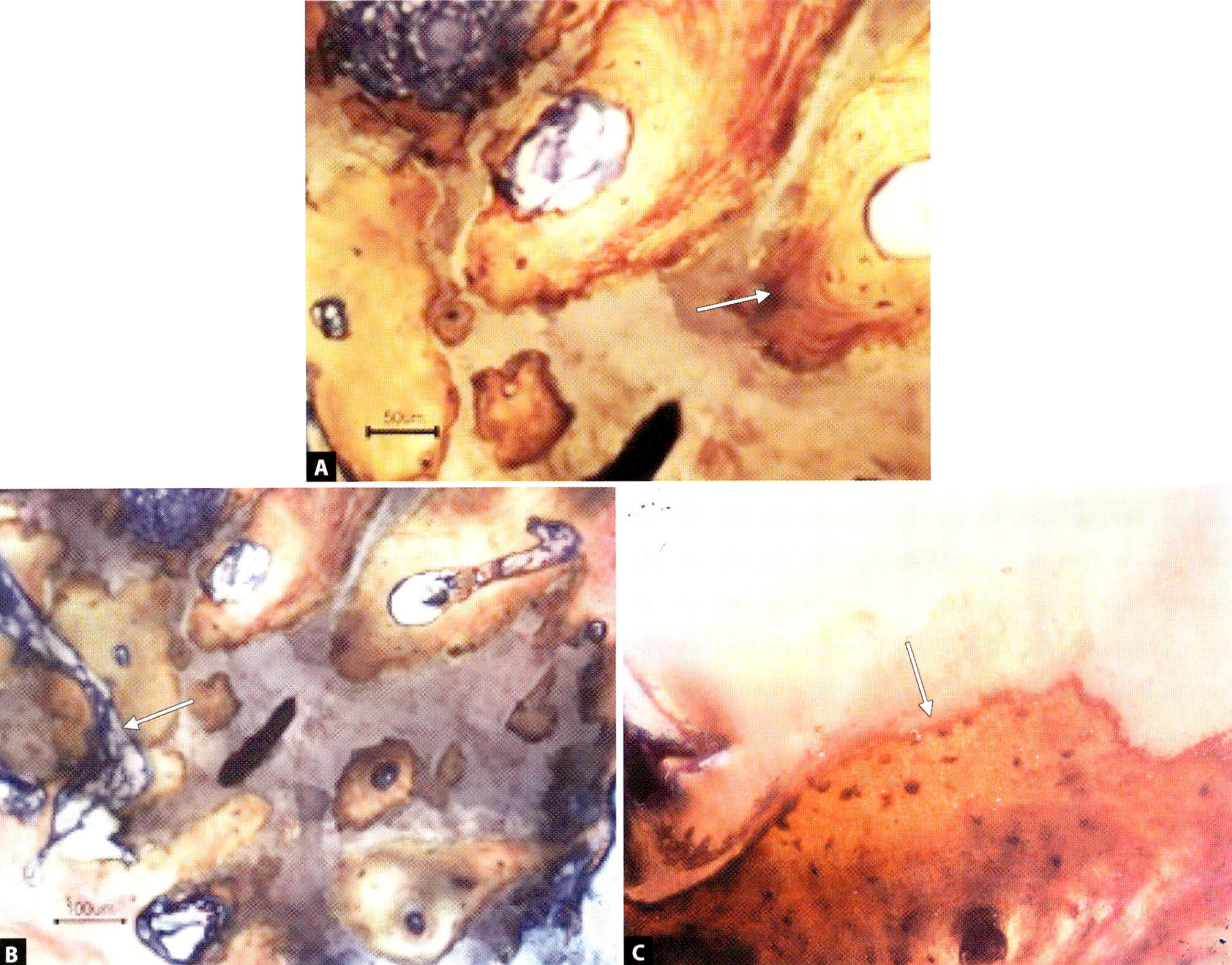

Figs. 8A to C: (A) Histology sample from the calcaneus demonstrating normal Haversian bone formation (white arrow); (B) Residual ceramic is seen as blue in this section (white arrow) amid well-formed bone trabeculae; (C) The ceramic–bone interphase is highlighted here showing fibrous tissue-free healing between the two (white arrow).

the bone and the residual ceramic is fibrous tissue free **(Figs. 8A to C)**. This feature has been established in other cancellous bone tissue as well.

It is indeed debatable whether the functional outcomes differ substantially or whether calcaneus fractures are grafted or not.[95-98] The limited evidence available does show some advantages in terms of structural restoration following bone grafting as demonstrated radiologically[13] by the various measures of calcaneal morphology. The authors are of the opinion that bone grafting does allow early partial and full weight-bearing following these devastating injuries.[14]

■ RECOMMENDATIONS

Controversy regarding the decision to use a void-filling material during the operative treatment of displaced, intra-articular calcaneal fractures continues to cloud the field of

evidence. Not every fracture benefits from the addition of a bone graft or substitute. However, particularly for those constructs that are less rigid and/or have larger bone defects (5–10 cc or larger), they may serve as a means to strengthen fixation and provide mechanical support. Despite the greater availability of increasingly rigid fixation, such as locking plates, certain fracture patterns and voids that extensively involve the neutral triangle may not be amenable to stable fixation without further augmentation. Additionally, these costly implants are not universally applied due to resource availability, economic constraints, or surgeon familiarity. Technical advancement and materials development have moved the choice of void fillers beyond traditional readily accessible autograft, which avoids unnecessary complications. Currently, the most appropriate choice appears to be injectable, bioresorbable ceramic cements, such as the most recent generation of calcium phosphate or HA. These possess the mechanical strength, osteoconductive, and osteointegrative characteristics required to complement fixation in maintaining reduction and allow for timely mobilization. If a graft material is being used to fill this defect, restricted weight-bearing usually is recommended for 8–12 weeks as the calcaneal height collapse may still occur with compressive loads applied prior to this point. Overall, the decision to use a bone graft or substitute during the treatment of these injuries is challenging and dependent on the patient's status, functional needs, fracture pattern, severity, and fixation type, as well as a thorough understanding of the available material options.

■ REFERENCES

1. Palmer I. The mechanism and treatment of fractures of the calcaneus. Open reduction with the use of cancellous grafts. J Bone Joint Surg Am. 1948;30A:2-8.
2. Sanders R, Fortin P, DiPasquale T, Walling A. Operative treatment in 120 displaced intraarticular calcaneal fractures. Results using a prognostic computed tomography scan classification. Clin Orthop Relat Res. 1993;(290):87-95.
3. Sanders R, Gregory P. Operative treatment of intra-articular fractures of the calcaneus. Orthop Clin North Am. 1995;26:203-14.
4. Sanders R. Current concepts review—displaced intra-articular fractures of the calcaneus. J Bone Joint Surg Am. 2000;82:225-50.
5. Schildhauer TA, Bauer TW, Josten C, Muhr G. Open reduction and augmentation of internal fixation with an injectable skeletal cement for the treatment of complex calcaneal fractures. J Orthop Trauma. 2000;14(5):309-17.
6. Barei DP, Bellabarba C, Sangeorzan BJ, Benirschke SK. Fractures of the calcaneus. Orthop Clin North Am. 2002;33:263-85.
7. Thordarson DB, Bollinger M. SRS cancellous bone cement augmentation of calcaneal fracture fixation. Foot Ankle Int. 2005;26:347-52.
8. Huber F, Hillmeier J, McArthur N, Kock HJ, Meeder PJ. The use of nanocrystalline hydroxyapatite for the reconstruction of calcaneal fractures: preliminary results. J Foot Ankle Surg. 2006;45(5):322-8.
9. Johal HS, Buckley RE, Le ILD, Leighton RK. A prospective randomized controlled trial of a bioresorbable calcium phosphate paste (α-BSM) in treatment of displaced intra-articular calcaneal fractures. J Trauma. 2009;67(4):875-82.
10. Böhler L. Diagnosis, pathology, and treatment of fractures of the os calcis. J Bone Joint Surg. 1931;13:75-89.
11. Benirschke SK, Sangeorzan BJ. Extensive intraarticular fractures of the foot. Surgical management of calcaneal fractures. Clin Orthop Relat Res. 1993;(292):128-34.
12. O'Farrell DA, O'Byrne JM, McCabe JP, Stephens MM. Fractures of the os calcis: improved results with internal fixation. Injury. 1993;24:263-5.
13. Parmar HV, Triffitt PD, Gregg PJ. Intra-articular fractures of the calcaneum treated operatively or conservatively. A prospective study. J Bone Joint Surg Br. 1993;75:932-7.
14. Sangeorzan BJ, Ananthakrishnan D, Tencer AF. Contact characteristics of the subtalar joint after a simulated calcaneus fracture. J Orthop Trauma. 1995;9:251-8.
15. Thordarson DB, Krieger LE. Operative vs. nonoperative treatment of intra-articular fractures of the calcaneus: a prospective randomized trial. Foot Ankle Int. 1996;17:2-9.
16. Geel CW, Flemister Jr AS. Standardized treatment of intra-articular calcaneal fractures using an oblique lateral incision and no bone graft. J Trauma. 2001;50:1083-9.
17. Tennent TD, Calder PR, Salisbury RD, Allen PW, Eastwood DM. The operative management of displaced intra-articular fractures of the calcaneum: a two-centre study using a defined protocol. Injury. 2001;32:491-6.
18. Buckley R, Tough S, McCormack R, Pate G, Leighton R, Petrie D, et al. Operative compared with nonoperative treatment of displaced intra-articular calcaneal fractures: a prospective, randomized, controlled multicenter trial. J Bone Joint Surg. 2002;84(10):1733-44.
19. Huang PJ, Huang HT, Chen TB, Chen JC, Lin YK, Cheng YM, et al. Open reduction and internal fixation of displaced intra-articular fractures of the calcaneus. J Trauma. 2002;52:946-50.
20. Sarkar MR, Stahl J, Wachter N, Schwamborn M, Schnettler RWW, Kinzl L. Defect reconstruction in articular calcaneus fractures with a novel calcium phosphate cement. Eur J Trauma. 2002;28:340-8.
21. Howard JL, Buckley R, McCormack R, Pate G, Leighton R, Petrie D, et al. Complications following management of displaced intra-articular calcaneal fractures: a prospective randomized trial comparing open reduction internal fixation with nonoperative management. J Orthop Trauma. 2003;17(4):241-9.
22. O'Brien J, Buckley R, McCormack R, Pate G, Leighton R, Petrie D, et al. Personal gait satisfaction after displaced intraarticular calcaneal fractures: a 2–8 year follow up. Foot Ankle Int. 2004;25:657-65.
23. Bajammal S, Tornetta 3rd P, Sanders D, Bhandari M. Displaced intra-articular calcaneal fractures. J Orthop Trauma. 2005;19(5):360-4.
24. Ibrahim T, Rowsell M, Rennie W, Brown AR, Taylor GJ, Gregg PJ. Displaced intra-articular calcaneal fractures: 15-year follow-up of a randomised controlled trial of conservative versus operative treatment. Injury. 2007;38:848-55.
25. Larsson S, Bauer TW. Use of injectable calcium phosphate cement for fracture fixation: a review. Clin Orthop Relat Res. 2002;(395):23-32.
26. Bibbo C, Patel DV. The effect of demineralized bone matrix-calcium sulfate with vancomycin on calcaneal fracture healing and infection rates: a prospective study. Foot Ankle Int. 2006;27(7):487-93.
27. Bajammal S, Zlowdozki M, Lelwica A, Tornetta 3rd P, Einhorn TA, Buckley R, et al. The use of calcium phosphate bone cement in fracture treatment. A meta-analysis of randomized trials. J Bone Joint Surg Am. 2008;90:1186-96.
28. Longino D, Buckley R. Bone graft in the operative treatment of displaced intraarticular calcaneal fractures: is it helpful? J Orthop Trauma. 2001;15(4):280-6.
29. Thordarson DB, Hedman TP, Yetkinler DN, Eskander E, Lawrence TN, Poser RD. Superior compressive strength of a calcaneal fracture construct augmented with remodelable cancellous bone cement. J Bone Joint Surg Am. 1999;81:239-46.

30. Buckley RE, Tough S. Displaced intra-articular calcaneal fractures. J Am Acad Orthop Surg. 2004;12(3):172-8.
31. Hak DJ. The use of osteoconductive bone graft substitutes in orthopaedic trauma. J Am Acad Orthop Surg. 2007;15(9):525-36.
32. Cassidy C, Jupiter JB, Cohen M, Delli-Santi M, Fennell C, Leinberry C, et al. Norian SRS cement compared with conventional fixation in distal radial fractures. A randomized study. J Bone Joint Surg Am. 2003;85:2127-37.
33. Horstman WG, Verheyen CC, Leemans R. An injectable calcium phosphate cement as a bone-graft substitute in the treatment of displaced lateral tibial plateau fractures. Injury. 2003;34:141-4.
34. Goodman SB, Bauer TW, Carter D, Casteleyn PP, Goldstein SA, Kyle RF, et al. Norian SRS cement augmentation in hip fracture treatment. Laboratory and initial clinical results. Clin Orthop Relat Res. 1998;(348):42-50.
35. Kopylov P, Jonsson K, Thorngren KG, Aspenberg P. Injectable calcium phosphate in the treatment of distal radial fractures. J Hand Surg Br. 1996;21:768-71.
36. Stankewich CJ, Swiontkowski MF, Tencer AF, Yetkinler DN, Poser RD. Augmentation of femoral neck fracture fixation with an injectable calcium-phosphate bone mineral cement. J Orthop Res. 1996;14:786-93.
37. Kopylov P, Adalberth K, Jonsson K, Aspenberg P. Norian SRS versus functional treatment in redisplaced distal radial fractures: a randomized study in 20 patients. J Hand Surg Br. 2002;27:538-41.
38. Giannoudis PV, Dinopoulos H, Tsiridis E. Bone substitutes: an update. Injury. 2005;36:S20-7.
39. Hall RL, Shereff MJ. Anatomy of the calcaneus. Clin Orthop Relat Res. 1993;(290):27-35.
40. Milner P, Burke G. Isolated infarction of os calcis in an adult. Clin Nucl Med. 1993:18;530-1.
41. Andermahr J, Helling HJ, Tsironis K, Rehm KE, Koebke J. Compartment syndrome of the foot. Clin Anat. 2001;14:184-9.
42. Elsner A, Jubel A, Prokop A, Koebke J, Rehm KE, Andermahr J. Augmentation of intraarticular calcaneal fractures with injectable calcium phosphate cement: densitometry, histology, and functional outcome of 18 patients. J Foot Ankle Surg. 2005;44(5):390-5.
43. Leung KS, Chan WS, Shen WY, Pak PP, So WS, Leung PC. Operative treatment of intraarticular fractures of the os calcis—the role of rigid internal fixation and primary bone grafting: preliminary results. J Orthop Trauma. 1989;3:232-40.
44. Banerjee R, Nickisch F, Easley ME, DiGiovanni C. Foot injuries: calcaneal fractures. In: Browner BD, Jupiter JB, Levine AM, Trafton PG, Krettek C (Eds). Skeletal Trauma, 4th edition. Philadelphia: Expert Consult; 2019 [Chapter 61].
45. Csizy M, Buckley RE, Fennell C. Benign calcaneal bone cyst and pathologic fracture—surgical treatment with injectable calcium-phosphate bone cement (Norian®): a case report. Foot Ankle Int. 2001;22:507-10.
46. Dickson KF, Friedman J, Buchholz JG, Flandry FD. The use of BoneSource hydroxyapatite cement for traumatic metaphyseal bone void filling. J Trauma. 2002;53:1103-8.
47. Rammelt S, Barthel S, Biewener A, Gavlik JM, Zwipp H. Calcaneus fractures. Open reduction and internal fixation. Zentralbl Chir. 2003;128:517-28.
48. De Long Jr WG, Einhorn TA, Koval K, McKee M, Smith W, Sanders R, et al. Bone grafts and bone graft substitutes in orthopaedic trauma surgery. A critical analysis. J Bone Joint Surg Am. 2007;89:649-58.
49. Essex-Lopresti P. The mechanism, reduction technique, and results in fractures of the os calcis. Br J Surg. 1952;39:395-419.
50. Soeur R, Remy R. Fractures of the calcaneus with displacement of the thalamic portion. J Bone Joint Surg Br. 1975;57:413-21.
51. Burdeaux BD. Reduction of calcaneal fractures by the McReynolds medial approach technique and its experimental basis. Clin Orthop Relat Res. 1983;(177):87-103.
52. Eastwood DM, Langkamer VG, Atkins RM. Intra-articular fractures of the calcaneum. Part II: open reduction and internal fixation by the extended lateral transcalcaneal approach. J Bone Joint Surg Br. 1993;75:189-95.
53. Letournel E. Open treatment of acute calcaneal fractures. Clin Orthop Relat Res. 1993;(290):60-7.
54. Stephenson JR. Displaced fractures of the os calcis involving the subtalar joint: the key role of the superomedial fragment. Foot Ankle. 1983;4:91-101.
55. Stephenson JR. Surgical treatment of displaced intraarticular fractures of the calcaneus: a combined lateral and medial approach. Clin Orthop Relat Res. 1993;290:68-75.
56. Rush SM. Bone graft substitutes: osteobiologics. Clin Podiatr Med Surg. 2005;22:619-30.
57. Bae HW, Field JS. Bone grafting/bone graft substitutes. In: Lieberman JR (Ed). AAOS Comprehensive Orthopaedic Review. Rosemont, IL: American Academy of Orthopaedic Surgeons. pp. 111-5.
58. American Academy of Orthopaedic Surgeons Physician Task Force. Bone void fillers: a technology overview. [online] Available from http://osteosyntese.dk/wp-content/uploads/2014/11/AAOS-Bone-Void-Fillers-A-Technology-Overview.pdf [Last accessed December, 2010].
59. Gazdag AR, Lane JM, Glaser D, Forster RA. Alternatives to autogenous bone graft: efficacy and indications. J Am Acad Orthop Surg. 1995;3:1-8.
60. Urist MR. Bone transplants and implants. In: Urist MR (Ed). Fundamental and Clinical Bone Physiology. Philadelphia: Lippincott Williams and Wilkins; 1980. pp. 331-68.
61. Bauer TW, Muschler GF. Bone graft materials. An overview of the basic science. Clin Orthop Relat Res. 2000;(371):10-27.
62. Bloemers FW, Stahl JP, Sarkar MR, Linhart W, Rueckert U, Wippermann BW. Bone substitution and augmentation in trauma surgery with a resorbable calcium phosphate bone cement. Eur J Trauma. 2004;30:17-22.
63. Demers C, Hamdy CR, Corsi K, Chellat F, Tabrizian M, Yahia L. Natural coral exoskeleton as a bone graft substitute: a review. Biomed Mater Eng. 2002;12(1):15-35.
64. Lenormant C, Wilmoth P, Lecoeur P. A propos du traitement sanglant des fractures du calcanéum. Bull Mem Soc Nat Chir. 1928;54:1353-5.
65. Wilmoth P. Traitement de fractures du calcanéum. J Med Chir Prat. 1931;102:328-35.
66. Sandhu HS, Grewal HS, Parvataneni H. Bone grafting for spinal fusion. Ortho Clin North Am. 1999;30:685-98.
67. Banwart JC, Asher MA, Hassanein RS. Iliac crest bone graft harvest donor site morbidity. A statistical evaluation. Spine (Phila Pa 1976). 1995;20(9):1055-60.

68. Kurz LT, Garfin SR, Booth Jr RE. Harvesting autogenous iliac bone grafts. A review of complications and techniques. Spine (Phila Pa 1976). 1989;14:1324-31.

69. Auleda J, Bianchi A, Tibau R, Rodriguez-Cano O. Hernia through iliac crest defects. A report of four cases. Int Orthop. 1995;19:367-9.

70. Goulet JA, Senunas LE, DeSilva GL, Greenfield ML. Autogenous iliac crest bone graft. Complications and functional assessment. Clin Orthop Relat Res. 1997;(339):76-81.

71. Abidi NA, Dhawan S, Gruen GS, Vogt MT, Conti SF. Wound-healing risk factors after open reduction and internal fixation of calcaneal fractures. Foot Ankle Int. 1998;19:856-61.

72. Baumgaertel FR, Gotzen L. Two-stage operative treatment of comminuted os calcis fractures. Primary indirect reduction with medial external fixation and delayed lateral plate fixation. Clin Orthop Relat Res. 1993;(290):132-41.

73. Gauthier O, Müller R, von Stechow D, Lamy B, Weiss P, Bouler JM, et al. In vivo bone regeneration with injectable calcium phosphate biomaterial: a three-dimensional micro-computed tomographic, biomechanical and SEM study. Biomaterials. 2005;26:5444-53.

74. Goad MEP, Aiolova M, Tofighi A, et al. Resorbable apatitic bone substitute material, alpha- BSM, is associated with rapid bone regrowth in defects of rabbit tibias. J Bone Miner Res. 1997;12:s518.

75. Kiyoshige Y, Takagi M, Hamasaki M. Bone-cement fixation for calcaneus fracture: a report on 2 elderly patients. Acta Orthop Scand. 1997;68:408-9.

76. De Peretti F, Trojani C, Cambas PM. Le corail comme soutien d'un enfoncement articulaire traumatique: Étude prospective au membre inférieur de 23 cas. Rev Chir Orthop Reparatrice Appar. 1996;82:234-40.

77. De la Caffinière J, Viehweger E, Worcel E. Évolution radiologique à long terme du corail implanté en os spongieux au membre inférieur: Corail madréporique versus hydroxyapatite du corail. Rev Chir Orthop Reparatrice Appar. 1998;84:501-7.

78. Huber FX, Belyaev O, Hillmeier J, Kock HJ, Huber C, Meeder PJ, et al. First histological observations on the incorporation of a novel nanocrystalline hydroxyapatite paste OSTIM® in human cancellous bone. BMC Musculoskelet Disord. 2006;7:50.

79. Galois L, Mainard D, Delagoutte JP. Beta-tricalcium phosphate ceramic as a bone substitute in orthopaedic surgery. Int Orthop. 2002;26:109-15.

80. Knaack D, Goad ME, Aiolova M, Rey C, Tofighi A, Chakravarthy P, et al. Resorbable calcium phosphate bone substitute. J Biomed Mater Res. 1998;43:399-409.

81. Mickiewicz RA, Mayes AM, Knaak D. Polymer–calcium phosphate cement composites for bone substitutes. J Biomed Mater Res. 2002;61:581-92.

82. Wippermann BW, den Boer F, Schratt HE, et al. The resorbable calcium phosphate cement alpha BSM in a sheep tibia segmental defect. Presented at the 45th Annual Meeting, Orthopaedic Research Society, Anaheim, CA; 1999. p. 525.

83. Sarkar MR, Wachter N, Patka P, Kinzl L. First histological observations on the incorporation of a novel calcium phosphate bone substitute material in human cancellous bone. J Biomed Mater Res. 2001;58:329-34.

84. Trenholm A, Landry S, McLaughlin K, Deluzio KJ, Leighton J, Trask K, et al. Comparative fixation of tibial plateau fractures using alpha-BSM, a calcium phosphate cement, versus cancellous bone graft. J Orthop Trauma. 2005;19:698-702.

85. Varma HK, Sivakumar R. Preparation and characterization of free flowing hydroxyapatite powders. Phosphorus Res Bull. 1996;6:35-8.

86. Abiraman S, Varma HK, Kumari TV, Umashankar AJ, John A. Preliminary in vitro and in vivo characterizations of a sol–gel derived bioactive glass–ceramic system. Bull Mater Sci. 2002;25(5):419-29.

87. John A, Varma HK, Kumari TV, Nisha VR. Narayanan D. Cytocompatibility studies of a novel bioactive glass coated porous hydroxyapatite bioceramic for use as a bone substitute. Key Eng Mater. 2005;284-286:317-20.

88. Nair MB, Varma HK, Menon KV, Shenoy SJ, John A. Tissue regeneration and repair of goat segmental femur defect with bioactive triphasic ceramic-coated hydroxyapatite scaffold. J Biomed Mater Res A. 2009;91(3):855-65.

89. Acharya NK, Kumar RJ, Varma HK, Menon VK. Hydroxyapatite-bioactive glass ceramic composite as stand-alone graft substitute for posterolateral fusion of lumbar spine: a prospective, matched, and controlled study. J Spinal Disord Tech. 2008;21(2):106-11.

90. Menon KV, Varma HK. Tibial plateau fractures treated with percutaneously introduced synthetic porous hydroxyapatite granules. Eur J Orthop Surg Traumatol. 2015;15(3):205-13.

91. Dhanakodi N, Thilak J, Varghese J, Menon KV, Varma H, Tripathy SK. Ceramic Bone Graft Substitutes do not reduce donor-site morbidity in ACL reconstruction surgeries: a pilot study. SICOT J. 2019;5:14.

92. Menon KV. Optimisation of mechanical strength of ceramic composites used as bone substitutes. Dissertation submitted to the University of Cardiff UK towards the MSc Orth Engineering degree; 2003.

93. Nair MB, Varma HK, Menon KV, Shenoy SJ, John A. Reconstruction of goat femur segmental defects using triphasic ceramic-coated hydroxyapatite in combination with autologous cells and platelet-rich plasma. Acta Biomater. 2009;5(5):1742-55.

94. Acharya NK, Mahajan CV, Kumar RJ, Varma HK, Menon VK. Can iliac crest reconstruction reduce donor site morbidity?: a study using degradable hydroxyapatite-bioactive glass ceramic composite. J Spinal Disord Tech. 2010;23:266-71.

95. Singh AK, Vinay K. Surgical treatment of displaced intra-articular calcaneal fractures: is bone grafting necessary? J Orthop Traumatol. 2013;14(4):299-305.

96. Zheng W, Xie L, Xie H, Chen C, Chen H, Cai L. With versus without bone grafts for operative treatment of displaced intra-articular calcaneal fractures: a meta-analysis. Int J Surg. 2018;59:36-47.

97. Duymus TM, Mutlu S, Mutlu H, Ozel O, Guler O, Mahirogullari M. Need for bone grafts in the surgical treatment of displaced intra-articular calcaneal fractures. J Foot Ankle Surg. 2017;56(1):54-8.

98. Renovell-Ferrer P, Bertó-Martí X, Diranzo-García J, Barrera-Puigdorells L, Estrems-Díaz V, Silvestre-Muñoz A, et al. Functional outcome after calcaneus fractures: a comparison between polytrauma patients and isolated fractures. Injury. 2017;48(Suppl. 6):S91-5.

20

Complications of Calcaneus Fracture Other than Malunion

Mandeep S Dhillon, Devendra K Chouhan

"I have yet to see any problem, however complicated, which, when you looked at it in the right way, did not become still more complicated".

–Poul Anderson (1926–2001)

INTRODUCTION

Malunion is the most frequent complication seen in the fracture of this important weight-bearing bone, and other issues often complicate the situation. Modern orthopedics has to contend with patients who are living longer, have weaker bones, have limited ability to comply with rehabilitation regimens, and may have medical issues that potentially compound fracture treatment. Additionally, there is significant evidence that smoking interferes with healing of both the bones and the soft tissues, and in the foot, this is no less a problem. This chapter discusses the other major problems associated with calcaneus fractures (although to a lesser extent than malunion), namely wound infection, compartment syndromes, reflex sympathetic dystrophy (RSD), nonunions, and potential neural problems.

COMPARTMENT SYNDROME

Compartment syndrome of foot was first described in 1981 by Mubarak.[1] The foot compartments are less resilient and have limited capacity to expand, so minimal interstitial fluid or extravasated blood can lead to an increase in compartment pressures beyond the threshold. Being a large cancellous bone, there is enough extravasated blood following fractures of calcaneum to establish the cascade of compartment syndrome.[2] The literature documents an incidence of 1–17% of patients who develop compartment syndromes following calcaneal fracture;[1-4] unfortunately, only 50% of these compartment syndromes developing after calcaneal fractures are diagnosed early, while the rest are diagnosed late, usually when they present with "curly toes". Jeffers et al. reported a 6% incidence of compartment syndrome in cases with calcaneal fracture after motorcycle accident.[5] There is no documentation of the incidence of this complication from developing countries such as India, but

the incidence may be significant, and some think more than that published from the developed world, as the problems in many calcaneal fractures may often be unrecognized, and the resources to manage these complications are limited in many centers.

Anatomy, Mechanism, and Pathophysiology

Foot consists of nine compartments: Four interosseous, one medial, one lateral, two central (superficial and deep/calcaneal), and one adductor compartments. Each compartment consists of a neurovascular structure and muscle bound in these osseofascial compartments[6] **(Fig. 1 and Table 1)**.

Like compartment syndromes anywhere else in the body, the problem in the foot shares the same pathophysiological

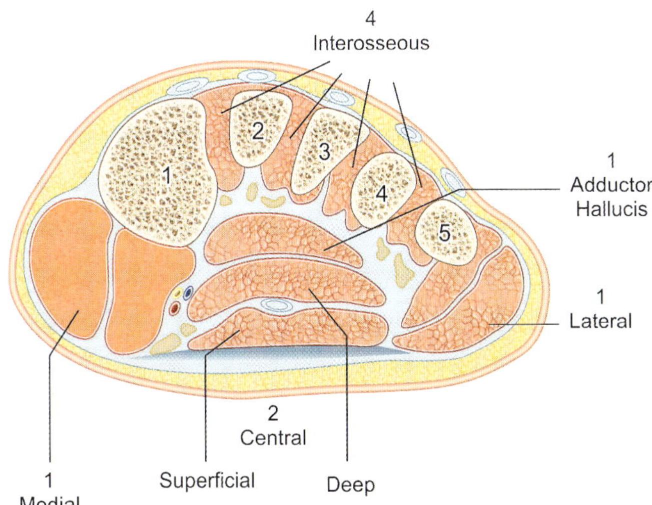

Fig. 1: Nine compartments of foot: Four interosseous compartments, one medial compartment, two central compartments, one lateral compartment, and one adductor compartment.

TABLE 1: Different compartments of foot and structures in each compartment.

Compartments	Muscles	Vessels	Nerves
Medial	Flexor hallucis brevis		
	Abductor hallucis		
Lateral	Abductor digiti quinti		
	Flexor digiti minimi		
Superficial	Flexor digitorum brevis		Medial plantar nerve
	Lumbricals		
	Flexor digitorum longus tendons		
Interosseus (×4)	Interossei		
Adductor	Adductor		
Calcaneal	Quadratus plantae	Posterior tibial artery	Posterior tibial nerve
		Posterior tibial vein	
		Lateral plantar artery	Lateral plantar nerve
		Lateral plantar vein	

pathway. Edema and hemorrhage consequent to primary trauma lead to an increase in interstitial pressure within the soft tissues, lowering capillary perfusion and creating ischemia and potential necrosis. Increasing pressure further hampers tissue perfusion; tissue perfusion ceases once the compartment pressure is within 10–30 mm Hg of diastolic blood pressure. Increased compartment pressure >30 mm Hg leads to insult of both muscle metabolism and neural dysfunction. The decreased perfusion pressure and not mechanical compression causes nerve dysfunction in compartment syndrome. As most calcaneus fractures occur due to high-velocity trauma (described as fall from >8 m in height), the subsequent injury creates pressures inside the foot compartments that are >40 mm Hg.[3,6] Initial neglect following injury can establish the cascade even after low-velocity trauma.

Clinical Presentation

Awareness of its existence, along with a high index of suspicion in cases of calcaneal fractures, are the main factors that guide us toward the diagnosis of foot compartment syndromes. High velocity of injury and associated injury to pelvis (which makes patient hemodynamically unstable) add to the risk. The most important clue for evolving compartment syndrome is pain out of proportion to the injury. Pain on passive dorsiflexion of the toes stretches the intrinsic musculature of the foot in the central compartment (which is commonly involved), exacerbating the pain; however, concurrent metatarsal fractures and midfoot injuries need to be ruled out. The foot is invariably swollen **(Fig. 2)** with shiny skin, and significant bruising along the planter side may be noted. An absent pulse or complete

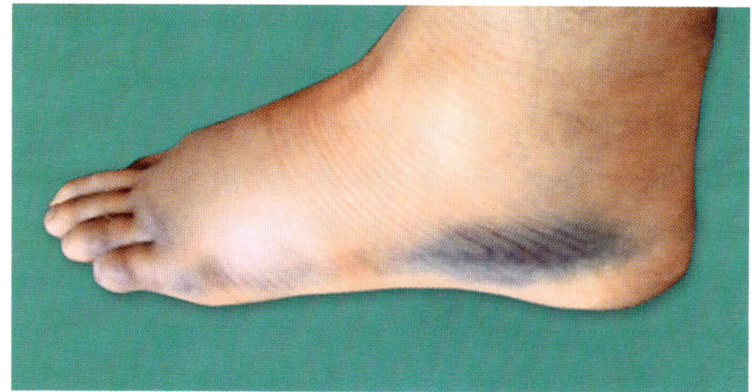

Fig. 2: Swollen foot with bruising over the lateral aspect of heel and toes.

sensory loss are late findings in compartment syndrome and may be difficult to diagnose in the presence of massive swelling. In one series, just 1 in 17 patients with diagnosed compartment syndrome had an absent pulse.[3] Measurement of compartment pressures using specific tools is diagnostic, but it cannot replace a high index of suspicion for early detection of the problem; waiting may establish irreversible damage to myoneural tissues.

Late-presenting patients with established compartment syndrome of foot are seen with clawing of the lesser toes, stiffness, chronic pain, motor weakness, neurovascular injury, and fixed deformities of the foot **(Fig. 3)**.

Treatment

Elevation to the level of the heart is the gold standard to prevent and treat compartment syndromes in the very early stage. Studies suggest that elevation above this level lowers the mean arterial pressure, thus reducing oxygen perfusion.

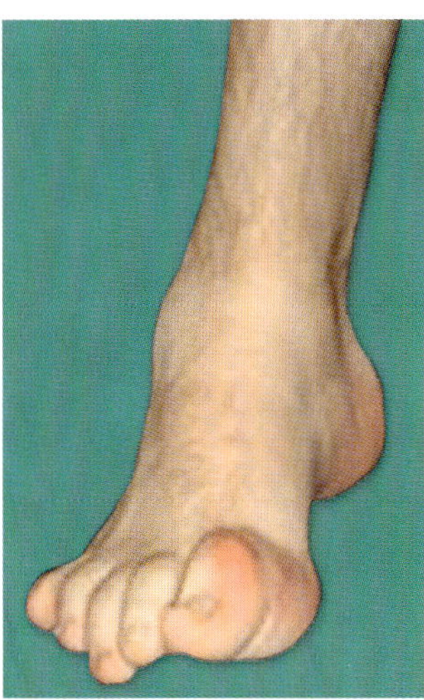

Fig. 3: Clawing of toes following neglected compartment syndrome of foot.

There is some role of modalities to improve venous return, such as pneumatic intermittent impulse compression devices, but these are usually not available routinely in developing countries.

Indications for Fasciotomy

- Patients presenting within 24 hours of developing the signs of compartment syndrome are the best candidates for fasciotomy. Studies suggest that after this time, ischemic changes become irreversible. In fact, recommendations concerning fasciotomy in patients who are seen after 24 hours of injury become less defined. Infection risk from fasciotomy incisions potentially outweighs the risks of further neural or muscle ischemia, and most suggest that fibrosis due to ischemia is inevitable in patients with delayed presentation. The patient's own skin provides the best biologic dressing and should not be violated under these circumstances.[3]
- Fasciotomy should be performed when compartment pressures are 30 mm Hg or greater or 10–30 mm Hg below the diastolic blood pressure in hypotensive trauma patients.[3,4]

Fasciotomy Incisions of Foot

There are multiple algorithms given for fasciotomy in cases with compartment syndrome of the foot. We could use a two-incision (two dorsal incisions) or three-incision (two dorsal and one medial) approach.[6] Whichever approach is used, the aim should be to decompress all the compartments, and to limit the consequences related to wound breakdown.

Dorsal—two incisions, overlying the second and fourth metatarsals. Maintain the widest skin bridge possible and make a blunt approach directly to the metatarsal bones. Do not undermine any skin, due to its tenuous nature. Continue blunt dissection into the web spaces, and deeper spaces decompress the hematoma **(Fig. 4A)**.

Medial—one incision, along the inferior border of the first metatarsal but superior to the abductor muscle. Expose the muscle by incising the fascia from its superior portion and enter the central compartment with further lateral penetration. Retract the abductor muscle superiorly (along with a fascial release, if necessary) and enter the quadratus compartment through the medial intermuscular septum **(Fig. 4B)**.

In general, multiple incisions need to be used if all compartments are involved. The medial approach is sufficient for isolated calcaneus fractures and subsequent central or calcaneal compartment syndrome. All fasciotomy incisions are left open for at least 5 days to enable sufficient dissipation of edema and swelling; at this stage, it is determined whether direct closure is possible or whether a split-thickness skin graft is required. Some authors have suggested applying a split-thickness skin graft at the time of initial compartment decompression to serve as both a biologic dressing (allowing drainage simultaneously) and long-term coverage[3,6] **(Fig. 4C)**.

Outcome

In a series of 14 patients, Myerson et al.[6] described four patients returning to work and resuming preoperative exercise activities. While six patients had occasional symptoms with daily activities or mild discomfort with normal shoe wear, three patients developed contractures with claw toes. In no patient was an amputation necessary. Frink et al.[7] found this in 15 of 33 patients with severe foot injury and associated other severe injuries. Eight of 33 patients had impaired range of motion of the toes or ankle, while three patients needed a free flap, resulting in decreased motor function. Paresthesia and numbness of the scars or distal to the affected compartments were common long-term sequelae in eight patients.

■ NONUNION

Malunion of the calcaneus is the most common problematic issue, and nonunion is fortunately rarely reported in these fractures.[8-11] It is seen more often with nonoperative management. A total of 13 cases were reported in seven publications. However, the problem exists after operative management, and in a series of 157 intra-articular fractures of the calcaneum treated by open reduction and internal fixation (ORIF), Zwipp et al. had a 1.3% rate of nonunion.[8] The problem becomes complex, as nonunion of calcaneum leads to severe deformity of foot, flattening of arches,

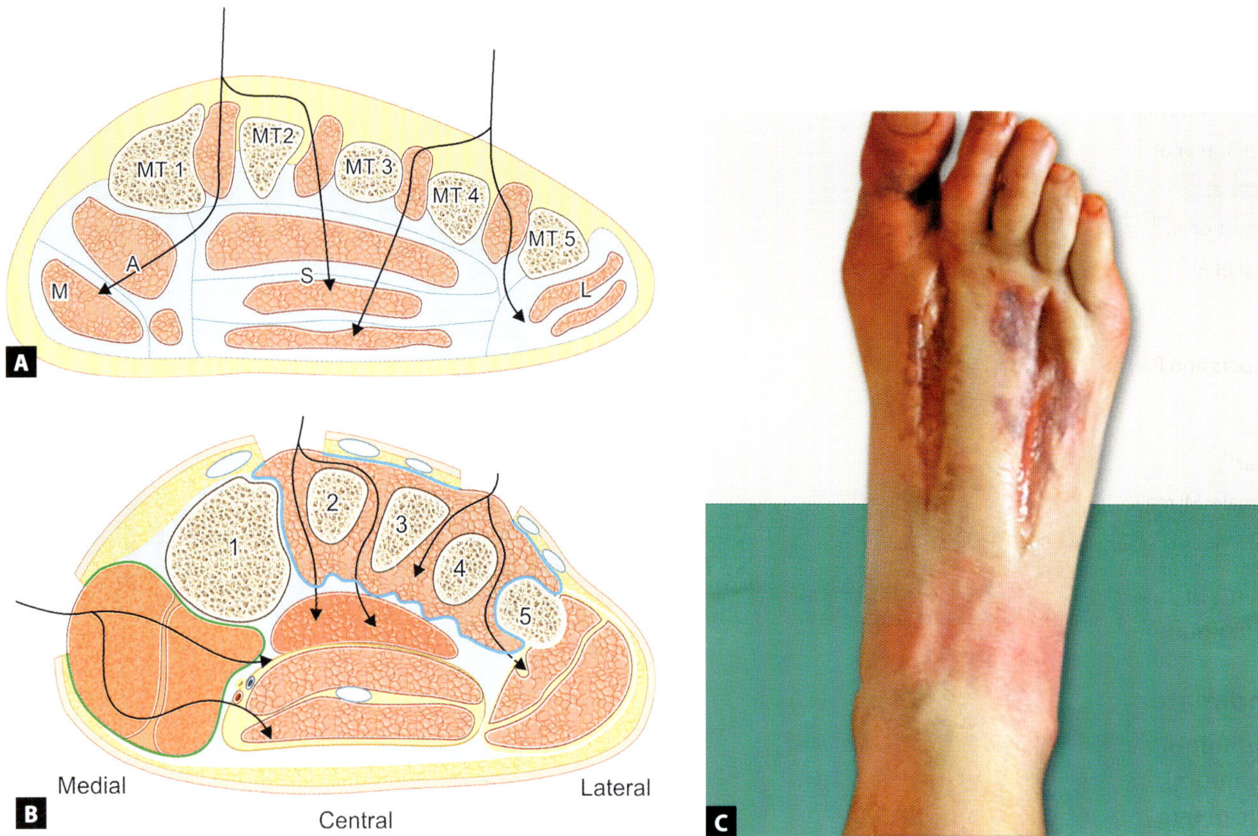

Figs. 4A to C: (A) Two dorsal incision approach; (B) one dorsal and medial incision approach; (C) dorsal compartment fasciotomy. (MT: metatarsal)

widening of heel, and loss of Bohler's angle. The problem is similar to that of a malunion, with the added issue that the bone has not united. Reconstruction of calcaneal nonunions thus becomes challenging, as there is not only difficulty in reconstituting the bony anatomy, but also difficulty in fixation of the fracture, and disuse fragility of the bone does not allow optimum fixation. Added to this is the fact that degenerative arthritis of the subtalar joint may compound the problem; this makes for a challenging situation where all factors have to be taken into account to get a good outcome.

In the senior author's experience over a 1-year period, two cases of nonunion were seen out of 37 calcaneal fractures; one patient was referred from another hospital where he was initially treated conservatively, and the other patient was a grade-2 open fracture, where minimally invasive fixation was attempted using K-wires as stabilizing devices. Following the initial management, both patients had persistent pain even 5 months after injury. Both the patients were diabetic for >10 years, while one of them was an occasional smoker as well.

Risk Factors

Smoking, diabetes, open fractures, and higher severity of injury have all been identified as independent risk factors for wound complications after internal fixation of calcaneal fractures, and it seems reasonable that they would also be risk factors for nonunion.[8-15] In a study by Molloy et al., half of the patients in their series were smokers, and they have identified smoking as a significant risk factor. However, the most significant risk factors for nonunion of a calcaneal fracture appear to be the quality of reduction and the appropriateness of fixation. In 86% of patients in the series mentioned above, the initial reduction and quality of fixation were poor, and the overall alignment gradually deteriorated over time **(Table 2)**.[9]

In a prospective evaluation over 1 year, in a series of 37 patients seen by us, we found both diabetes and inadequate fixation to be important risk factors, as both of our cases with nonunion were diabetic, and both had been less than optimally stabilized.

Nonunion of extra-articular fractures of calcaneum has also been reported; nonunion of the fracture anterior process is somewhat more common as compared to that of sustentaculum tali. Nonunion of the anterior process of calcaneum is documented to be a consequence of missed diagnosis at the initial presentation; the mechanism of injury and clinical presentation may mimic an ankle sprain,[12,13] and

TABLE 2: Nonunion cases: Review of literature.

Author	n	Age/gender	Initial treatment	Comorbidity	Treatment
Thomas and Wilson[12]	1	36/F	Conservative		Osteotomy, bone graft, plate fixation
Thermann et al.[13]	4	49 (mean)/2M, 2F	Conservative		Subtalar fusion
Gehr et al.[14]	1	42/M	ORIF		Osteotomy, bone graft
Karakurt et al.[10]	1	61/M	Conservative	Smoker	Bone graft
Zwipp et al.[8]	2	61 and 45/F	Conservative Percutaneous fixation		Subtalar fusion
Schepers and Patka[11]	2	47 (mean)/1F, 1M	Percutaneous fixation Conservative		Subtalar fusion
Kumar[15]	1	29/F	Conservative	Diabetes mellitus	Subtalar fusion with bone graft

(F: female; M: male; ORIF: open reduction and internal fixation)

the patient may present initially with an established and painful nonunion.

Pathoanatomy

Nonunion of calcaneal fractures can be subdivided into nonunion of intra-articular and extra-articular fractures of calcaneum. Management of nonunion of intra-articular fracture depends on the associated subtalar arthritis and location of fracture site. The more distal the fracture inside the joint, the more difficult the fixation will be. Less than 2 cm of available distal fragment can be considered as cutoff length for sparing the midfoot joints.[9] However, the presence of subtalar joint arthritis makes it difficult to leave the midfoot untouched while considering salvage procedures following nonunion of calcaneus. Deformities secondary to nonunion at the fracture site need to be assessed on preoperative X-rays; importantly, the Bohler's and talar tilt angle need to be addressed while planning the surgery, along with any residual lateral wall widening and tuberosity varus.

Clinical Presentation

Persistent heel pain and an inability to bear weight on the affected limb even after 4–6 months of conservative management or ORIF should raise suspicions of a calcaneal nonunion. However, the clinical diagnosis of malunion and consequent peroneal impingement always stay at the forefront, being much more common, and the nonunion may often be masked, unless specifically looked for. Nonunions of calcaneum are very rare but are more severe issues because of the associated severe deformities of foot, e.g., flattening of arches, widening of the heel, and varus of the heel **(Figs. 5A to C)**. The presence of visible cortical discontinuity on radiograph confirms the diagnosis, and often multiple views in different planes are necessary to pick this up.[10-15]

Management

Radiological confirmation of diagnosis and description of pathoanatomy require various radiographic views supplemented by computed tomography (CT) scans, all of which are important in planning surgery. Lateral radiograph of the ankle is helpful for measurement of Böhler's angle and talar tilt **(Fig. 6)**, while axial views of the calcaneum are required to evaluate the subtalar joint for arthritis changes **(Figs. 7A and B)**. CT scan has been proven to be the best imaging tool for demonstrating calcaneal nonunion and identifying subtalar and calcaneocuboid arthritis **(Figs. 7C and D)**.

Surgical Approach

The surgical procedure is usually similar to that for open reduction or malunion fixation (Chapters 9 and 22). As described in Chapter 9, the lateral extensile approach can be used to address the nonunion. The aim is to obtain subtalar fusion with correction of malunion and fracture healing.

The basic surgical steps are enumerated below:
- Removal of hardware (if any) from previous surgery
- Lateral wall ostectomy if widening of heel is present (Chapter 22).
- Preparation of subtalar joint—fusion with or without bone block to be decided as per talar tilt angle. If significant, distraction subtalar arthrodesis needs to be done using an adequate thickness graft to regain Bohler's angle. If bone block arthrodesis of the subtalar joint is to be performed, a laminar spreader is inserted into the subtalar joint and on to the calcaneal tuberosity, which

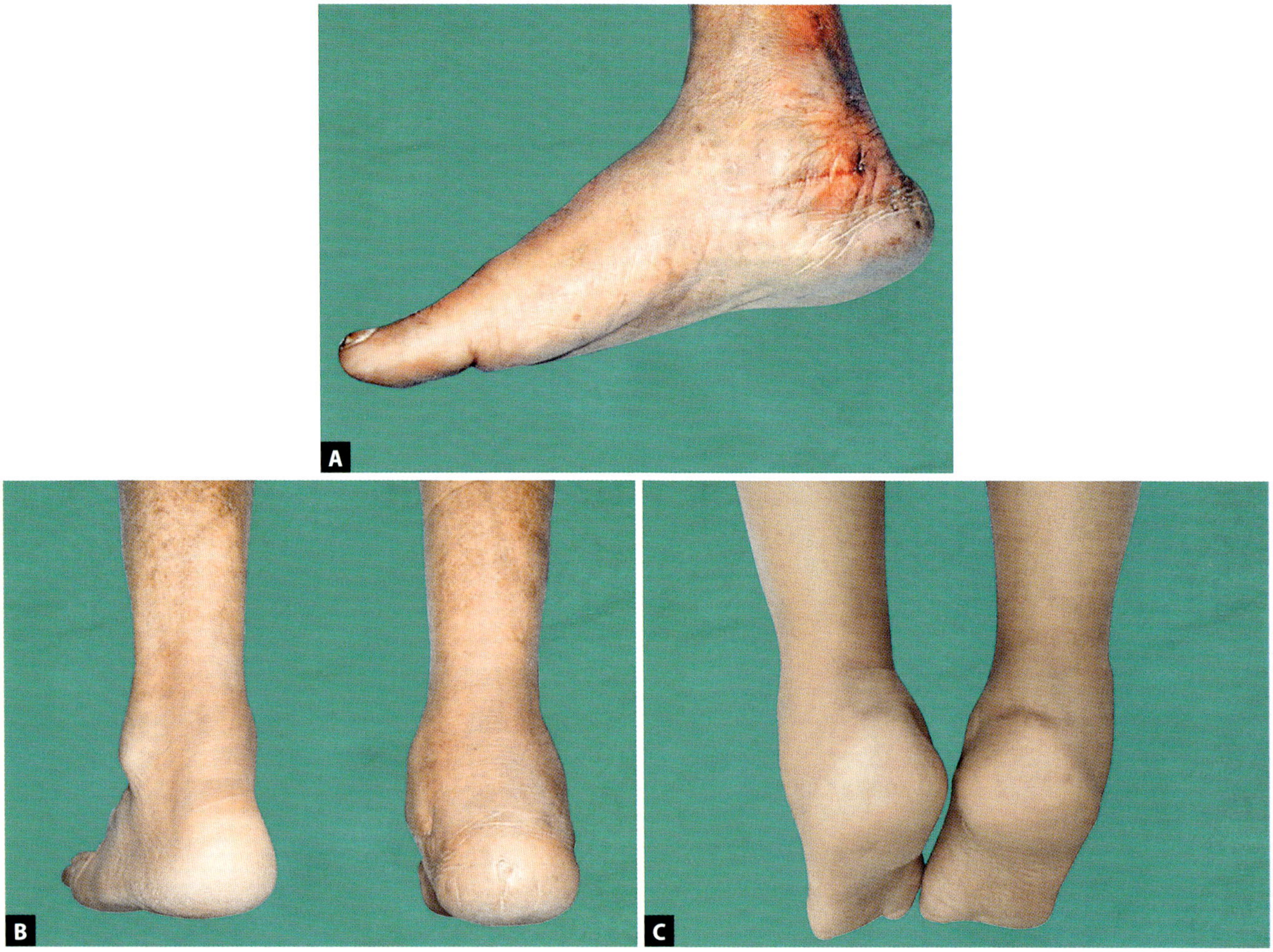

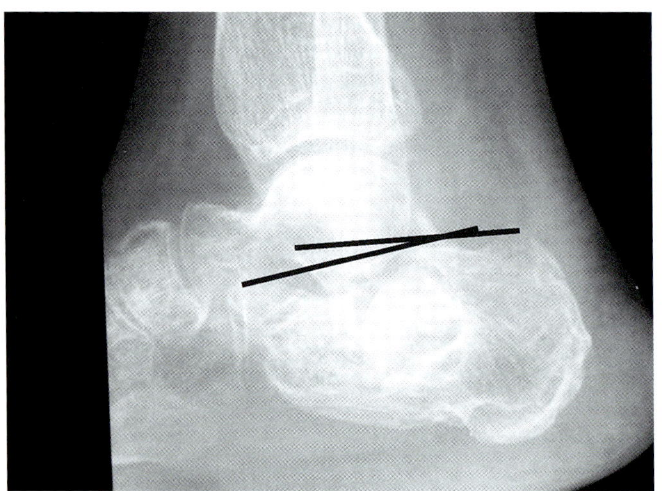

Figs. 5A to C: (A) Nonunion calcaneus with flattening of arches; (B) Nonunion calcaneus showing widening of heel; (C) Varus of heel.

Fig. 6: Loss of Böhler's angle after calcaneal fracture.

percutaneous or open lengthening of the tendo-achilles is often necessary. At this stage, the true size of the defect becomes evident. It is then filled with bicortical structural bone graft, depending on its size and the deformity.

- Preparation of nonunion site—freshening of the nonunion site is required till healthy and bleeding bone is seen; removal of avascular bone pieces, fibrous tissue, etc., is essential. The distal part of calcaneal nonunion is usually very small; so instead of cutting or nibbling, it is better to make multiple drill holes to expose healthy bone. After debridement, we can make a decision about use of bone graft blocks.
- Fixation of the subtalar joint and fracture site can be done using 6.5 mm partially threaded screws (**Fig. 7E**).
- A postoperative below-knee cast is required till healing of subtalar joint and nonunion site.

■ TARSAL TUNNEL SYNDROME

Tarsal tunnel syndrome is described as a sensation of paresthesia, dysesthesia, or hypoesthesia inferior to medial

is then depressed toward a more anatomical position. This corrects the altered angle of talar declination. To enable this relative lengthening of the calcaneum, a

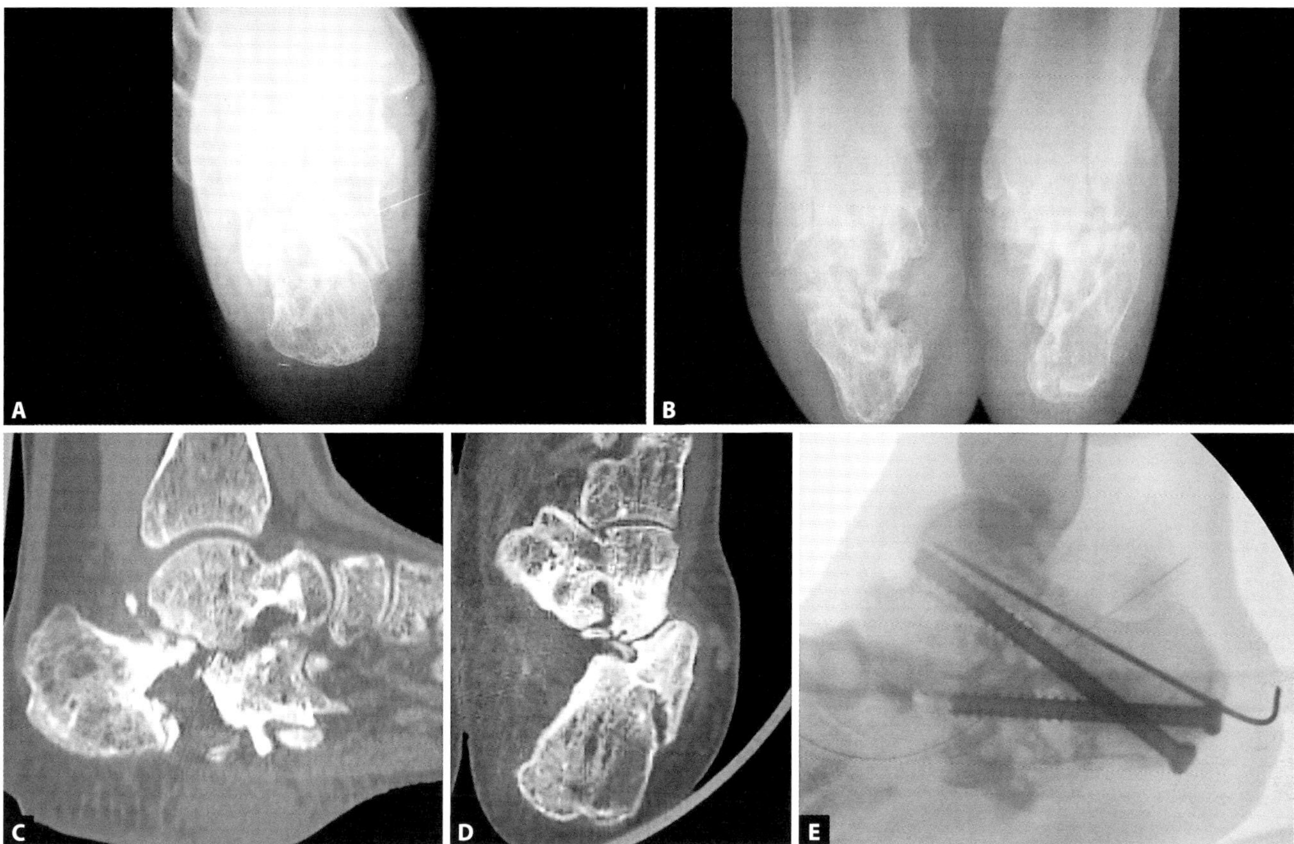

Figs. 7A to E: (A) Axial view clearly defines the ununited fracture line; (B) Bilateral nonunion calcaneus heel in varus; (C and D) Computed tomography (CT) scan showing fracture nonunion; (E) Postoperative images.

malleolus radiating to the heel, medial side of the foot and sole. It is caused by entrapment of the tibial nerve or its branch in flexor retinaculum. Calcaneum forms the medial wall of this fibro-osseous tunnel **(Fig. 8A)**.[16]

Medially open injury or medially displaced fragment, nonunion of sustentaculum tali, or prominent hardware can cause symptoms such as tarsal tunnel syndrome **(Figs. 8B and C)**, either because of direct injury at the time of trauma or secondary irritation.[17,18] Diagnosis can be confirmed by clinical demonstration of Tinel's sign and dorsiflexion eversion test. A radiologically axial view of the calcaneum can demonstrate bony piece or spur in this area. Removal of inciting cause relieves the symptom, but sensory recovery usually lags behind or may not recover.[17]

■ REFLEX SYMPATHETIC DYSTROPHY

Reflex sympathetic dystrophy, or the newer synonym complex regional pain syndrome (CRPS type I), is a pain disorder that develops unpredictably and can follow a minor injury. CRPS type I is not limited to a single peripheral nerve distribution and is associated with edema, changes in skin blood flow, abnormal sudomotor activity in the region of pain, and allodynia or hyperalgesia. In CRPS type II or

causalgia, there is a history of peripheral nerve injury; thus, the pain and autonomic disturbance can be identical to CRPS type I but have a nerve-specific distribution.[19-25] RSD can occur following foot injury with or without bony injury. There is very limited published literature on this subject, so the exact incidence of the problem is not well documented. Both types of CRPS can occur in association with fracture of calcaneum. CRPS type II is more commonly seen in association with open surgery or open injury causing injury to sural nerve on the lateral side or tibial nerve on the medial side.

Diagnosis of this condition is basically clinical. Routine radiography shows soft-tissue swelling and demineralization, which is nonspecific and a late manifestation; to confirm the diagnosis, bone scintigraphy provides a good and effective noninvasive method. In adults, bone scintigraphy demonstrates increased uptake on both blood pool and delayed images, and in children, a decreased uptake in all the phases.[19,24] Magnetic resonance imaging (MRI) can provide supportive evidence for CRPS type I. Soft-tissue changes and bone marrow edema are early changes, and muscle atrophy is present in the disorder at late stages. MRI may also be helpful in follow-up.[23,25]

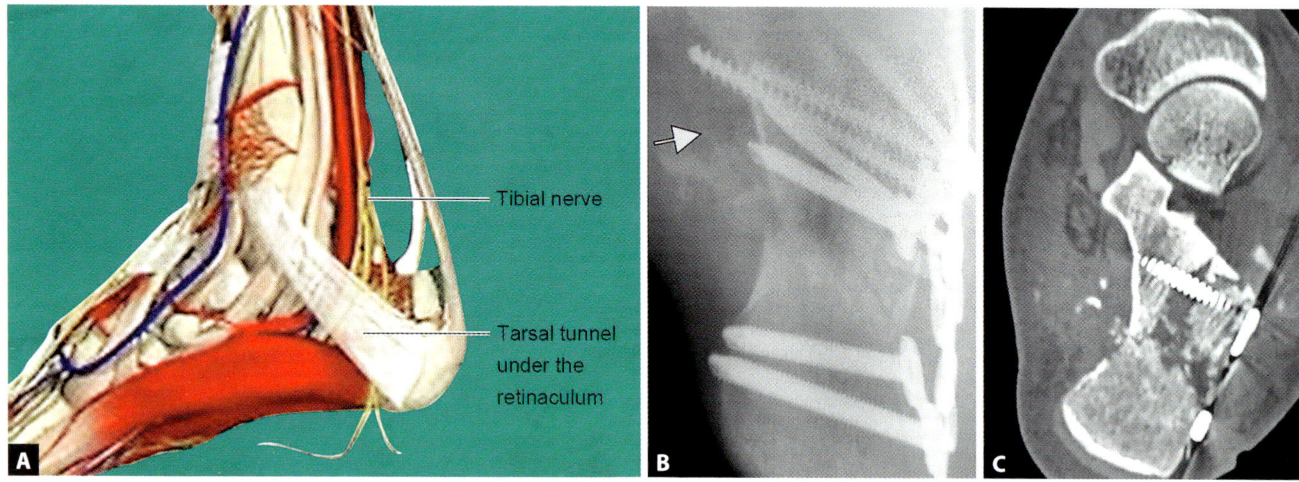

Figs. 8A to C: (A) Anatomy of flexor retinaculum and relation of tibial nerve to calcaneum; (B) Iatrogenic tarsal tunnel prominent screw tip marked with arrow; (C) Postoperative computed tomography (CT) scan after removal of prominent screw.

Treatment

The treatment of CRPS type I includes physiotherapy, drugs (analgesia, antidepressants, anticonvulsants), and sympathetic blockade.

■ INFECTION AND WOUND COMPLICATIONS

In 1958, conservative treatment was advocated for calcaneal fractures following a critical report by Lindsay and Dewar highlighting the complications of surgery and better results with conservative treatment.[27] This viewpoint remained unchanged until the 1980s and 1990s, when a swing toward operative intervention was noted,[28] mainly due to an improved implant profile, better surgical skills, and evolution of surgical techniques. However, postoperative infection and wound breakdown remain a constant worry, inhibiting many surgeons from performing surgical reconstruction for fractures of os calcis.

Review of Gold Standard Evidence

Following ORIF for closed calcaneus fracture, the surgical site infection (SSI) is reported to be as high as 2–25%. The spectrum of infection could range widely from simple marginal necrosis to exposed bone and implant requiring major surgical intervention **(Figs. 9 to 11)**. The consequences of infection after calcaneus fracture are more serious in open fractures, and the reported SSI ranges from 10 to 39%, and some of them land up with amputation. Stephenson reported marginal wound necrosis in 27% of cases.[29,30] Zwipp et al. reported wound margin necrosis in 8.5% of cases, hematomas requiring decompression in 2.6%, and a 2% "deep" infection rate, with a 1% calcanectomy rate.[8] Sanders et al., in a series of 120 surgically managed patients, reported eight wound dehiscences, three below-knee amputations, and five myocutaneous free flaps to cover wounds.[31] Folk et al., in a series of 190 fractures, noted that 25% developed some forms of wound complications, 40 of whom (21%) developed a wound complication that required surgical treatment. Out of this group of 40 surgically treated wound complications, 36 required surgical wound debridement, 22 required hardware removal, and 11 eventually required free myocutaneous flap coverage of the wound. Four went on to amputations.[32] On the other hand, Benirschke and Sangeorzan reported only two deep infections requiring hardware removal in a series of 80 surgically managed calcaneus fractures.[33] In the experience of Macey et al.,[34] skin loss at the wound margin is the most common complication and occurs in approximately 10% of patients. This problem responds well to daily dressing changes on an outpatient basis. The incidence of superficial wound infection was <2%, and deep infection requiring hardware removal was not encountered. Familiarity with the surgical technique and the demand for meticulous handling of soft tissues during this approach are critical factors in achieving a successful result and avoiding postoperative complications.[34] Howard et al. reported that infections and wound breakdown are the most devastating complications of displaced intra-articular calcaneal fracture (DIACF) surgery.[35] Letournel had 3% of wound-related issues in their series.[36]

Prevention of wound complications needs planning right from the start and begins with choosing the management plan. Folk et al. identified smoking, diabetes, and open injury as the three risk factors; our experience has also been somewhat similar. The presence of more than one risk factor increases the relative risk of wound complication requiring surgery. For diabetic smokers, the relative risk of a

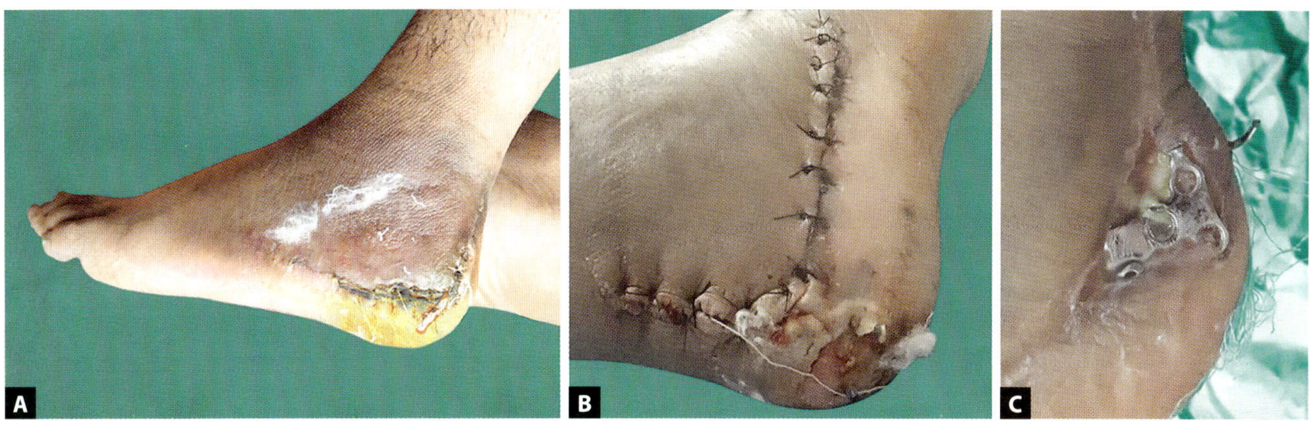

Figs. 9A to C: (A) Blackening of skin margins, and some discharge at the corner of the wound; (B) Suture line necrosis; (C) Exposed implant.

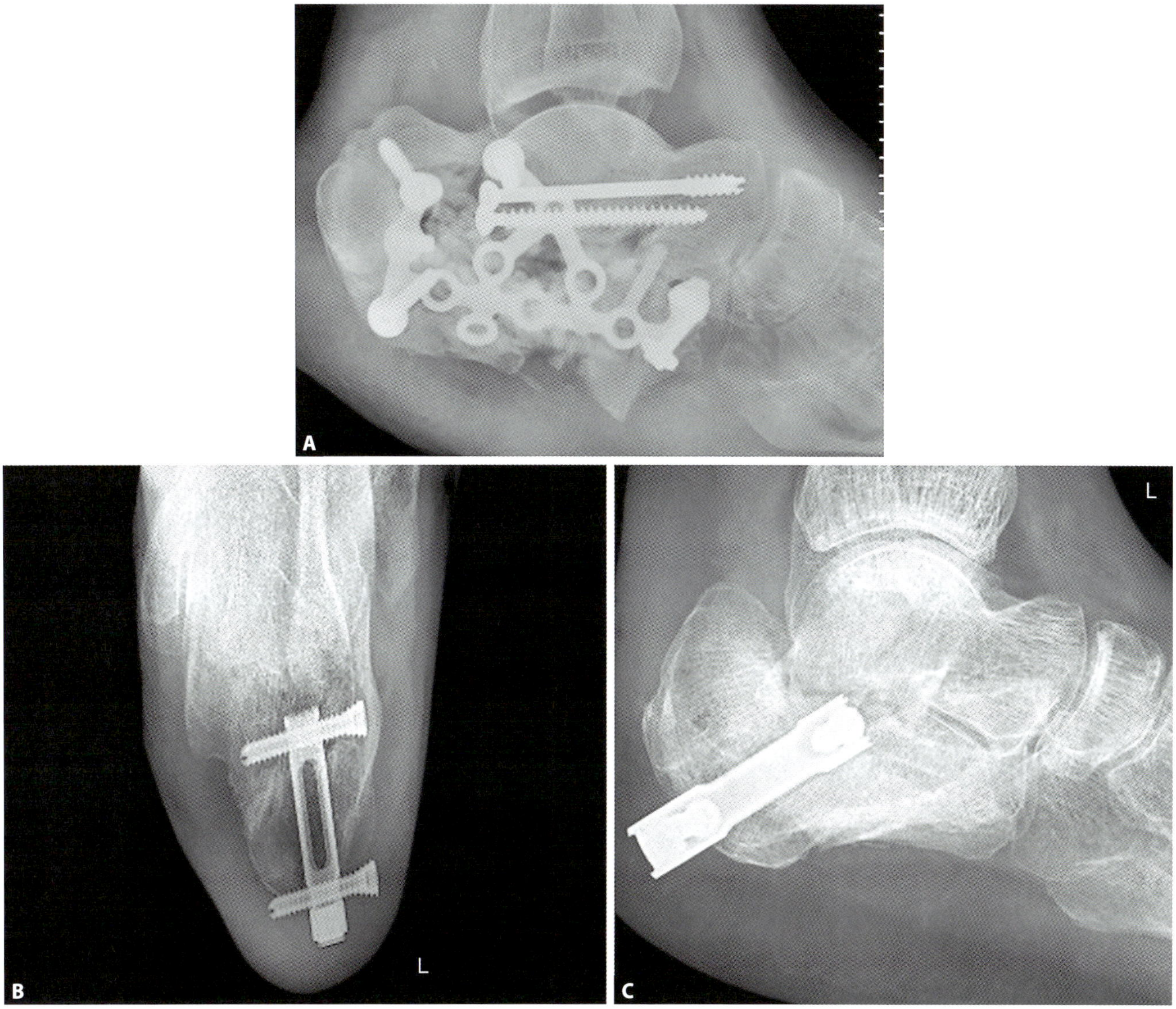

Fig. 10A to C: (A) Non union after fixation of complex calcaneus fracture; (B and C) Axial and lateral view of failed interlocking nailing of calcaneus and nonunion.
Courtesy: J Hermus.

wound complication has been noted to be 3.6; for smokers with open fractures, the relative risk is 3.1. For diabetics with open fractures, the relative risk was documented to be 3.3, and for diabetic smokers with open fractures, the relative risk was 3.2.[31]

Clinical Presentation and Management

Surgical steps and preoperative planning to reduce wound complications are already described in the previous chapters. Wound complications are categorized as follows:

- Wound that responded to nonsurgical management:
  - Wounds with erythema and swelling
  - Wounds with persistent serous drainage 2 weeks after surgery **(Fig. 9A)**
  - Superficial wound dehiscence <1 cm of widening of the surgical incision, with no exposed hardware **(Fig. 9B)**.

These cases can be managed with oral antibiotics for 10 days, daily or twice-a-day dressing on an outpatient basis, and extremity elevation. Vacuum-assisted wound closure (VAC) can be used.

- Wound complications that require immediate surgical intervention:
  - Wound dehiscence with exposed hardware **(Fig. 9C)**
  - Wounds that have drained grossly purulent fluid
  - Wounds that had persistent serous drainage, erythema, and swelling, in spite of a 10-day course of oral antibiotics.

These cases need surgery on an urgent basis. Surgical treatment includes a sequence of procedures as per clinical presentation, e.g., surgical irrigation and debridement, hardware removal, debridement of necrotic bone and cement spacer **(Figs. 10 and 11)**, free myocutaneous flap wound coverage, calcanectomy, and amputation.

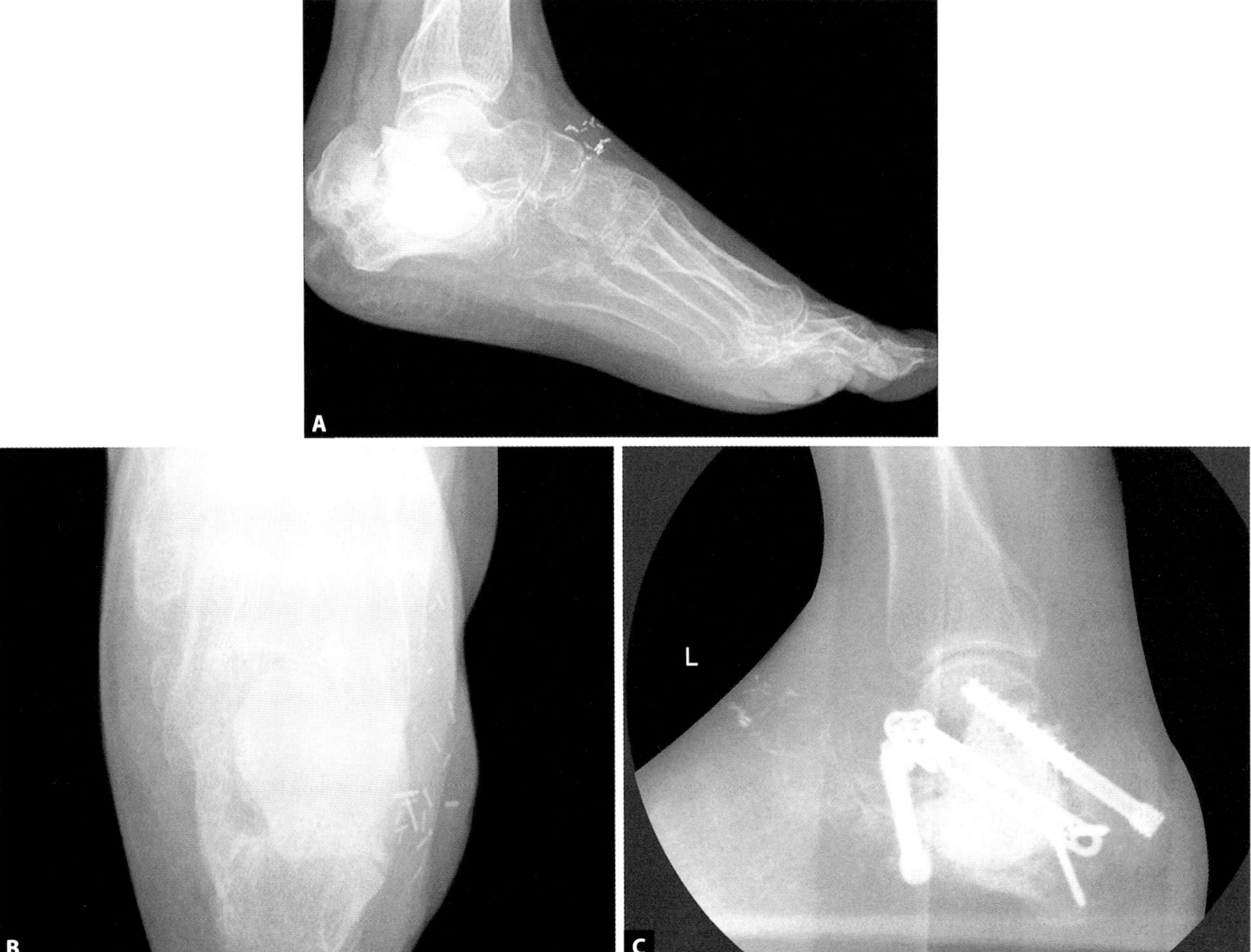

Figs. 11A to C: (A) Lateral and axial view of case (B) With postoperative infection after implant removal addressed by debridement and antibiotic loaded cement spacer; (C) After subtalar fusion.
Courtesy: Joris Hermus.

■ REFERENCES

1. Mubarak SJ. Lower extremity compartment syndromes: treatment. In: Mubarak SJ, Hargens AR (Eds). Compartment syndromes and Volkmann's contracture. Philadelphia: WB Saunders; 1981. pp. 163-4.
2. Mittlmeier T, Mächler G, Lob G, Mutschler W, Bauer G, Vogl T. Compartment syndrome of the foot after intraarticular calcaneal fracture. Clin Orthop Relat Res. 1991;(269):241-8.
3. Steven LH. Managing risk: compartment syndromes of foot. AAOS Now. 2007.
4. Kalsi R, Dempsey A, Bunney EB. Compartment syndrome of the foot after calcaneal fracture. J Emerg Med. 2012;43(2): e101-6.
5. Jeffers RF, Tan HB, Nicolopoulos C, Kamath R, Giannoudis PV. Prevalence and patterns of foot injuries following motorcycle trauma. J Orthop Trauma. 2004;18:87-91.
6. Myerson MS. Management of compartment syndromes of the foot. Clin Orthop Relat Res. 1991;(271):239-48.
7. Frink M, Hildebrand F, Krettek C, Brand J, Hankemeier S. Compartment syndrome of the lower leg and foot. Clin Orthop Relat Res. 2010;468:940-50.
8. Zwipp H, Tscherne H, Thermann H, Weber T. Osteosynthesis of displaced intra-articular fractures of the calcaneus. Clin Orthop Relat Res. 1993;(290):76-86.
9. Molloy AP, Myerson MS, Yoon P. Symptomatic nonunion after fracture of the calcaneum. J Bone Joint Surg Br. 2007;89(9):1218-24.
10. Karakurt L, Erhan Y, Oktay B, Incesu M, Serin E. Pseudarthrosis of a calcaneus fracture: a case report. Acta Orthop Traumatol Turc. 2004;38(4):288-90.
11. Schepers T, Patka P. Calcaneal nonunion: three cases and a review of the literature. Arch Orthop Trauma Surg. 2008;128:735-8.
12. Thomas P, Wilson LF. Non-union of an os calcis fracture. Injury. 1993;24:630-2.
13. Thermann H, Hüfner T, Schratt HE, Held C, Tscherne H. Subtalar fusion after conservative or surgical treatment of calcaneus fracture: a comparison of long-term results. Unfallchirurg. 1999;102:13-22.
14. Gehr J, Schmidt A, Friedl W. Calcaneus pseudarthrosis: a clinical rarity. Unfallchirurg. 2000;103:499-503.
15. Kumar N. Non-union of calcaneum: a rare complication of calcaneal fracture—a case report with brief review of literature. J Clin Orthop Trauma. 2015;6:187-9.
16. Lui TH. Endoscopic excision of symptomatic nonunion of anterior calcaneal process. J Foot Ankle Surg. 2011;50:476-9.
17. Manasseh N, Cherian VM, Abel L. Malunited calcaneal fracture fragments causing tarsal tunnel syndrome: a rare cause. Foot Ankle Surg. 2009;15:207-9.
18. Myerson MS, Berger BI. Nonunion of a fracture of the sustentaculum tali causing a tarsal tunnel syndrome: a case report. Foot Ankle Int. 1995;16(11):740-2.
19. Blombery PA. A review of reflex sympathetic dystrophy. Aust Fam Physician. 1995;24:1651-5.
20. Walker SM, Cousins MJ. Complex regional pain syndromes including "reflex sympathetic dystrophy" and "causalgia". Anaesth Intensive Care. 1997;25:113-25.
21. Phelps GR, Wilentz S. Reflex sympathetic dystrophy. Int J Dermatol. 2000;39:481-6.
22. Murray CS, Cohen A, Perkins T, Davidson JE, Sills JA. Morbidity in reflex sympathetic dystrophy. Arch Dis Child. 2000;82:231-3.
23. Schweitzer ME, Mandel S, Schwartzman RJ, Knobler RL, Tahmoush AJ. Reflex sympathetic dystrophy revisited: MR imaging findings before and after infusion of contrast material. Radiology. 1995;195(1):211-4.
24. Zyluk A, Birkenfeld B. Quantitative evaluation of three-phase bone scintigraphy before and after the treatment of post-traumatic reflex sympathetic dystrophy. Nucl Med Commun. 1999;20:327-33.
25. Botha SH. Reflex sympathetic dystrophy/complex regional pain syndrome, type 1. SA J Radiol. 2004;8:38-40.
26. Degan TJ, Morrey BF, Braun DP. Surgical excision for anterior-process fractures of the calcaneus. J Bone Joint Surg Am. 1982;64(4):519-24.
27. Lindsay WR, Dewar FP. Fractures of the os calcis. Am J Surg. 1958;95:555-76.
28. Ibrahim T, Rowsell M, Rennie W, Brown AR, Taylor GJS, Gregg PJ. Displaced intra-articular calcaneal fractures: 15-year follow-up of a randomised controlled trial of conservative versus operative treatment. Injury. 2007;38: 848-55.
29. Stephenson JR. Treatment of displaced intra-articular fractures of the calcaneus using medial and lateral approaches, internal fixation, and early motion. J Bone Joint Surg Am. 1987;69:115-30.
30. Tscherne H, Zwipp H. Calcaneal fracture. In: Tscherne H, Schatzker J (Eds). Major Fractures of the Pilon, the Talus and the Calcaneus: Current Concepts of Treatment. Berlin: Springer-Verlag; 1993. pp. 153-74.
31. Sanders R, Fortin P, DiPasquale T, Walling A. Operative treatment in 120 displaced intraarticular calcaneal fractures. Results using a prognostic computed tomography scan classification. Clin Orthop Relat Res. 1993;(290): 87-95.
32. Folk JW, Starr AJ, Early JS. Early wound complications of operative treatment of calcaneus fractures: analysis of 190 fractures. J Orthop Trauma. 1999;13(5):369-72.
33. Benirschke SK, Sangeorzan B. Extensive intra-articular fractures of the foot: surgical management of calcaneus fractures. Clin Orthop. 1993;292:128-34.
34. Macey LR, Benirschke SK, Sangeorzan BJ, Hansen ST. Acute calcaneal fractures: treatment options and results. J Am Acad Orthop Surg. 1994;2:36-43.
35. Howard JL, Buckley R, McCormack R, Pate G, Leighton R, Petrie D, et al. Complications following management of displaced intra-articular calcaneal fractures: a prospective randomized trial comparing open reduction internal fixation with nonoperative management. J Orthop Trauma. 2003;17(4):241-9.
36. Letournel E. Open reduction and internal fixation of calcaneus fractures. In: Spiegel P (Ed). Topics in Orthopaedic Trauma. Baltimore: University Park Press; 1984. pp. 173-92.

21

Malunion Calcaneus: Understanding It, Classification, and Treatment Planning

Rajiv Shah, Shivam Shah

"As to diseases, make a habit of two things—to help, or at least, to do no harm".

–Hippocrates (460–377 BC)

■ INTRODUCTION

The calcaneus joins the midfoot and forefoot with the axial skeleton. A fracture of the calcaneus is associated with multidirectional deformations. If these deformities are not understood and not appropriately addressed in the first instance, then malunion will be inevitable. Once malunion sets in, correcting all the elements of malunion are very daunting and with unpredictable end result.[1]

Traditionally, fracture of the calcaneus is treated conservatively either due to fear of complications or due to lack of operative expertise.[2] This results in malunion leading to multiple problems. More often than not, the fracture of the calcaneus is intra-articular and needs accurate reduction as at other places in the body.[3]

Understanding of surgical anatomy of calcaneus and anatomy of the malunion is apt for the successful planning of the treatment.

▌SURGICAL ANATOMY AND ANATOMY OF THE MALUNION

The calcaneus has three articular facets: anterior, middle, and posterior. The anterior facet lies anterolaterally and articulates with the cuboid. The small middle facet articulates with the head of the talus. In contrast, the more significant and most crucial posterior facet articulates with the body of talus superiorly, forming the subtalar joint **(Fig. 1)**. Fractures extending into these articular facets need to be aligned accurately to preserve joint motion and prevent subsequent arthrosis. Malunion of a calcaneus fracture can lead to arthritis of both, calcaneocuboid and talocalcaneal joints **(Fig. 2)**.

The body of the calcaneus has a subcutaneous lateral surface, which is in close relation with peroneal tendons and has the attachment of the calcaneofibular ligament. Burst

fractures cause outward blasting of the lateral surface, which, if uncorrected, will impinge peroneal tendons, resulting in friction and restriction of tendon excursion, which may cause

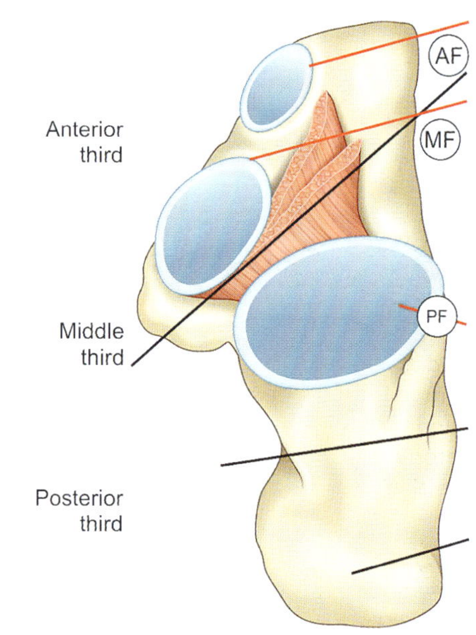

Fig. 1: Calcaneus bone showing the relationship of facets with three parts. (AF: anterior facet; MF: middle facet; PF: posterior facet)

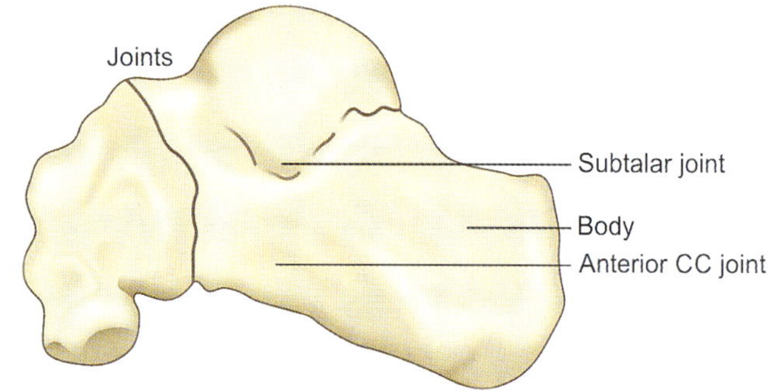

Fig. 2: Articulation of calcaneus forms calcaneocuboid (CC) joint anteriorly and subtalar joint posteriorly.

tenosynovitis and tear. The tendon of flexor hallucis longus (FHL) and branches of the posterior tibial nerve are in close relationship with the medial surface of the bone **(Fig. 3)**. Any fracture involving the medial surface, if not repositioned precisely, can lead to tendinitis of FHL and posterior tibial nerve impingement, resulting in secondary tarsal tunnel syndrome. The posterior end of the calcaneus gives insertion to tendoachilles tendon. Posteriorly displaced fragments can impinge upon the insertion of tendoachilles, leading to painful tendinitis. In severely shattered fractures, there may be a significantly displaced fragment pointing plantarward. This fragment, if not reduced back to its original position, will give pain on walking.[4]

With the vertical compression force, malunion results in a reduction of calcaneus height, shortening of tendoachilles, and relative dorsiflexion of the talus, which in turn leads to restricted ankle dorsiflexion **(Figs. 4A and B)**. In some long-standing cases, the presence of a talar osteophyte may be seen on X-rays due to persistent impingement of the dorsiflexed talus onto the anterior lip of the tibia **(Fig. 5)**. Fractures of the calcaneus may also lead to the deviation of the heel axis due to malposition of calcaneal body fragments, leading to either heel varus or heel valgus. With malpositioned heel, the weight-bearing axis of the body shifts, posing abnormal stresses on the joints above **(Figs. 6 and 7)**.[1]

■ MALUNION—CLINICAL EVALUATION

A thorough clinical evaluation of the deformed hindfoot is the first step toward the planning of the treatment. The patient who presents with significant malunion will complain of pain on locomotion, with restriction of day-to-day activities due to stiffness. Pain while walking on uneven surfaces is the most common complaint and is due to subtalar joint stiffness and arthrosis. Patients also complain of difficulty in wearing shoes due to the deformed and broadened heel, and the lowered malleoli will impinge on regular shoes. Limp, if noted, is usually due to heel shortening. Pain at the first toe may suggest FHL tendinitis.

Location of pain is essential as it will help focus on the problem areas. Pain at the lateral aspect of hindfoot can be due to subfibular impingement and peroneal tendon problems.[5] Pain at the posterior heel is often due to the impingement of tendoachilles by bone. Symptoms such as burning pain may be due to tarsal tunnel compression **(Fig. 8)**.

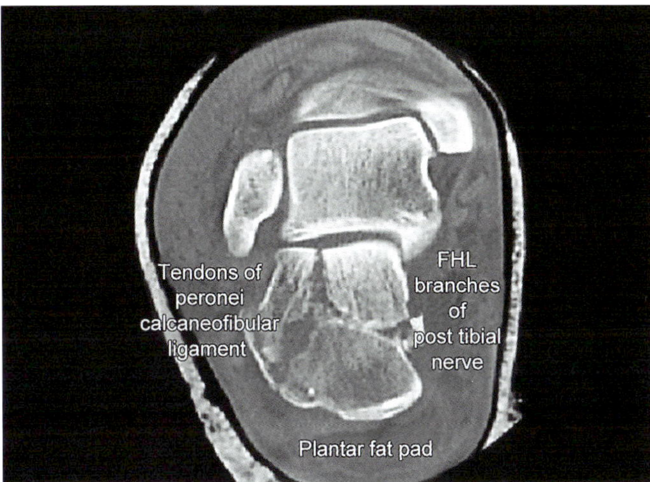

Fig. 3: Computed tomography (CT) scan showing the relationship of calcaneal fracture with surrounding structures. Flexor hallucis longus (FHL) tendon and branches of posterior tibial nerve lie medially. Tendons of peronei and calcaneofibular ligaments are located laterally, and the plantar fad pad is located inferiorly.

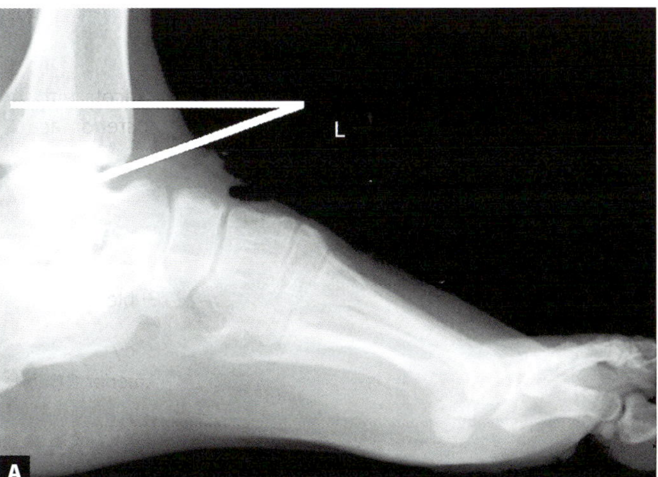

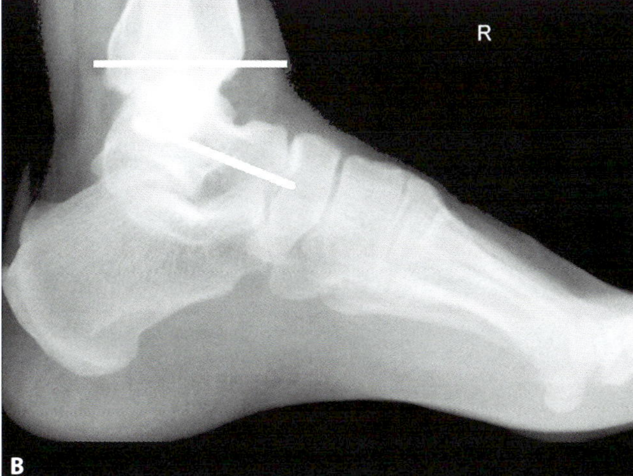

Figs. 4A and B: Radiographs demonstrating reduced dorsiflexion on the left side because of dorsiflexed talus in a malunited fracture of the calcaneus.

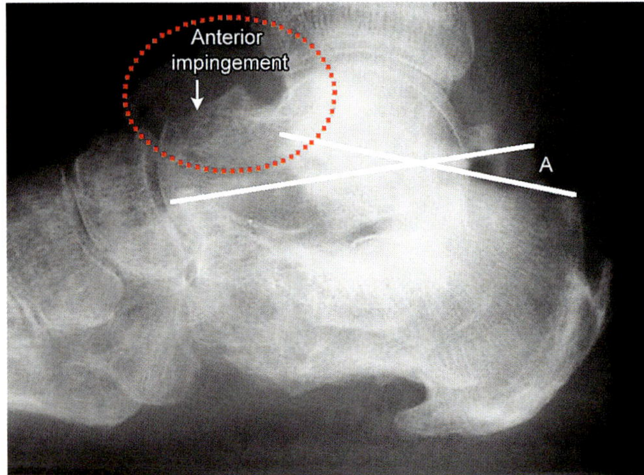

Fig. 5: Malunited fracture of the calcaneus with talar osteophyte due to dorsiflexed talus.

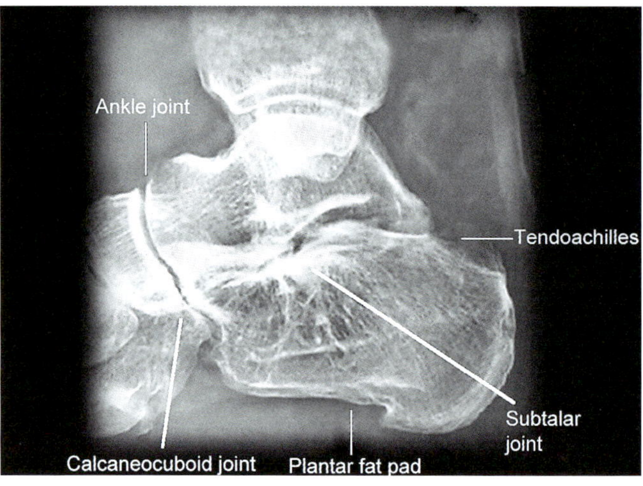

Fig. 8: Possible pain generators in the case of malunion of the calcaneus.

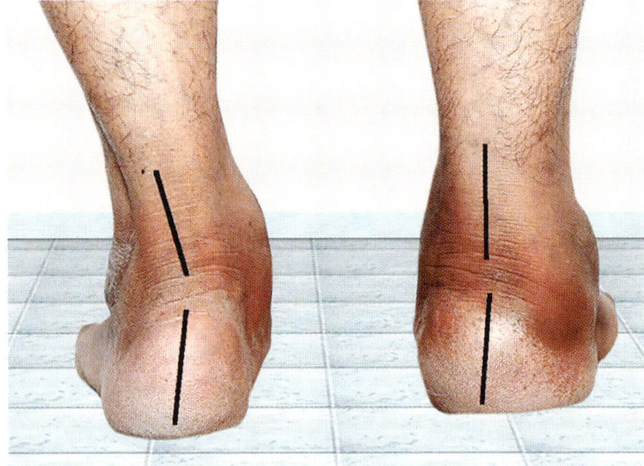

Fig. 6: Clinical photograph of a patient with a right-sided malunited fracture of the calcaneus. Note the position of the right heel, which is in varus. Because of the flatfoot on the left side, that heel is in more valgus.

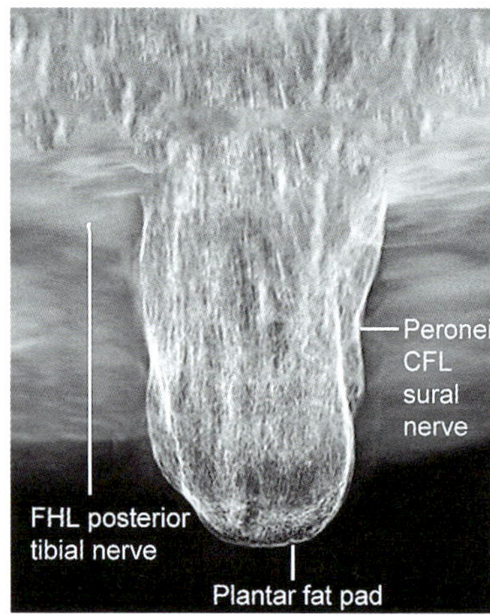

Fig. 9: Axial image of the malunited fracture of the calcaneus showing possible pain generators. (CFL: calcaneofibular ligament; FHL: flexor hallucis longus)

On clinical examination, specific attempts should be made to identify areas of impingement. It is essential to look for the presence of any swellings around the heel and palpate them for bony consistency and tenderness. The bony prominences can be all around the calcaneus, e.g., on the medial, plantar, posterior side, but are encountered most commonly on the lateral side **(Fig. 9)**. The size and shape of the calcaneus are assessed; any scars around the heel and its location and type of healing are noted. The scars could be due to previous surgery or sequelae of open wounds. The tendons surrounding the heel are scrutinized. These are tibialis posterior (TP), FHL, and tendoachilles. The excursion of these tendons is assessed. Any signs of impingement or thickening are also assessed. The examination proceeds toward diagnosing tarsal tunnel compression; when properly looked for, Tinel's sign may be positive in some, and there is a specific history of pain and paresthesia.[6]

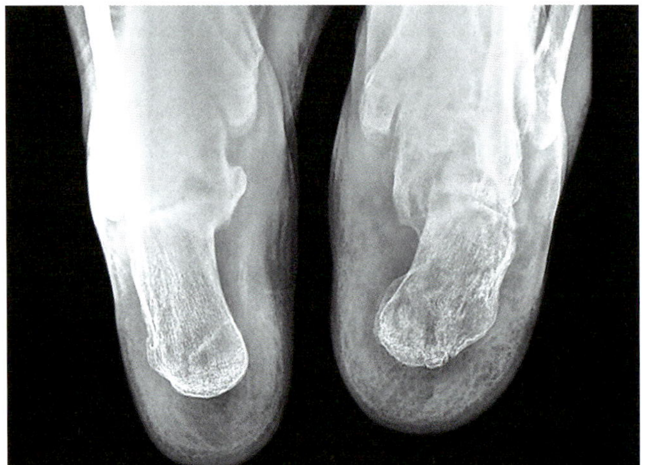

Fig. 7: X-ray picture of the same patient as in **Figure 6** showing an axial image of both calcanei. Note the broadening and shortening of the right-sided calcaneus with varus position.

Evaluation of motion of all the surrounding joints follows next. These include the ankle, subtalar, and transverse tarsal joints. There could be extreme restriction of movements at one or all joints with pain, depending on the time since fracture and duration of malunion. The weight-bearing and nonweight-bearing posture of the forefoot, midfoot, and hindfoot are then assessed to note for deformities such as forefoot abduction or adduction, hindfoot varus or valgus, and also the development of secondary flatfoot **(Fig. 10)**. Physical examination may demonstrate reduced dorsiflexion of the ankle due to tibiotalar impingement. Analysis of gait, surrounding areas such as knee, hip, and back, and evaluation of the patient's footwear cannot be overemphasized. For differentiation of pain arising from adjoining areas,

infiltration with a local anesthetic is needed.[7] For previously operated cases, prominence and impingement by the implant are evaluated. The presence of discharging sinus suggests underlying postoperative infection. The critical positive and negative findings at the clinical examination are recorded, and subsequent correlation with radiological findings is done. The senior author compares the evaluation of a case of a calcaneus malunion with the evaluation of a case of back pain. The essence of clinical evaluation is to find out every possible "pain generators" for a given case, like in a case of back pain.

■ MALUNION—RADIOLOGICAL EVALUATION

Radiology, like clinical evaluation, also forms the essential tool for planning of the treatment. The X-rays include routine foot and ankle series such as anteroposterior (AP), lateral, and mortise views of the ankle and AP and oblique views of the foot. A specific note is made of various bony protrusions, quality of bone, and joint surfaces **(Figs. 11A and B)**. There could be arthritis at various joints such as the subtalar and calcaneocuboid joints **(Fig. 12)**. Long-standing cases may also show an element of disuse osteoporosis.[4] The position and stability of any previously placed implants are noted. The bony prominences are evaluated as this can help for a better understanding of the pressure symptoms caused by the malunion. On the lateral radiographic view, Böhler's angle, talocalcaneal angle, talar declination angle, and the height of the calcaneus are assessed. Böhler's angle indicates the level of posterior facet depression or flattening of calcaneus; the talocalcaneal angle and talar declination angle indicate the deformity of the calcaneus and suggest tibiotalar impingement **(Fig. 13)**.[8] The Harris axial view of

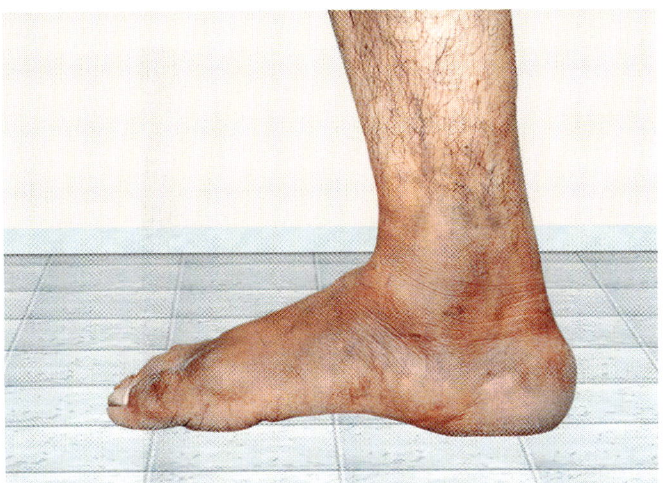

Fig. 10: Clinical photograph of weight-bearing feet showing flattened medial longitudinal arch secondary to malunited fracture of the calcaneus.

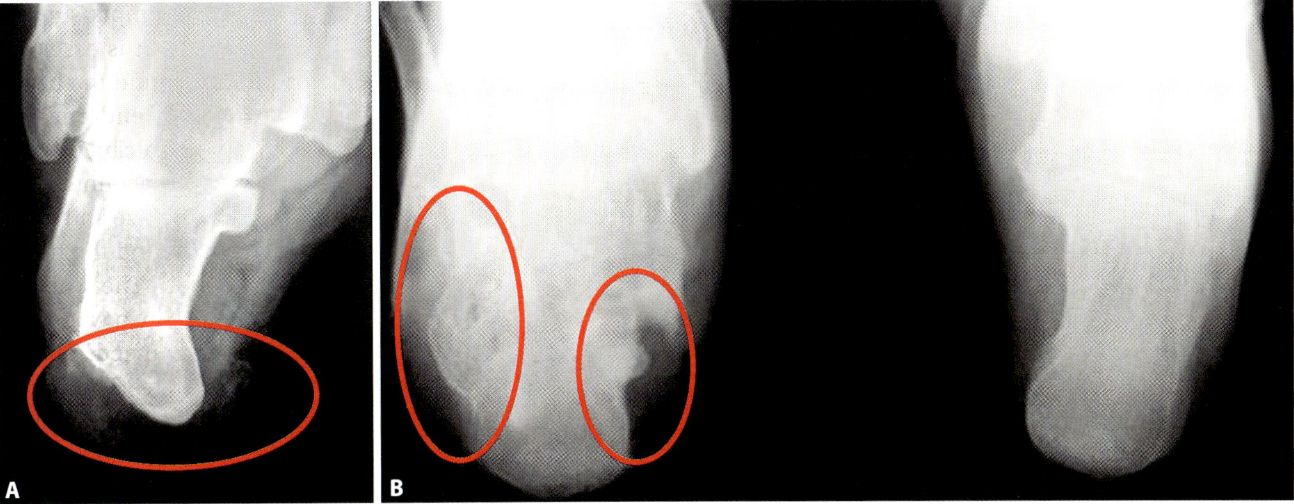

Figs. 11A and B: (A) Axial view showing a plantar bump in a case of malunited fracture of the calcaneus; (B) Similar axial images showing medial and lateral bumps on the right-sided malunited calcaneus fracture.

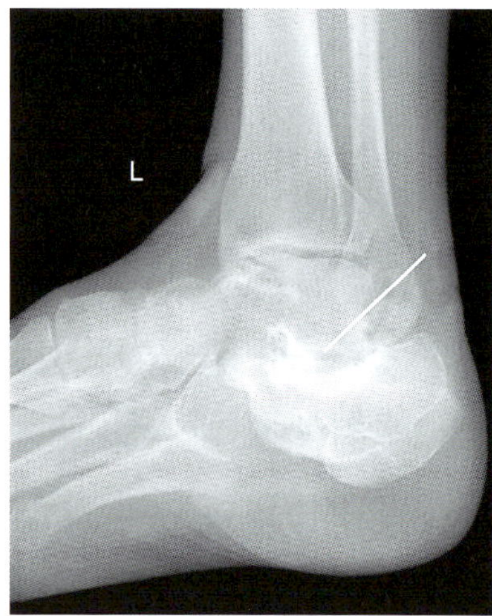

Fig. 12: Subtalar arthritis in the case of malunited fracture of the calcaneus.

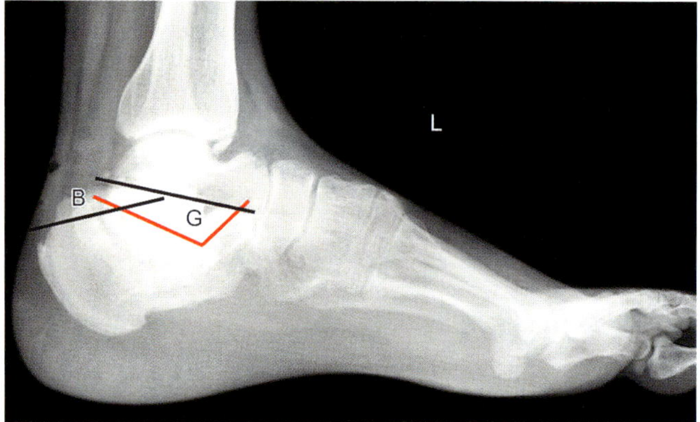

Fig. 13: Both Böhler's (B) and Gissane's (G) angles are abnormal in this case of malunited fracture of the calcaneus.

both heels in one film should be taken for better evaluation of heel height and width; this view defines the relative varus/valgus of the calcaneus and shows the widening of the bone in different directions. It also shows the extent of arthritis of the subtalar joint.[4] This is vital for planning treatment in the absence of computed tomography (CT) scans. Subsequent weight-bearing lateral views of the foot and ankle will demonstrate the position of the medial longitudinal arch and also the amount of talar dorsiflexion. Weight-bearing AP and oblique views of the foot are essential to evaluate the overall structure of the foot and to see for any deformities of the forefoot and the midfoot. These views also help to evaluate the calcaneocuboid and talonavicular joints and show evidence and details of any arthrosis. Hindfoot alignment view helps in delineating the axis of the tibia, talus, and calcaneus. When in doubt, comparative views of the opposite ankle and foot should be taken to evaluate better the status of the joints, deformities, and malunion.[6,8] Broden's view demonstrates posterior facet concerning its depression and any resultant arthritis of the subtalar joint **(Figs. 14A to D).**[7]

Computed tomography scan with three-dimensional (3D) reconstructions has revolutionized our understanding of calcaneal malunions **(Figs. 15A and B).**[8] It has evolved into the most useful and reliable tool. Coronal images at the level of posterior facet were used to develop a specific classification of these malunions **(Figs. 16 and 17).**[5,6,8]

■ CLASSIFICATIONS

Stephens and Sanders, in 1996,[6,8] classified calcaneus malunions based on coronal CT scan images. They described three types of calcaneus malunion **(Fig. 18).**[6,8,9]

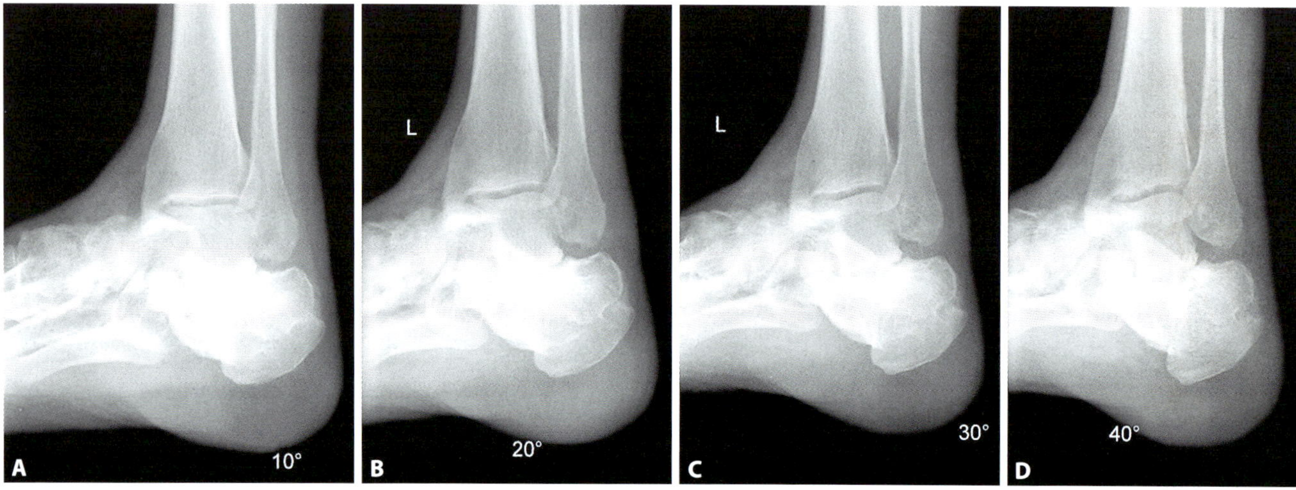

Figs. 14A to D: Broden's views at 10°, 20°, 30°, and 40° showing status of subtalar joint and posterior articular facet.

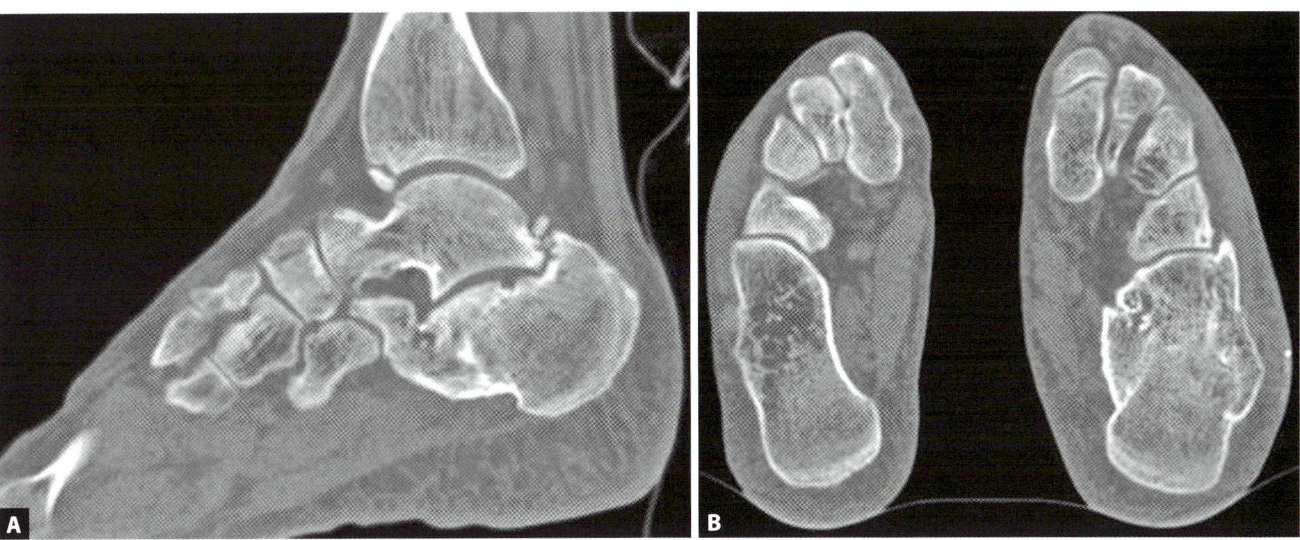

Figs. 15A and B: Two-dimensional computed tomography (CT) scan pictures of the malunited calcaneus. Pictures show heel broadening, shortening with subtalar arthritis, and lateral protrusion.

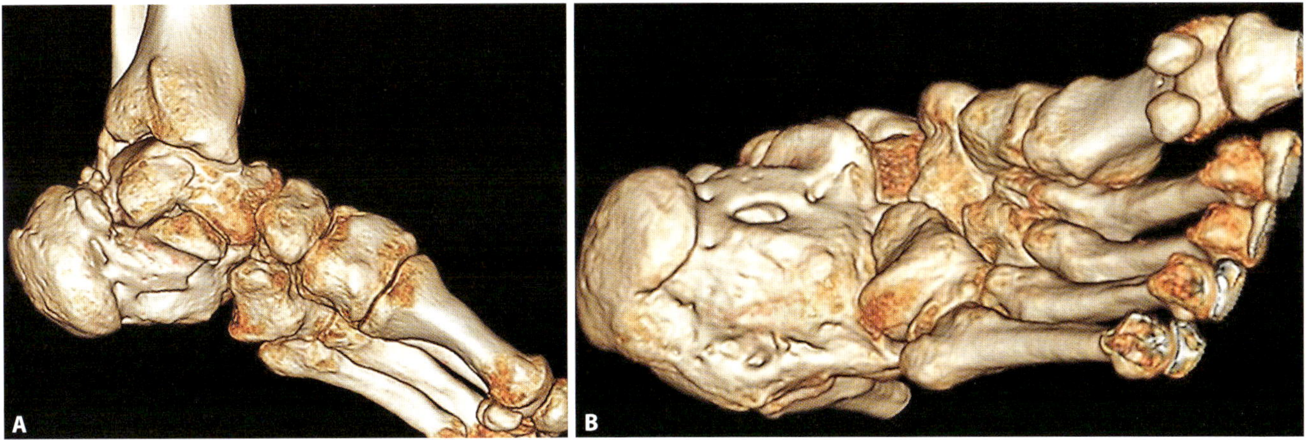

Figs. 16A and B: Three-dimensional reconstruction of the same case showing lateral and plantar views.

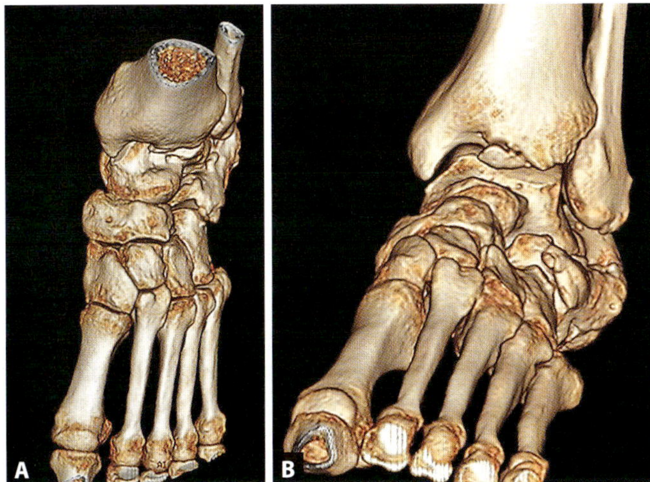

Figs. 17A and B: Three-dimensional reconstruction views of the same case showing projections of foot and subfibular broadening of the heel.

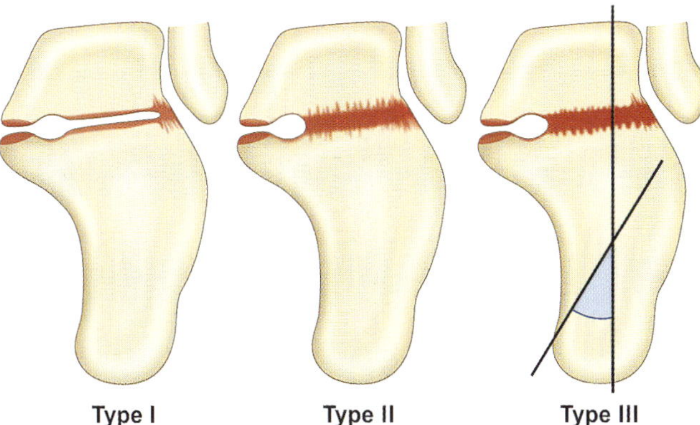

Fig. 18: Stephens and Sanders proposed computed tomography (CT) based classification of malunited fracture of the calcaneus. Types I, II, and III are diagrammatically represented in figures.

Type I: In this subtype, there is no or marginal subtalar joint arthrosis, and there is just protrusion or broadening of the lateral wall of calcaneum.

Type II: In this subtype, over and above lateral wall expansion, there is subtalar joint arthritis involving the whole of the subtalar joint.

Type III: In this subtype, all features of type II are found with an additional feature of malpositioned heel in either varus or valgus.

Stephens and Sanders also suggested a treatment algorithm based on this classification **(Figs. 19 and 20)**.[6,8]

In 2003, Zwipp and Rammelt proposed a deformity-based classification of calcaneus malunions,[10] dividing calcaneus malunion cases into six types, type 0 to type V. Type 0 covered extra-articular malunion cases. Authors also proposed management guidelines **(Figs. 21 and 22)**.

Type 0: Extra-articular malunion without subtalar joint involvement

Type I: Arthritis of subtalar joint

Type II: This subtype has every feature of type I with an additional feature of malposition of a heel in either a varus or valgus

Type III: Additional loss of height of the heel

Type IV: Lateral and upward translation of the tuberosity

Type V: Irregular deformity with deep impaction of the talus into the calcaneus leading to the tilt of the talus in the ankle mortise.

Shortcomings of Classification

The senior author did a retrospective exercise in the form of classifying 65 cases of calcaneus malunion under both

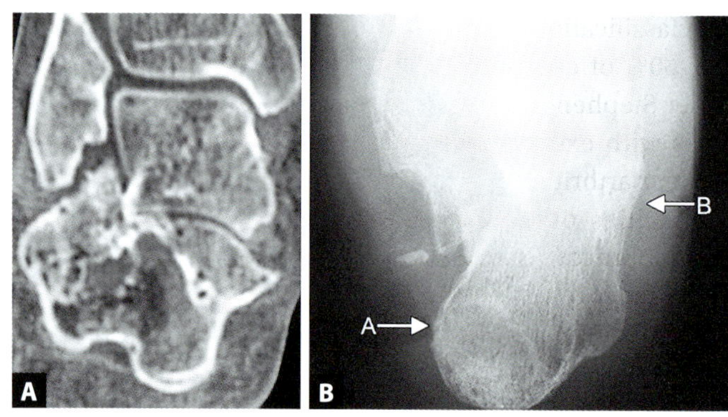

Figs. 20A and B: (A) Computed tomography (CT Scan) and axial x-ray view of patient having type II calcaneal malunion. (B) Arrow A is pointing towards heel valgus deformity and arrow B is pointing towards lateral wall exostosis.

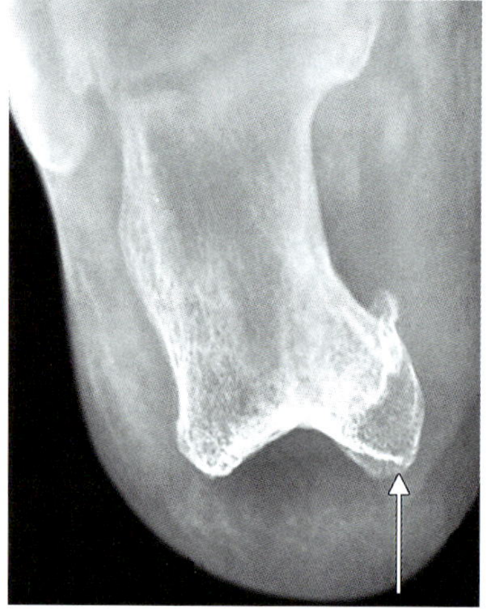

Fig. 21: The axial radiograph of an extra-articular calcaneus malunion classified as type 0 of Zwipp and Rammelt classification. The arrow points at plantar medial exostosis.

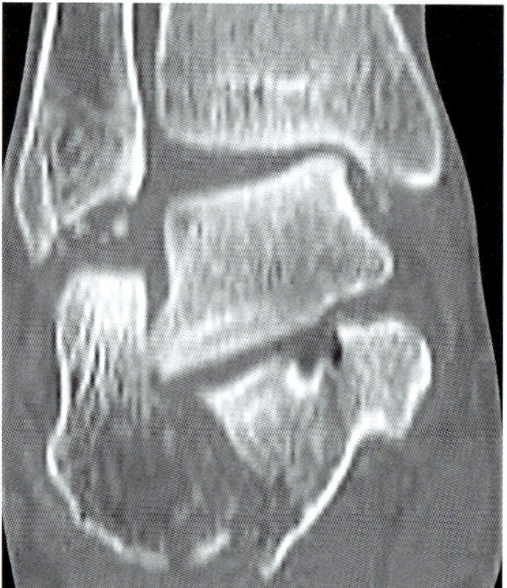

Fig. 22: Coronal computed tomography (CT) scan of type IV calcaneus malunion as per Zwipp and Rammelt classification demonstrating fracture–dislocation of the calcaneus.

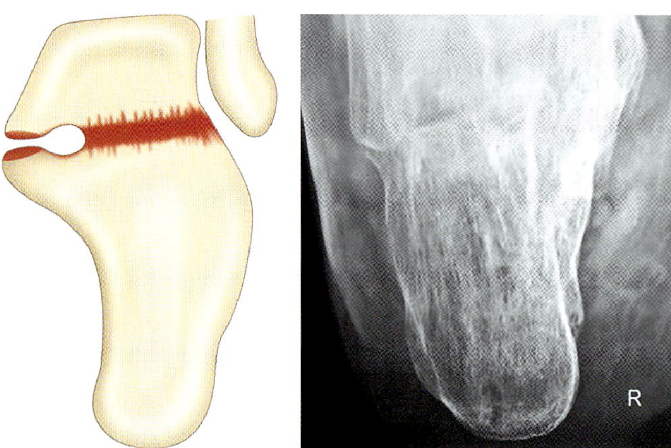

Figs. 19: Example of axial view of a patient having type II malunion of the calcaneus.

the classifications. In an unpublished study, it was noticed that 60% of cases (39 out of 65) could not be classified under Stephens and Sanders classification. These were the cases with extra-articular malunion, arthritis other than subtalar arthritis, exostosis other than lateral wall exostosis, deformities other than coronal plane deformities, and nerve injuries. Cases with claw and hammertoe deformities secondary to healed compartment syndrome and cases with infection and impingement associated with retained implants were also left uncovered by this classification. **Figures 23 and 24** demonstrate two such example cases.

It was further noticed that Zwipp and Rammelt classification also failed to cover 37% of cases (24 cases out of 65). Though this classification did address extra-articular malunion and most of the deformities, it failed to cover cases with arthritis other than subtalar arthritis, deformities such as claw and hammertoes, nerve problems, and problems of infection and impingement associated with the retained implant. **Figures 25 to 27** demonstrate three such example cases.

Till the time an ideal classification system to guide toward treatment is available, it would be worthwhile to document

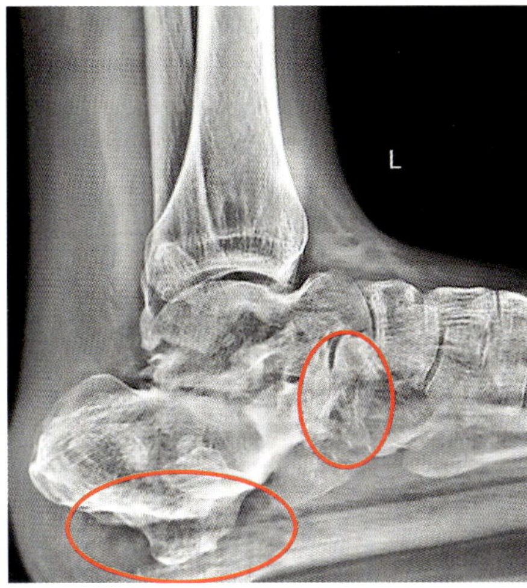

Fig. 23: Lateral radiograph of a patient with calcaneus malunion demonstrating plantar exostosis and calcaneocuboid joint arthritis, elements that are not described in Stephens and Sanders classification.

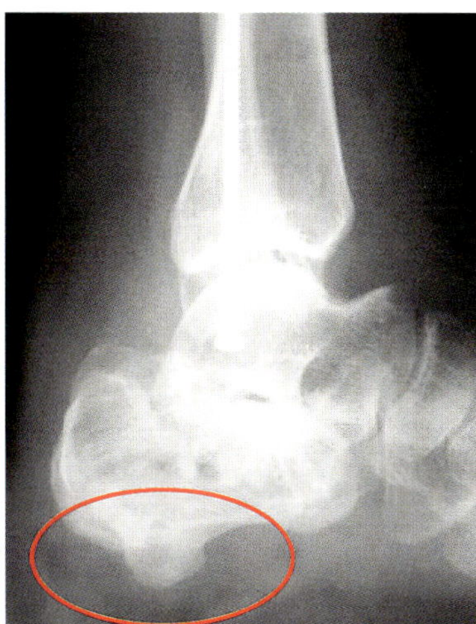

Fig. 24: The plantar exostosis seen in a lateral radiograph of a case of calcaneus malunion is not described in Stephens and Sanders classification.

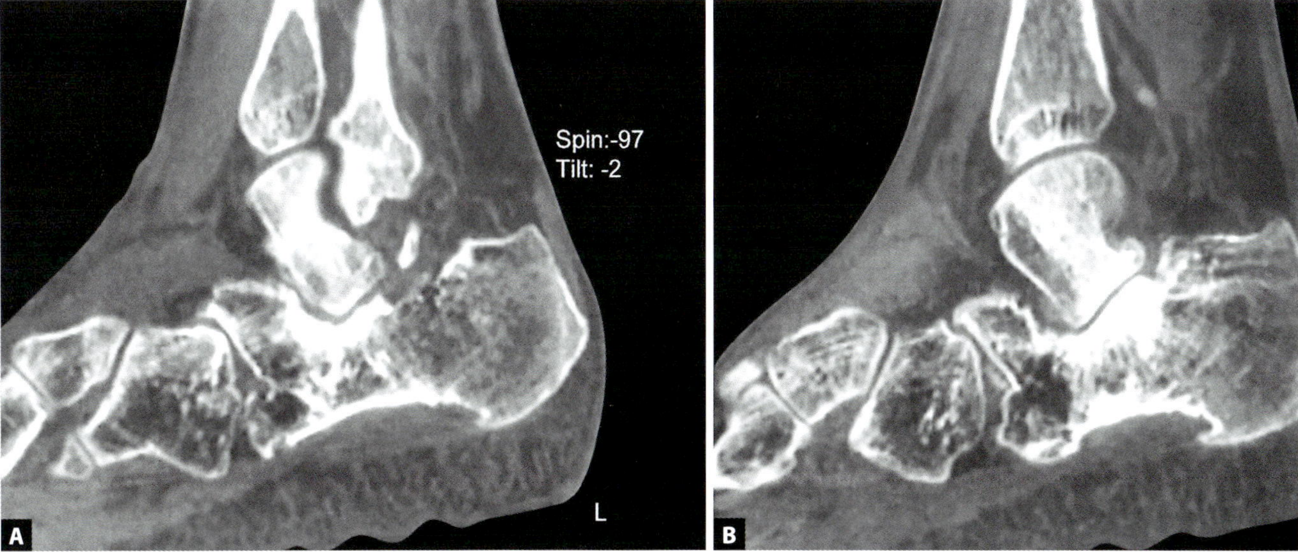

Figs. 25A and B: Sagittal computed tomography (CT) scan pictures of a case of calcaneus malunion demonstrating calcaneocuboid joint arthritis, uncovered under Zwipp and Rammelt classification.

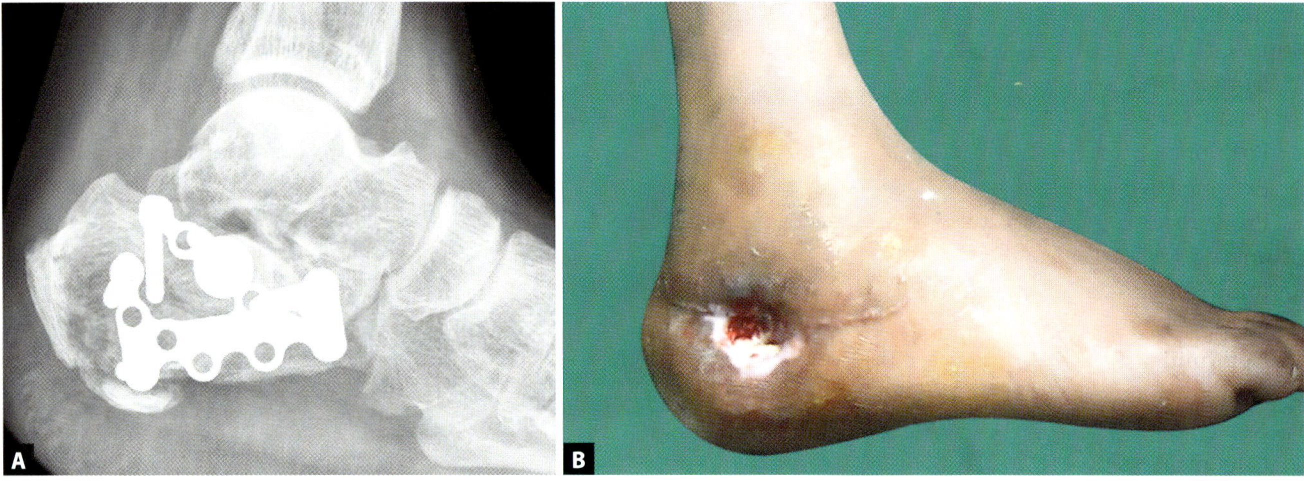

Figs. 26A and B: (A) The lateral radiograph of a patient with calcaneus malunion demonstrating presence of malunion with implants in situ; (B) The clinical picture of the same patient showing wound dehiscence. Issues related to infection and implant are uncovered under Zwipp and Rammelt classification.

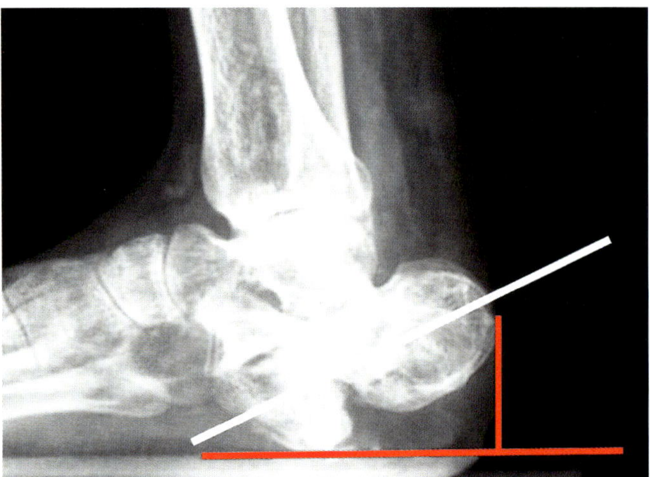

Fig. 27: The lateral radiograph of a patient with a calcaneus malunion demonstrating marked tendoachilles contracture uncovered under Zwipp and Rammelt classification.

TABLE 1: Issues found in calcaneus malunion cases under six groups represented by six alphabets.

A	Arthritis	Subtalar joint
		Calcaneocuboid joint
		Other hindfoot joints
D	Deformity	Heel varus
		Heel valgus
		Shortening
		Talar dorsiflexion
E	Exostosis	Lateral
		Posterior
		Plantar
		Medial
I	Infection and implant	
N	Nerve problems	Sural nerve
		Posterior tibial nerve
		Other nerves
O	Other soft-tissue problems	Tendoachilles contracture
		Toe deformities
		Fat pad atrophy
		RSD
		Others

(RSD: reflex sympathetic dystrophy)

problems noticed in a clinical setting on a paper and to plan treatment addressing each one of them. The senior author proposes to document elements of malunion under six groups, represented by six alphabets. **Table 1** shows the details of such segregation. We have observed that such segregation of pain generators helps in precise planning of treatment where no problem remains unaddressed.

PLANNING OF THE SURGICAL TREATMENT FOR CALCANEAL MALUNION

Every case of calcaneus malunion, to begin with, must be treated conservatively. Failure of all conservative modalities for 4–6 months only sets an indication for surgical management. For a successful planning of surgical management, all significant points in the history, clinical examination, and radiological evaluation should be taken into consideration. It would be worthwhile to document every problem and plan solutions for the same. Our checklist comprises 10 points of significance:

1. Duration of malunion
2. Prior treatment(s) taken
3. Position of previous scars
4. Presence of implants
5. Pressure areas and problems: Medial/lateral/posterior/ anterior/plantar
6. Joint status: Calcaneocuboid/subtalar/talonavicular/ ankle
7. Deformities: Forefoot/midfoot/hindfoot
8. Status of tendons: TP/FHL/tendoachilles
9. Nerve pressure: Sural/posterior tibial/others
10. Quality of the bone.

Before devising a final operative plan, four points of significance are taken into consideration:

1. Approach and incisions
2. Soft-tissue procedures
3. Bony procedures
4. Order and staging of the procedures.

Arthritis of joints is managed with osteotomy, fusion, or osteotomy with fusion. Deformities require corrective procedures in the form of osteotomies or corrective fusions.[8,9] Exostosis is addressed with either the same or separate incisions for decompressive exostectomy. Infection requires serial debridement and implant removal. Nerve problems may necessitate releases, neurolysis, and neurectomy.[11] Soft-tissue procedures need issue-based management. Such management may be in the form of tendon lengthening or correction of deformities. An operative plan must be discussed with the patient as outcomes after surgical management of calcaneus malunion may not be optimum.[9,11]

Case Studies

Here are three example case studies for the exercise for the planning of the treatment of calcaneus malunion.

Case 1 (Figs. 28 and 29)

History and clinical examination: A 49-year-old lady sustained fall and an intra-articular fracture of the calcaneus. She was treated in a plaster cast and subsequently presented after 4 years with complaints of pain and difficulty in walking on smooth as well as uneven surfaces. She also had difficulty sitting on the floor. She felt a bump in her heel, with pain on the outer aspect of the affected heel.

Clinical examination revealed swelling, with tenderness below the fibula and severe restriction of inversion and eversion.

X-ray findings: X-rays showed loss of both Böhler's and Gissane angles, with broadening and shortening of the heel, with prominence on the lateral side. The subtalar joint showed subchondral sclerosis with joint space narrowing, suggesting full-length subtalar arthritis.

Problems: The patient has a calcaneal malunion, giving rise to impingement of the peronei on the lateral aspect with subtalar arthritis. The posterior tuberosity is in a neutral position. Heel shape and heel height are maintained. This case falls in type II malunion as per Sanders classification. Problems are A (arthritis of subtalar joint) and E (lateral exostosis). Treatment is planned accordingly.

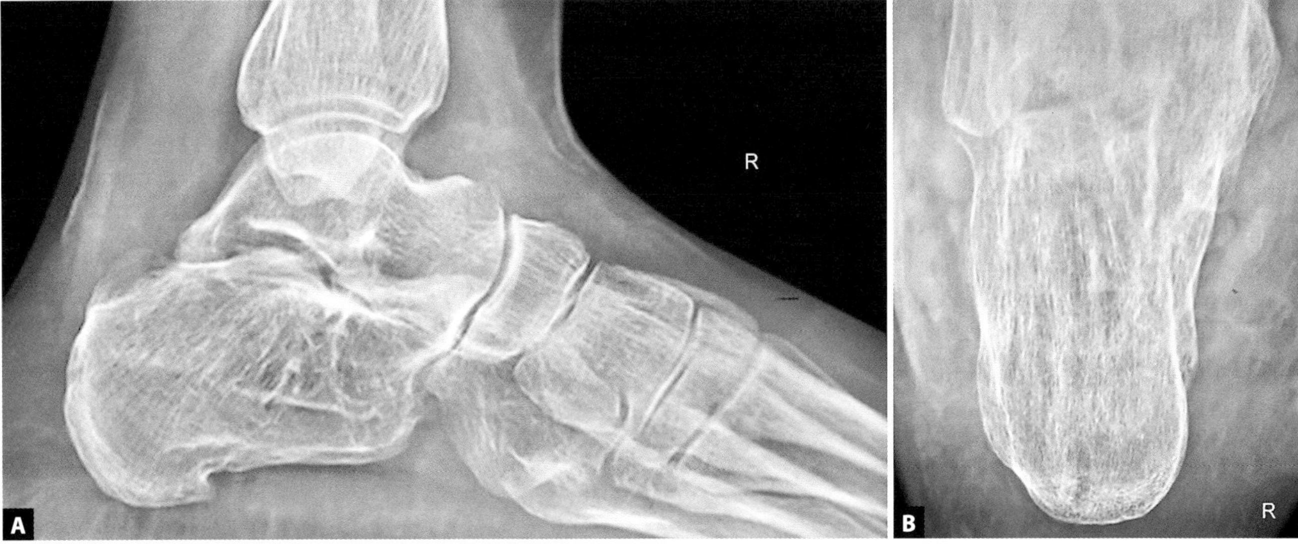

Figs. 28A and B: Axial and lateral images of a patient with malunion of calcaneus showing subtalar arthritis with lateral wall exostosis. Note that the height of calcaneus is preserved, and there is no heel varus or valgus.

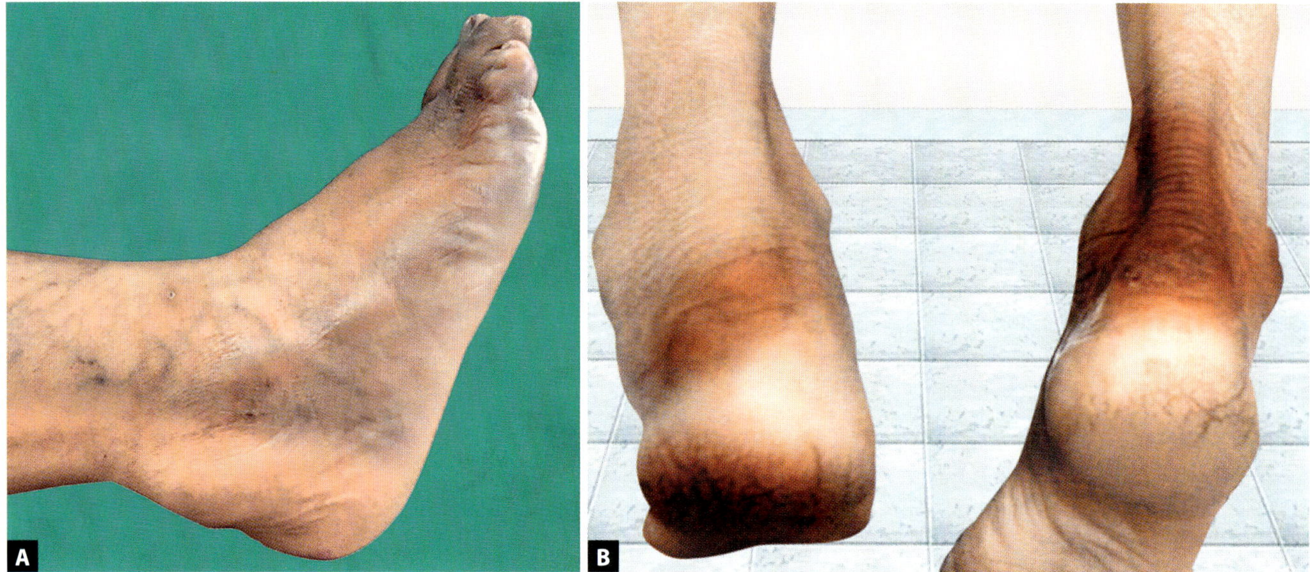

Figs. 29A and B: Clinical photograph of the same patient with soft-tissue swelling on the lateral aspect of the ankle. The comparative photograph shows broadened heel.

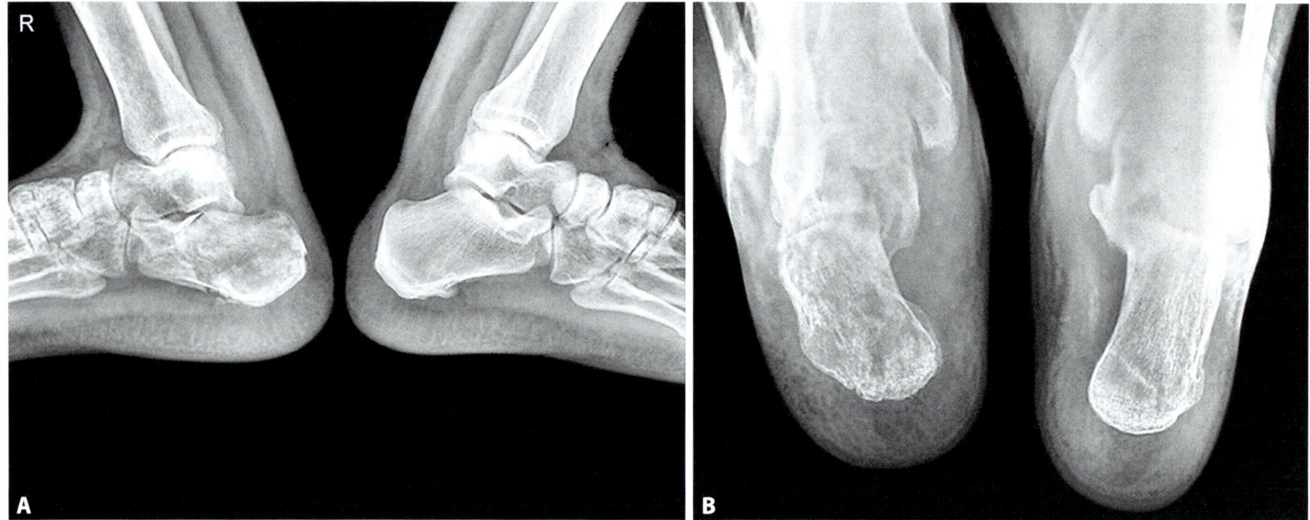

Figs. 30A and B: Lateral and axial images of the both heels of a patient with calcaneus malunion demonstrating heel varus and subtalar arthritis on the right side.

Case 2 (Figs. 30 to 32)

History and clinical examination: A 42-year-old male sustained fall from height and had an intra-articular fracture of the calcaneus. He was treated conservatively with a plaster cast. One year after the injury, he presented with complaints of the stiffness of heel with pain laterally.

On clinical examination, he revealed subtalar joint stiffness with peroneal tenosynovitis with heel varus.

X-ray findings: X-rays showed arthritis of the subtalar joint with the prominent lateral wall of the calcaneus with a heel varus.

Problems: The patient has arthritis of the subtalar joint (A), with heel in varus (D). Also, this patient has a lateral exostosis (E), giving rise to the impingement of the peronei. This case classically falls into Stephens and Sanders type III malunion.

Case 3 (Figs. 33A and B)

History and clinical examination: A 32-year-old male had a fall from height and sustained an open comminuted intra-articular fracture of the calcaneus. Debridement followed by the application of a plaster cast was done. The patient also had associated fracture of the lateral malleolus, which

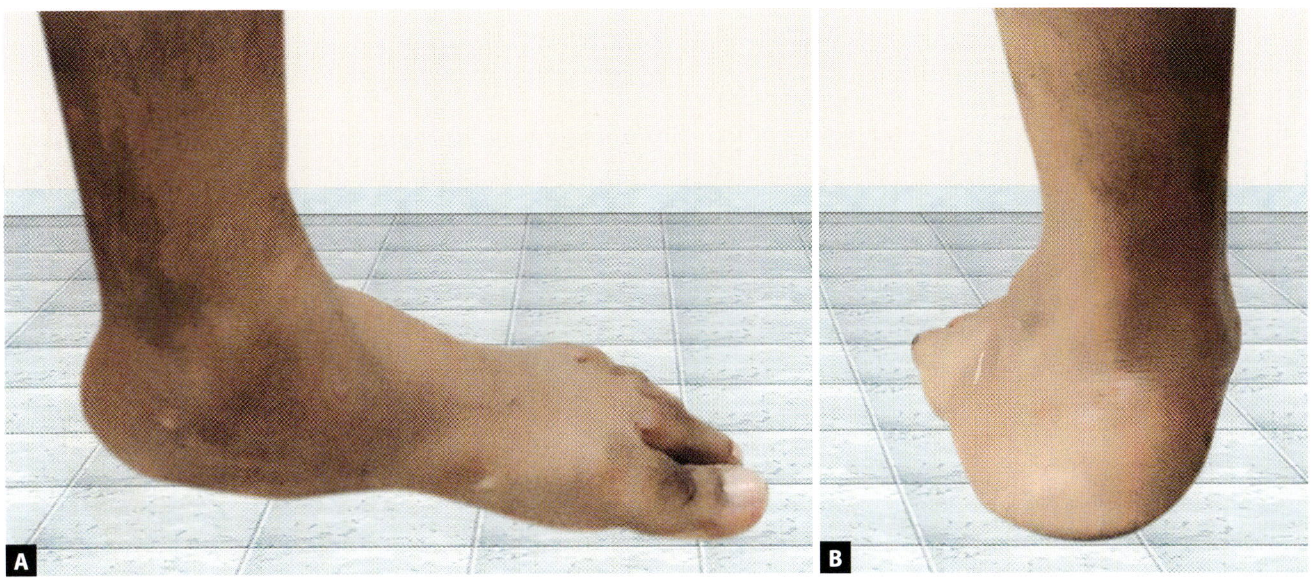

Figs. 31A and B: Standing clinical photographs of the same patient as in Figure 30, showing secondary flatfeet with heel valgus deformity.

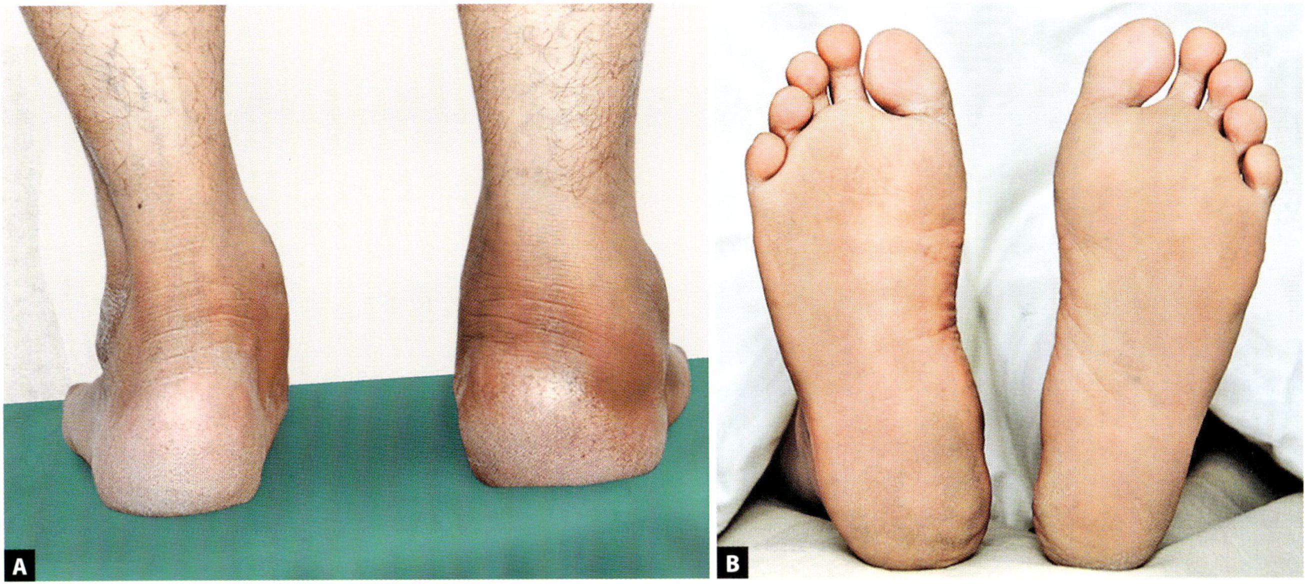

Figs. 32A and B: Clinical photographs of the same patient as in Figure 30, showing broadened and shortened right heel.

was fixed with a cancellous screw. Nine years after the injury, the patient presented with multiple problems. The patient complained of the stiffness of heel with difficulty in wearing shoes. He had pain laterally, medially, and on the plantar surface of the calcaneus. Walking on smooth and uneven surfaces as well as barefoot walking was almost impossible. He also had tingling and numbness of lateral two toes, which was continuous and unrelenting.

On clinical examination, there was flattening of the foot, with heel and forefoot diverted outward. The patient had neuralgic pain originating from the posterior tibial nerve with positive Tinel's sign. There were no movements at the subtalar joint, and dorsiflexion at the ankle was markedly restricted.

X-ray findings: X-rays showed the loss of both Böhler's and Gissane angles with broadening and shortening of the heel. Bony prominences were seen on medial and plantar aspects of the calcaneus. The subtalar joint and the calcaneocuboid joint were arthritic, and the medial arch was flattened. The forefoot was abducted while the heel was in valgus.

Problems: The present case has arthritis of subtalar and calcaneocuboid joints (A). The patient also has lateral, medial, and plantar exostosis (E). The heel is shortened

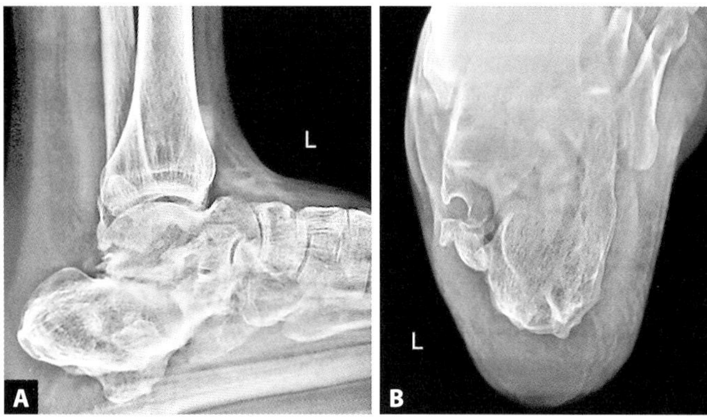

Figs. 33A and B: Lateral and axial images of a patient with calcaneal malunion. Medial and plantar exostosis is seen with arthritis of subtalar and calcaneocuboid joints.

and is in valgus malalignment. Talus is dorsiflexed in ankle mortise (D). The posterior tibial nerve is under compression due to sharp medial exostosis (N). Additionally, this patient also had claw toe deformity of all lesser toes (O). The case does not fall under any of the present classifications.

■ REFERENCES

1. Buckley R, Tough S, McCormack R, Pate G, Leighton R, Petrie D, et al. Operative compared with nonoperative treatment of displaced intra-articular calcaneal fractures: a prospective, randomized, controlled multicenter trial. J Bone Joint Surg. 2002;84(10):1773-44.
2. Rammelt S, Zwipp H. Calcaneus fractures: facts, controversies and recent developments. Injury. 2004;35(5):443-61.
3. James ET, Hunter GA. The dilemma of painful old os calcis fractures. Clin Orthop Relat Res. 1983;(177):112-5.
4. Myerson M, Quill Jr GE. Late complications of fractures of the calcaneus. J Bone Joint Surg. 1993;75(3):331-41.
5. Braly WG, Bishop JO, Tullos HS. Lateral decompression for malunited os calcis fractures. Foot Ankle. 1985;6(2):90-2.
6. Sanders R, Fortin P, DiPasquale T, Walling A. Operative treatment in 120 displaced intraarticular calcaneal fractures. Results using a prognostic computed tomography scan classification. Clin Orthop Relat Res. 1993;(290):87-95.
7. Isbister JF. Calcaneo-fibular abutment following crush fracture of the calcaneus. J Bone Joint Surg Br. 1974;56B(2):274-8.
8. Stephens HM, Sanders R. Calcaneal malunions: results of a prognostic computed tomography classification system. Foot Ankle Int. 1996;17(7):395-401.
9. Csizy M, Buckley R, Tough S, Leighton R, Smith J, McCormack R, et al. Displaced intra-articular calcaneal fractures: variables predicting late subtalar fusion. J Orthop Trauma. 2003;17(2):106-12.
10. Zwipp H, Rammelt S. Posttraumatische Korrekturoperationen am FuB. Zentralbl Chir. 2003;128:218-26.
11. Sanders R. Displaced intra-articular fractures of the calcaneus. J Bone Joint Surg Am. 2000;82:225-50.

Surgical Treatment of Calcaneal Malunion

Stephen W Pournaras III, Andrew Sands, Rahul Banerjee, Mandeep S Dhillon

> *"The sense of an entailed disadvantage—the deformed foot doubtfully hidden by the shoe, … easily turns a self-centered, unloving nature into an Ishmaelite".*
>
> **–George Eliot**

INTRODUCTION

Many patients with calcaneal malunion will improve with nonoperative treatment. Surgical treatment of calcaneal malunion is best reserved for active, healthy patients who have not responded to nonsurgical treatment. When operative treatment is chosen, thorough preoperative evaluation, including physical examination and radiographic imaging, is essential in order to determine the best surgical option for the patient.

PATHOANATOMY

Determining the optimal surgical treatment requires an understanding of the pathoanatomy associated with calcaneal malunion. Calcaneus fractures are usually produced by a high-energy axial load which results in a primary fracture line, separating the medial sustentaculum tali from the calcaneal tuberosity.[1] Additional secondary fracture lines traverse the calcaneus and result in comminution of the anterior process, posterior facet, and tuberosity. The axial load also impacts the talus into the calcaneus resulting in the "blowout" of the lateral wall. These fracture lines, in combination with the unique anatomy of the calcaneus and its surrounding soft tissues, result in the typical deformities seen in calcaneus fractures.

When left untreated, these deformities will result in the alteration of calcaneal morphology that is frequently seen in calcaneal malunion. This includes loss of height, heel widening and associated subfibular impingement, calcaneocuboid joint impingement, varus alignment of the heel, and post-traumatic arthrosis.

High-energy axial loads result in a flattening of the calcaneus with a loss of Böhler's angle at the time of injury **(Figs. 1 and 2)**. When the calcaneus heals in this position, the resultant malunion allows the talus to assume a horizontal or dorsiflexed position. This loss of height may result in a painful anterior impingement of the talar neck on the anterior tibial plafond.

Malunion of displacement of the lateral wall results in heel widening, which can affect the peroneal tendons and the sural nerve. With significant displacement, painful subfibular impingement **(Fig. 2C)** can occur as the displaced lateral wall abuts the distal fibula.[2] In addition, the peroneal tendons may be dislocated.

The calcaneocuboid joint is involved in 48% of calcaneus fractures.[3] Untreated displacement at this joint will result in impingement.

The fractured calcaneal tuberosity typically assumes a varus position at the time of the fracture. If this fragment heals, the malunion will result in an overall varus alignment to the hindfoot. A varus position to the hindfoot affects the function of the midfoot (transverse tarsal joint) and the ankle

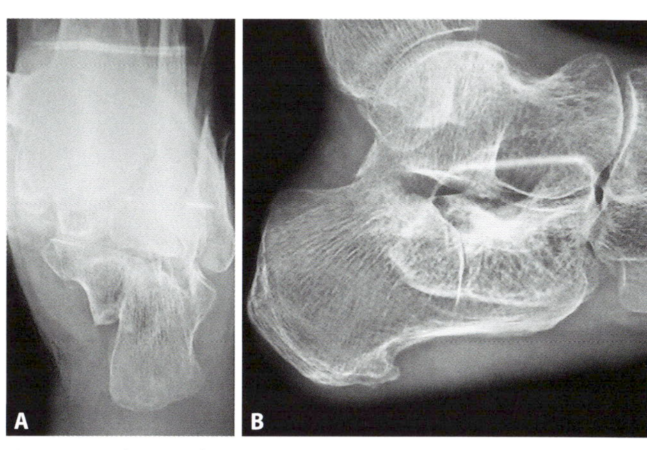

Figs. 1A and B: Axial view and lateral view of a calcaneus malunion.

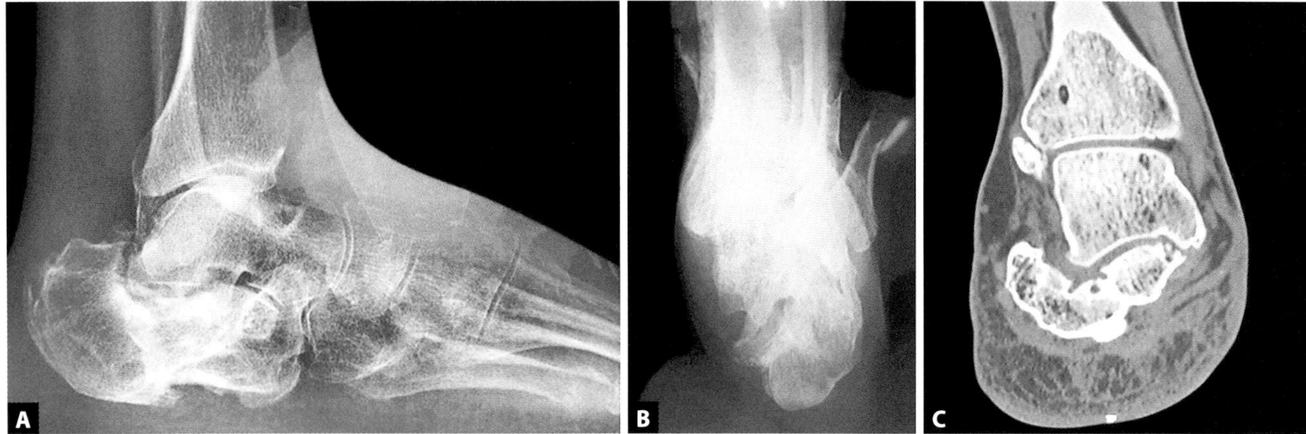

Figs. 2A to C: Lateral radiograph, axial view, and computed tomography (CT) scan of a calcaneus malunion showing severe deformity of calcaneus, with reversal of Böhler's angle, loss of heel height, and significant lateral impingement.

joint, which contributes to increased degenerative wear at these joints.

Even 2 mm of displacement has been shown to alter the contact pressures of the subtalar joint.[4] Untreated displacement contributes to the development of post-traumatic osteoarthrosis. In some cases, the arthrosis may be the result of irreversible damage to the articular surface that occurs at the time of injury.[5]

Some cases may be malunited even after surgery **(Figs. 3 and 4)**; these are more complex, and since surgery has already been done, soft-tissue compromise and often infection may be associated.

SURGICAL INDICATIONS AND CONTRAINDICATIONS

The surgeon can optimize surgical outcomes by careful patient selection and ensuring that the planned surgical correction will specifically address the patient's symptoms and underlying pathology. The goal of surgical treatment of calcaneal malunion is to relieve pain and restore function. Often, the simplest technique to achieve this goal is the best.

Surgical treatment is reserved for symptomatic patients who have not improved with nonoperative methods. Almost all patients with symptomatic calcaneal malunion warrant a trial of nonoperative treatment including activity modification, shoewear modification, orthotic devices and braces, injections, medical pain control, and functional rehabilitation. The exception to this may be the young, active, healthy patient with gross deformity or severe lateral impingement who may benefit from early surgical intervention.

Patients with symptoms and complications of calcaneal malunion that cannot be treated surgically should be identified and excluded. Patients with complex regional pain syndrome or heel pad pain will not improve with surgical treatment, and surgery may instead worsen the patient's condition.

Additional patient factors such as age, profession, activity level, workers' compensation status, smoking history, and medical comorbidities also influence the decision to pursue operative treatment. Many of these factors have been shown to impact the outcomes of acute treatment of calcaneus fractures.[6] Patient expectations and outcomes are affected by factors such as profession, activity level, and workers' compensation status. Wound healing after surgical treatment of calcaneus fractures is precarious in patients who smoke and have medical problems such as diabetes, and similar risks may apply in patients undergoing surgical treatment of calcaneal malunion.[7] Nonunion rates for reconstructive hindfoot fusions are 2.7 times higher in patients who smoke.[8]

It is very important that the planned surgical correction will specifically address the patient's symptoms. Preoperative assessment of the patient helps to determine the best surgical option. A thorough history and physical examination enable the surgeon to determine the extent and precise location of the patient's symptoms. Diagnostic injections with local anesthetic are very useful in determining the source of pain in patients with calcaneal malunion.[9]

Analysis of radiographs, in conjunction with examination of the patients, enables the surgeon to choose the best operation to relieve pain and restore function. Preoperative radiographic evaluation includes weight-bearing anteroposterior (AP), lateral, and oblique X-rays of the affected foot and AP, mortise, and lateral views of the ipsilateral ankle. In addition, an axial or Harris heel view and a hindfoot alignment view[10] are also helpful. Images of the contralateral foot are useful to describe the normal anatomy for the patient. Computed tomography (CT) scan

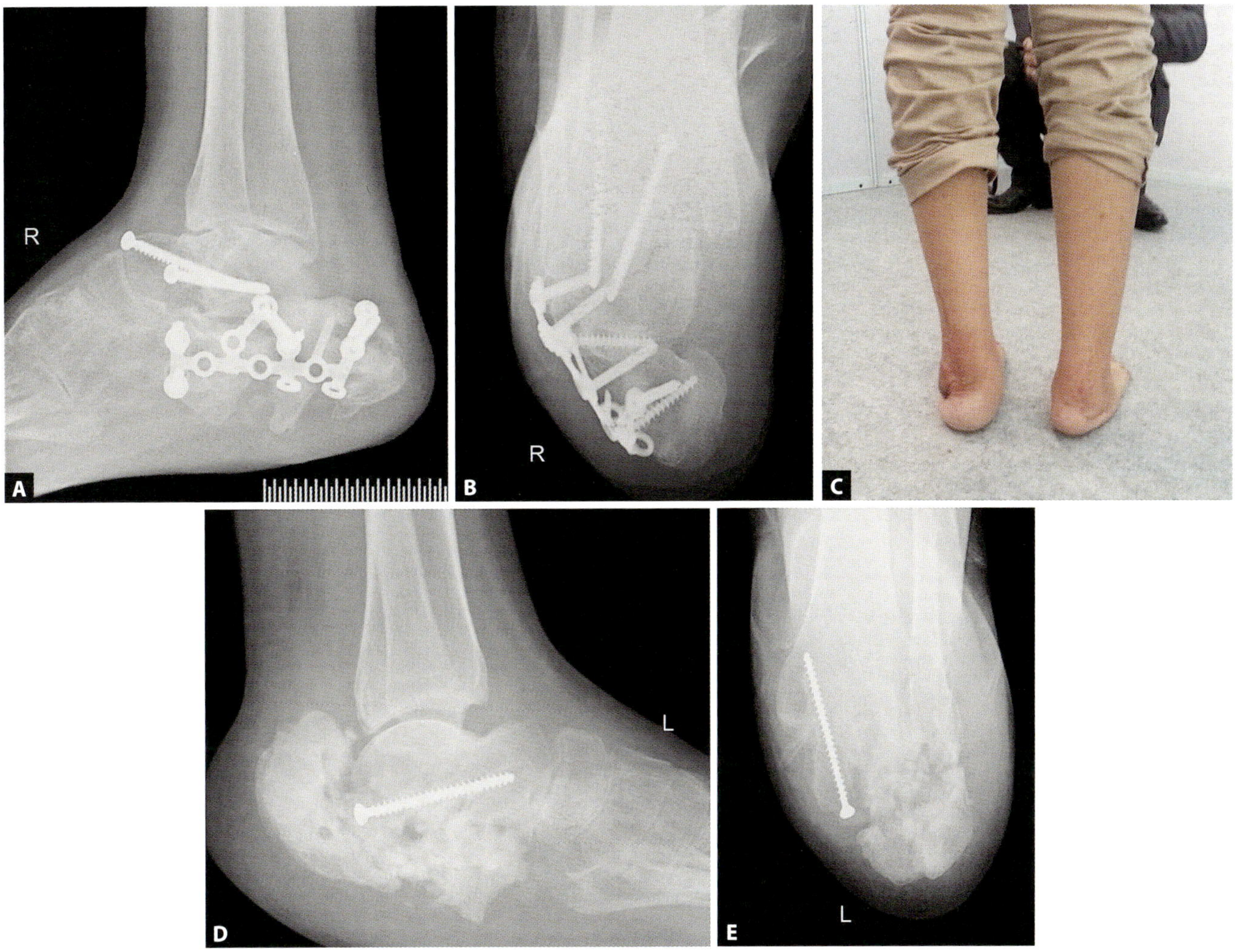

Figs. 3A to E: (A and B) Lateral and axial views of an operated case of calcaneus fracture, with implants in situ and presence of infection. (C) This was a bilateral case, with associated ipsilateral talus fracture. (D and E) Opposite side with a malunion/nonunion with severe collapse and failed multiple operations.

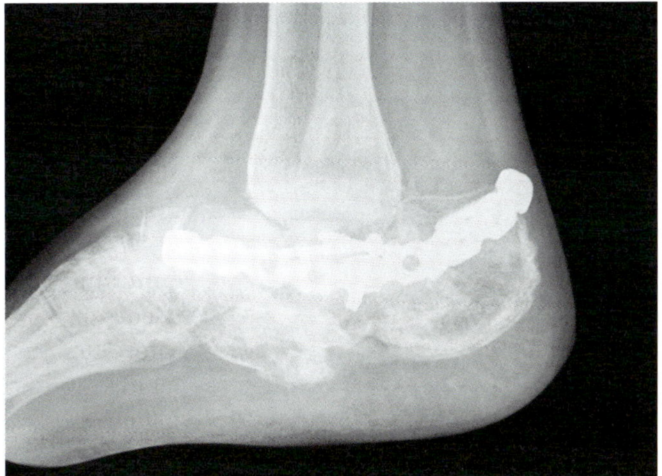

Fig. 4: Lateral view of another malunion despite an attempt at reduction and fixation, with plate in situ. These cases do not fit into the standard cases of malunion defined in the literature, with the patterns of displacement and deformities being different.

with coronal and sagittal reconstructions of the ankle and hindfoot is generally recommended in order to further assess the condition of the subtalar and calcaneocuboid joints, the location of the peroneal tendons, and the overall deformity of the malunited calcaneus.

General Principles of Surgical Treatment

Prior to surgery, the patient and surgeon should work together to optimize conditions for a successful outcome. This includes assessment of the patient's medical comorbidities and nutritional status. Wound healing complications are not uncommon and patients should be strongly encouraged to stop smoking. Diabetic patients should be educated as to the importance of controlling pre- and postoperative blood glucose.

Depending on the surgeon's preference and the chosen technique, the patient is usually positioned in a prone or lateral position on a radiolucent operating table. It is important for the patient to be positioned with the operative foot as close to the end of the surgical table as possible as this allows for better access during the procedure. If the surgical plan calls for autologous bone grafting (e.g., iliac crest or proximal tibia), care should be taken to position and appropriately drape these areas.

Preoperative prophylactic antibiotics are provided, and surgical treatment is performed under thigh tourniquet in order to minimize blood loss.

During surgery, extreme care is taken when managing the skin and soft tissues. Careful handling of the skin during exposure and closure is essential to avoid wound healing complications.

■ LATERAL WALL DECOMPRESSION

Lateral wall decompression is indicated in cases with large lateral wall exostoses and heel widening with minimal or no subtalar arthrosis.[11] The surgery provides relief for patients with symptoms related to the deformity, such as pain from subfibular impingement, and symptoms due to the overlying peroneal tendons and sural nerve. Lateral wall decompression alone does not address advanced subtalar arthrosis or more complex deformities affecting the remainder of the calcaneus.

Technique

A number of different surgical approaches have been utilized to perform a lateral exostectomy including a Kocher lateral curvilinear approach, an extensile lateral approach, a subtalar Ollier approach, or a posterolateral longitudinal incision. If there are incisions from previous surgery, these should be utilized, if possible. The displaced lateral wall is carefully dissected subperiosteally and then excised using an osteotome (**Figs. 5 and 6**). The site of excision is carefully

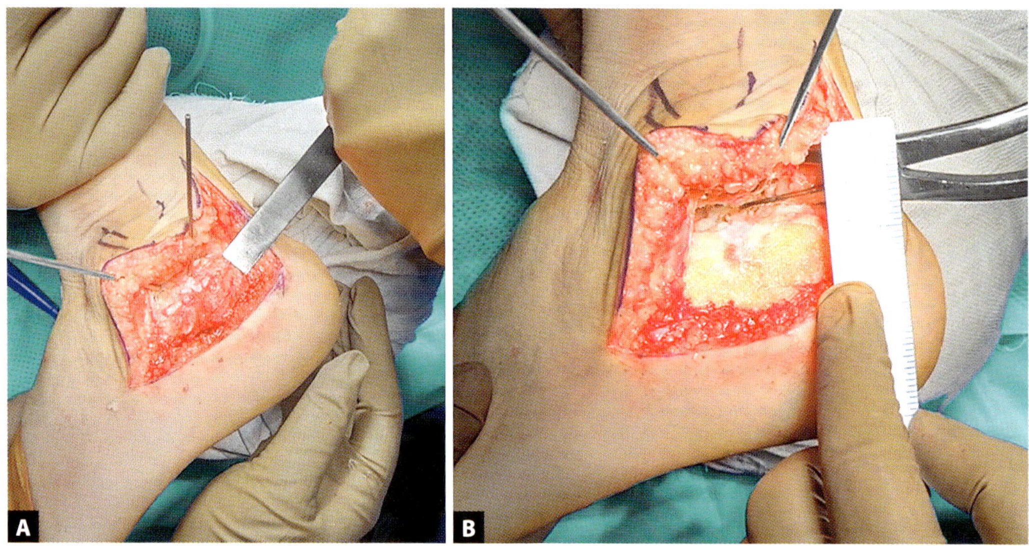

Figs. 5A and B: Intraoperative picture of the exostosis being shaved off with a curved osteotome. Same case after excision showing size of exostosis being taken off.

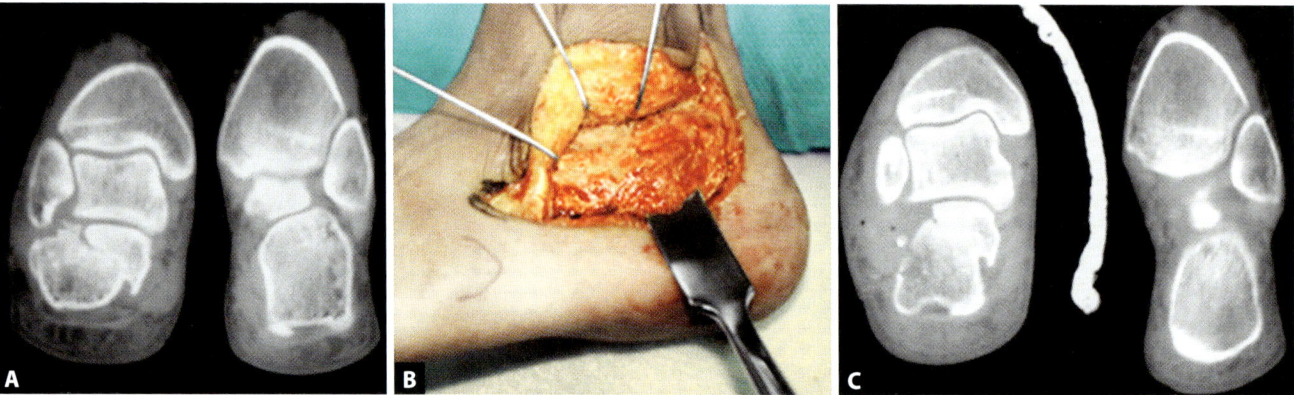

Figs. 6A to C: (A) Computed tomography (CT) scan showing calcaneal malunion with fibular abutment; (B) Intraoperative photograph showing lateral wall exostosis; (C) CT scan after lateral wall exostectomy.

smoothed using a bone rasp. Bone wax is applied to the site to help control bleeding. The skin is closed carefully in layers, with care taken to avoid handling the skin edges.

This technique was designed primarily to address symptoms caused by the displaced lateral wall. However, the surgical approach may also be used to address peroneal tendonitis, sural nerve problems, or arthrosis involving the lateral aspects of the subtalar joint or calcaneocuboid joint. Excision of the displaced lateral wall alone may be sufficient to relieve peroneal nerve symptoms, but exploration and peroneal tenolysis can also be performed through the same approach.[12] Sural neurolysis or neuroma excision will relieve sural nerve symptoms.[12] In patients with arthritis involving the lateral aspect of the subtalar joint or calcaneocuboid joint, excision of the lateral wall along with the lateral aspect of the involved joint may help to relieve symptoms related to the arthrosis.[13]

Outcomes

Braly et al. treated 11 patients with lateral decompression combined with release or lengthening of the peroneal tendons and sural nerve release or transection. A satisfactory result was obtained in 9 of 11 patients.[12] Stephens and Sanders described the results of this technique in seven patients.[11] There were six excellent results and one good result. Approximately 50% of patients noted an improved range of motion with lateral wall decompression. Clare et al. reported an average postoperative American Orthopaedic Foot and Ankle Society (AOFAS) hindfoot score of 68.2 in five patients treated with this technique at 2 years follow-up.[13]

◼ POSTERIOR EXOSTECTOMY

Posterior exostectomy is indicated in cases where posterior or superior displacement of the calcaneal tuberosity has resulted in a malunion with a prominent posterior exostosis. The surgical procedure relieves posterior pain over the tuberosity and pain at the Achilles tendon insertion. In addition, the surgery may provide relief from painful shoes wear.

Case Example

A 61-year-old female sustained bilateral calcaneus fractures in a fall. She underwent primary surgical treatment of both fractures. She presented 1 year after her surgery with a chief complaint of a painful posterior heel bump on her right and trouble wearing shoes. She noted recurrent ulceration over her calcaneal tuberosity. X-rays demonstrated a prominent posterior exostosis **(Fig. 7A)**. The patient underwent resection of the exostosis through a posterior midline incision with partial elevation of the Achilles tendon. The elevated portion of the tendon was repaired with a suture anchor **(Fig. 7B)**. The patient's symptoms improved and were resolved at 3 months follow-up.

Technique

The patient is positioned prone to allow a posterior approach to the calcaneal tuberosity. The skin may be incised in the midline or slightly medially. The exostosis is approached by splitting the Achilles tendon in its midline or by elevating the tendon at its medial edge. The exostosis is dissected subperiosteally and excised using osteotomes and a rongeur. A variable portion of the Achilles tendon insertion may need to be elevated to fully decompress the exostectomy; if a large portion of the tendon is elevated, we recommend reattachment using suture anchors. If a midline incision was made in the Achilles tendon, it is repaired with nonabsorbable suture. The skin is closed carefully in layers.

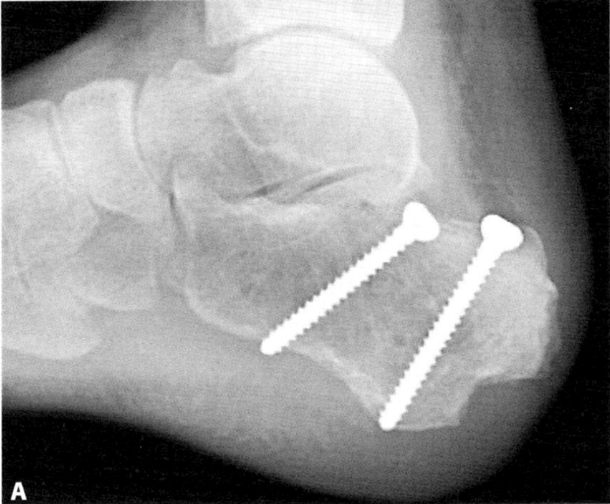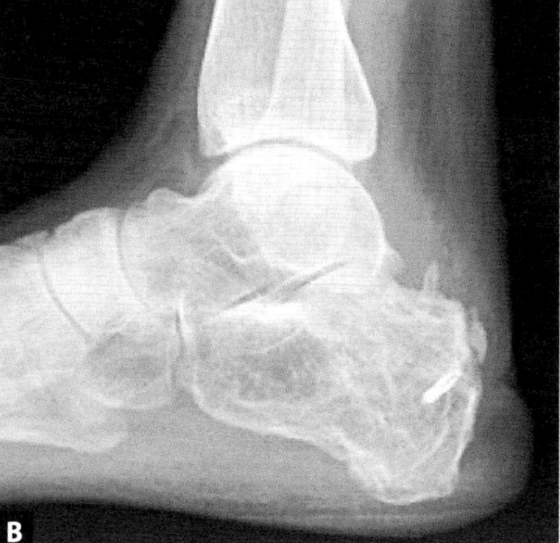

Figs. 7A and B: (A) Lateral radiograph of a 61-year-old female with painful prominent posterior exostosis after surgical treatment of calcaneus fracture; (B) Lateral radiograph after posterior exostectomy.

The patient is immobilized in a short-leg splint for 1–2 weeks at which time the wound is examined and the sutures are removed. Early range of motion is important to preserve subtalar motion. If a large portion of the Achilles insertion was elevated and subsequently repaired, weight-bearing is restricted for 6 weeks, followed by progressive increase to full weight-bearing over a course of 2–4 weeks.

■ IN SITU SUBTALAR ARTHRODESIS

In situ subtalar arthrodesis is best utilized for patients with symptomatic calcaneal malunion with minimal deformity but significant painful subtalar arthrosis. As this procedure does not change the morphology of the calcaneus or hindfoot, it is not indicated for patients with significant loss of height or varus or valgus deformities.[9,11,13,14] This procedure may be combined with lateral decompression if symptoms of lateral impingement are present in addition to the subtalar arthrodesis.

Technique

The subtalar joint is approached through a sinus tarsi incision that extends from the tip of the lateral malleolus to the base of the fourth metatarsal. Branches of the sural nerve and superficial peroneal nerve are identified and protected. The subtalar joint is exposed and distracted using a bone spreader or joint distractor and the articular surfaces of the joint are denuded of cartilage using osteotomes, curettes, and high-speed burrs. The subchondral bone is perforated with a drill to establish viability and to provide vascularity to the region of fusion. Sclerotic, avascular bone is excised to improve fusion.[15]

After irrigation and removal of all debris, the subtalar joint is bone grafted. Bone graft may be obtained locally if the procedure is combined with a lateral wall exostectomy. Alternatively, autograft may be obtained from the calcaneus, proximal tibia, or iliac crest. The subtalar joint is then reduced into approximately 5° of valgus and stabilized with two partially threaded large fragment screws inserted from the posteroinferior aspect of the heel perpendicular to the posterior facet and into the talus. Intraoperative fluoroscopy is used to confirm correct screw position and to ensure proper alignment of the heel. Additional bone graft is placed in any remaining space in the subtalar joint (**Figs. 8A and B**).

Patients are immobilized in a short leg splint for approximately 2 weeks after surgery until the incisions are healed. Sutures are removed and the patient is placed into a short leg cast. Weight-bearing is restricted for 6–8 weeks. The patient is then placed into a walking boot with a rocker sole and weight-bearing is progressively advanced over the next 6 weeks. Radiographic union is observed after 10–14 weeks but may take longer in more complex cases.

Outcomes

In situ subtalar fusion results in high rates of union (>90%) and patient satisfaction with low reported complication rates.[13,16,17] Patients who smoke, diabetic patients, and elderly patients are at risk for nonunion and worse outcomes.[15,18]

■ SUBTALAR DISTRACTION BONE BLOCK ARTHRODESIS

Subtalar distraction bone block arthrodesis is indicated in patients with calcaneal malunion that develops painful subtalar arthrosis, loss of hindfoot height, and symptomatic anterior ankle impingement. The procedure may be combined with a lateral wall exostectomy in patients with the

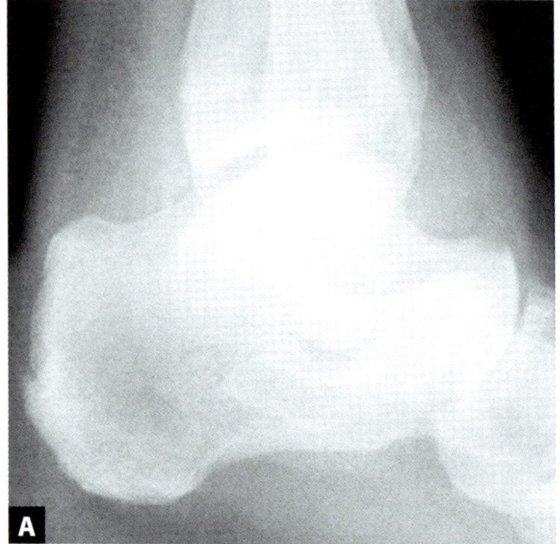
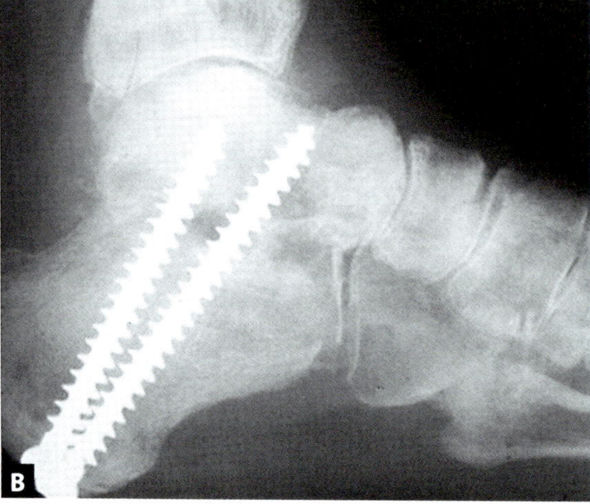

Figs. 8A and B: Lateral radiographs before and after in situ subtalar fusion fixed with two fully threaded screws.

above symptoms in combination with lateral wall blowout. Chandler et al. recommended this procedure in patients with disabling ankle pain and <10° of ankle dorsiflexion.[16] This procedure is not indicated to correct major varus or valgus deformity.

Case Example 1

An 18-year-old male was involved in a high-speed motor vehicle accident and sustained bilateral femur fractures, a right open tibia fracture, and a displaced right intra-articular calcaneus fracture. His calcaneus fracture was treated nonoperatively. Six months after injury, he presented with right foot pain with an antalgic slow gait. On examination, he was noted to have minimal subtalar motion with pain. Radiographs and CT scan demonstrated calcaneal malunion with loss of hindfoot height, subtalar arthrosis, and subfibular impingement **(Fig. 3)**. The patient underwent distraction bone block subtalar arthrodesis. The excised lateral wall was used as the bone block. Radiographs at 6 months demonstrate restoration of hindfoot height and talar declination **(Fig. 4)**. The patient reported resolution of symptoms.

Technique

The subtalar joint is approached through a posterolateral longitudinal incision. Although a lateral incision may be utilized, wound closure may be problematic after joint distraction is performed.[19] Use of an extensile lateral approach is another option but should be done with care to avoid wound problems; care should be taken to identify the peroneal tendons, which may be dislocated from their normal position.

If a lateral wall exostectomy is required, the procedure is performed as above, but the excised bone is saved to be used as the bone block.[13] The subtalar joint is exposed and distracted. Distraction may be performed by placing a large distractor spanning from the medial distal tibia to the calcaneal tuberosity which helps to correct varus malalignment. Alternatively, the joint may be distracted by utilizing a Hintermann retractor or a laminar spreader applied directly to the joint. If a laminar spreader is used, it must not be placed on the lateral aspect of the joint as lateral distraction will result in varus malposition of the heel **(Figs. 9A to E)**. An appropriately sized graft from the iliac crest is inserted and the joint is fixed by screws.

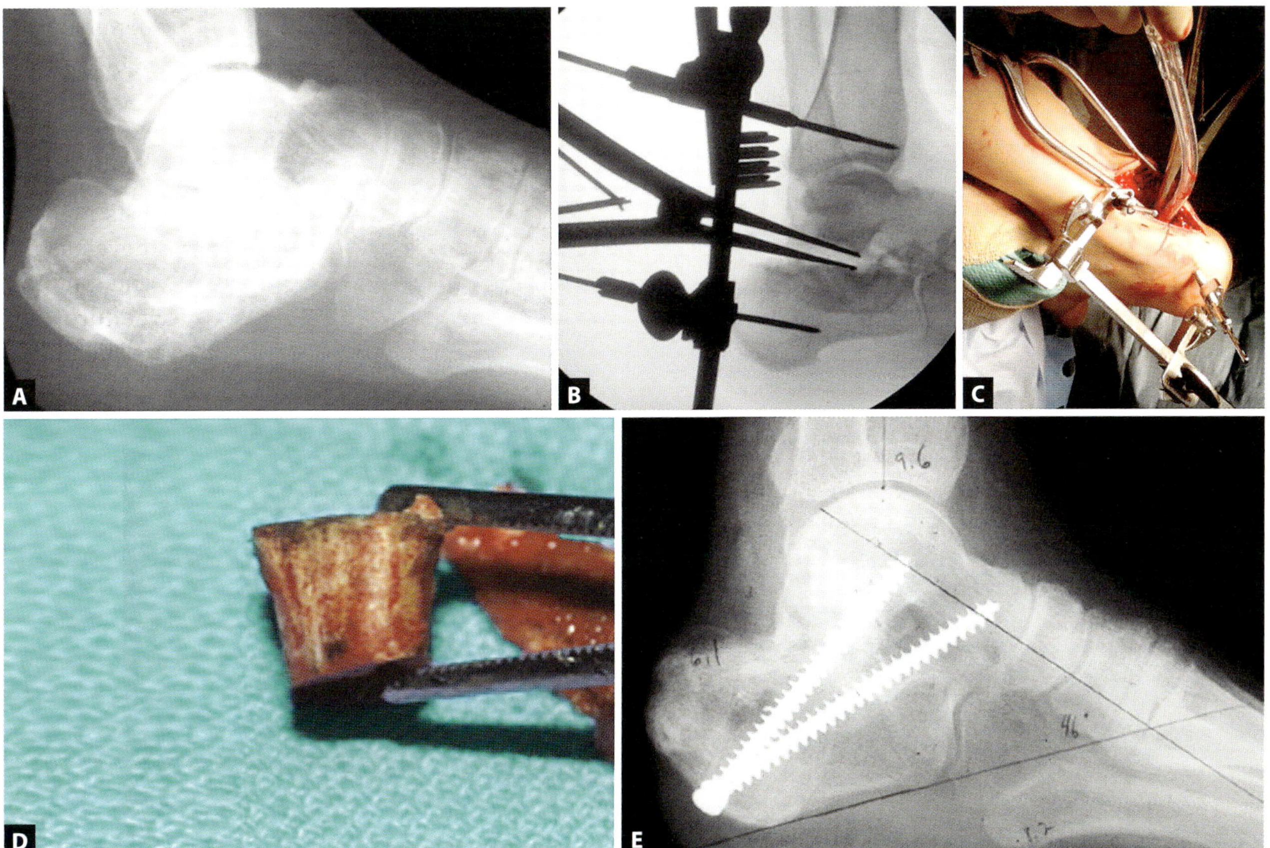

Figs. 9A to E: (A) Lateral radiograph showing calcaneal malunion; (B) Intraoperative lateral radiograph demonstrating correction after subtalar distraction; (C) Positioning of distractors and laminar spreader; (D) Bone graft harvested from iliac crest; (E) Lateral radiograph demonstrating fusion in corrected position.

Case Example 2

Surgical Technique (Figs. 10A to G)

Patients may have scarring and contracted tissues medially which may prevent correction of varus. In these cases, careful subperiosteal dissection of the medial calcaneal wall through the distracted joint is required to enable correction of varus.

Once the joint is exposed, the articular surface is prepared similar to the procedure described above for in situ subtalar arthrodesis. The joint is held in a distracted, corrected position and fluoroscopy is used to confirm adequate correction of hindfoot height, talar declination, and heel varus.

A tricortical bone graft is harvested from the ipsilateral iliac crest and shaped to ensure that the height is appropriate. The block should be of adequate size to gain a press fit into the distracted, corrected subtalar joint. The usual size is about 1.5 cm; this graft tends to collapse a bit over time, so one should take a few millimeters of thicker graft. The bone block is then placed in the distracted joint and stabilized with a K-wire. In cases where the procedure is combined with a lateral wall exostectomy, the excised bone is further added to the corrected joint; this bone is never enough in isolation to be able to maintain the joint in adequate distraction.[13] The bone block should be placed slightly medially in order to avoid varus malalignment. Two bone blocks of different sizes may also be placed side by side in order to correct varus or valgus malalignment.[14]

After placement of the block(s), the distraction is removed, and additional bone graft is placed in any remaining space in the subtalar joint. The joint is then stabilized with one, ideally two large fragment screws as described above for in situ subtalar arthrodesis. For this procedure, the more anterior screw is directed into the talar neck in order to further correct the talar declination. Use of a fully threaded screw placed into the talar body is recommended to maintain hindfoot height **(Figs. 11A and B)**. The graft may be too small to allow a screw to pass through it; to avoid dislocation of the graft, a 2 mm K-wire could replace the second screw, and this can be removed after 6–8 weeks.

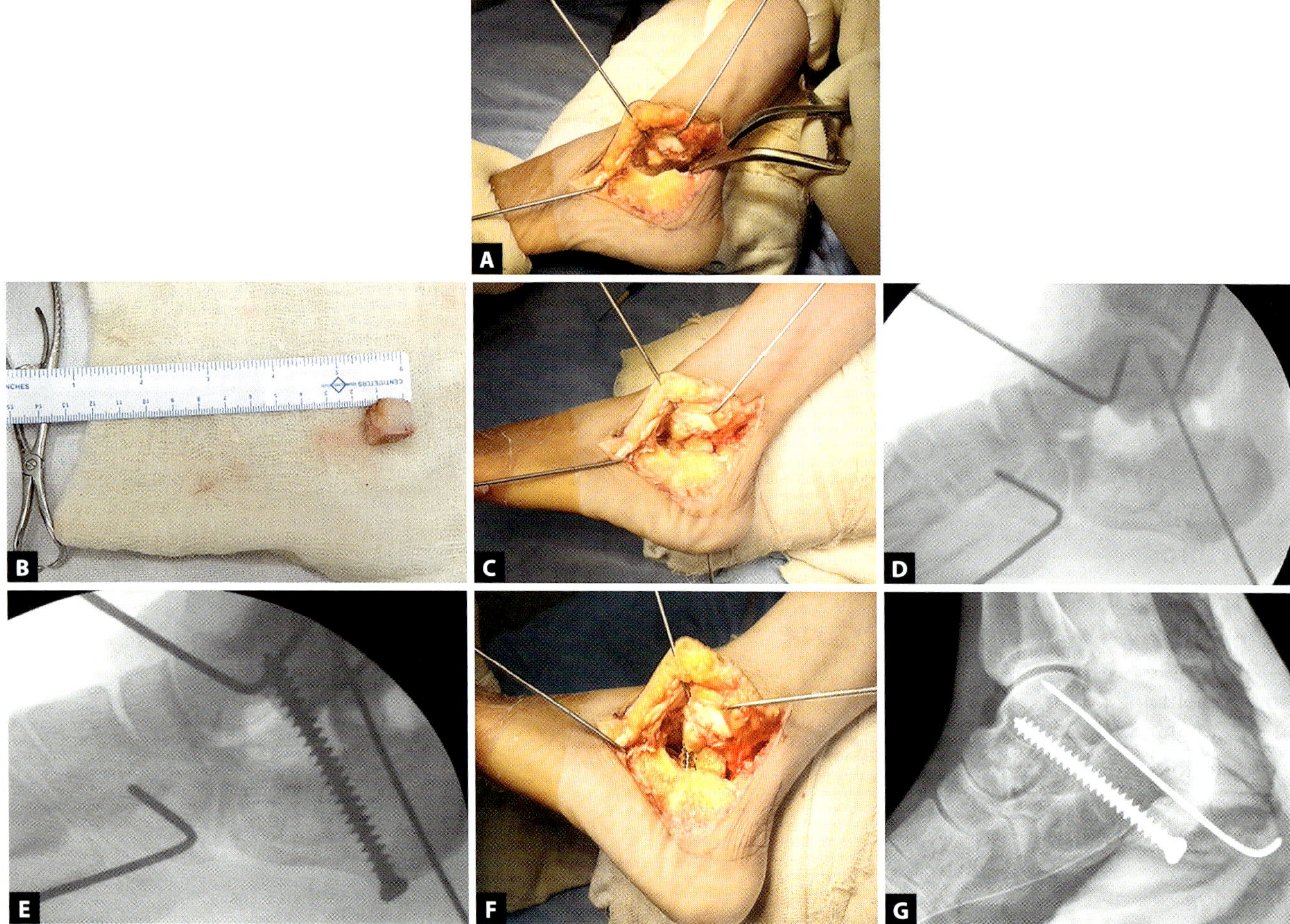

Figs. 10A to G: (A) Exposed calcaneus with laminar spreader in position; (B) Sizing of harvested iliac bone tricortical bone graft; (C) Graft in position; (D to G) Stabilization with one K-wire through the graft and one fully threaded screw to maintain the position.

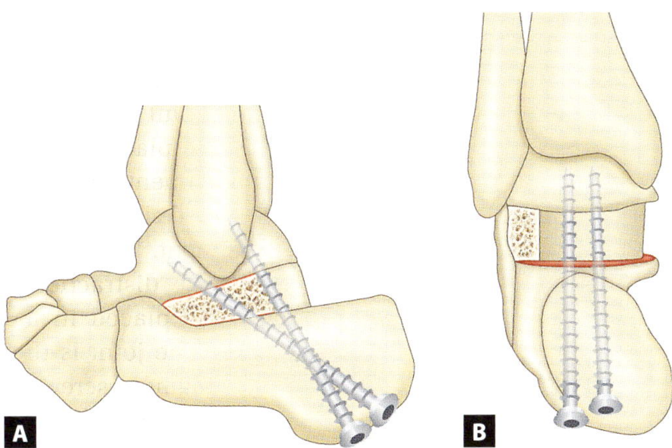

Figs. 11A and B: Line diagrams showing graft positioning to correct both heel varus and loss of heel height. Screws do not need to be parallel and should be fully threaded to maintain distraction of the joint.

The postoperative plan is like that described above for in situ subtalar arthrodesis.

Outcomes

The nonunion rate after distraction bone block arthrodesis is up to 14%,[19,20] but the outcomes are similar to those reported with in situ subtalar arthrodesis.[20-22] Complications include dislocation of the bone block, malunion, painful hardware, infection, and nerve problems.[19]

CORRECTIVE OSTEOTOMY AND ARTHRODESIS

Deformity due to calcaneal malunion may also be corrected by means of corrective calcaneal osteotomies combined with subtalar fusion. Although these techniques can achieve powerful correction of deformity, these techniques should be reserved for more severe deformity and applied with care.

Vertical Sliding Calcaneal Osteotomy and Arthrodesis

Huang et al. described a vertical sliding corrective calcaneal osteotomy combined with subtalar fusion.[23] The authors recommended this procedure primarily for patients with impingement of the ankle malleoli on the shoes counter due to loss of height. Although this procedure restores hindfoot height, it does not address correction of talar declination and therefore will not address symptoms of anterior ankle impingement.

Technique

The calcaneus is approached through a vertical incision just posterior to the posterior facet of the subtalar joint, taking care to identify and protect the sural nerve. The technique was originally described with an extensile lateral approach, but as noted above, since the procedure increases the height of the hindfoot, this approach may be difficult to close or result in wound complications.

A vertical osteotomy is made in the calcaneal tuberosity immediately posterior to the articular surface. The osteotomy is started with an oscillating saw but completed medially with an osteotomy in order to protect the medial neurovascular structures. The tuberosity is shifted in a plantar direction. Lengthening of the Achilles tendon may be required to allow for adequate mobilization. The osteotomy is then fixed with large fragment screws placed perpendicular to the osteotomy. Subtalar arthrodesis is performed as described above.

The postoperative plan is similar to that described above for in situ subtalar arthrodesis.

Outcomes

Huang et al. treated 12 patients with this procedure.[23] Excellent results were obtained in 11 of 12 patients based on physical examination and radiographic findings.

Osteotomies and Arthrodesis to Correct Varus or Valgus Deformity

For calcaneal malunions with subtalar arthrosis and >10° of axial hindfoot malalignment, subtalar arthrodesis (in situ or distraction bone block) may be combined with calcaneal osteotomy to correct the alignment.[11,13] Varus deformity is more common than valgus deformity.

Technique

The surgical technique is similar to that described above for in situ or distraction bone block subtalar arthrodesis, but in these cases, calcaneal osteotomy is performed prior to completion of the subtalar arthrodesis. For severe varus deformity, a lateral closing wedge osteotomy (Dwyer) is performed. For less common valgus deformity, a medializing calcaneal osteotomy with or without rotation of the tuberosity is performed.[13] In these procedures, the osteotomy and the fusion are simultaneously stabilized with two large fragment screws.

The postoperative plan is similar to that described above for in situ subtalar arthrodesis.

Outcomes

Clare et al. treated 10 feet with calcaneal malunion with significant (>10°) varus or valgus deformity with this protocol.[13] The average Maryland foot score and AOFAS ankle and hindfoot score were 83.1 and 76.1, respectively.

ROMASH OSTEOTOMY

Romash described a corrective calcaneal osteotomy through the plane of the primary fracture line combined with a subtalar arthrodesis.[24] The osteotomy allows for restoration of calcaneal height and length, narrows the heel, and decompresses the lateral structures, while the arthrodesis addresses subtalar arthrosis.

Technique

The calcaneus and subtalar joint are approached through an oblique incision in line with the sinus tarsi. The peroneal tendons are retracted distally, and the subtalar joint is exposed. The lateral calcaneal wall is exposed with subperiosteal dissection. The joint is distracted utilizing a bone spreader. The subtalar joint is prepared as described above for subtalar arthrodesis.

The primary fracture line is then identified by means of direct visualization and intraoperative fluoroscopy. A thick K-wire or Steinmann pin is then placed along the plane of primary fracture line. Positioning of this wire is confirmed with fluoroscopy. The wire is used as a guide and a calcaneal osteotomy is performed along the plane.

After completion of the osteotomy, the tuberosity fragment is displaced along the plane of the osteotomy in a posterior and medial direction **(Figs. 12A to C)**. A Schanz pin placed into the tuberosity can help with this mobilization. After correction is achieved, the tuberosity fragment is temporarily fixed with K-wires and intraoperative fluoroscopy is used to verify adequate correction of the deformity.

The subtalar joint is prepared as described above. The arthrodesis is then performed with two large fragment screws placed from the posteroinferior aspect of the calcaneal tuberosity, through the sustentaculum, into the talus. Bone graft is packed into the subtalar joint and the lateral gap is created by this osteotomy.

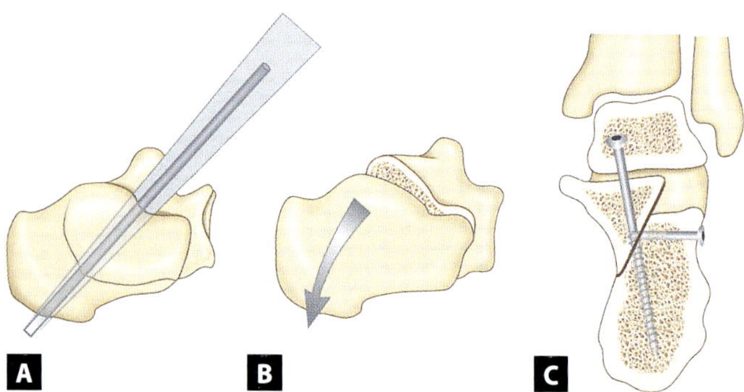

Figs. 12A to C: Diagrammatic demonstration of displacement osteotomy described by Romash.
Source: Adapted from Romash (1993).[24]

The postoperative plan is similar to that described above for in situ subtalar arthrodesis.

Outcomes

Romash reported 9 out of 10 satisfactory results in patients treated with this osteotomy.[24]

SUMMARY

Surgical treatment of calcaneal malunion is best reserved for active, healthy patients who have not responded to nonoperative treatment. A careful understanding of the patient's symptoms and pathoanatomy is necessary to select the best surgical treatment option. Although a variety of surgical procedures are available to correct calcaneal malunion, the simplest technique that addresses the patient's specific problems is often the best.

REFERENCES

1. Böhler L. Diagnosis, pathology, and treatment of fractures of the os calcis. J Bone Joint Surg Am. 1931;13:75-89.
2. Isbister JF. Calcaneo-fibular abutment following crush fracture of the calcaneus. J Bone Joint Surg Br. 1974;56(2):274-8.
3. Silhanek AD, Ramdass R, Lombardi CM. The effect of primary fracture line location on the pattern and severity of intraarticular calcaneal fractures: a retrospective radiographic study. J Foot Ankle Surg. 2006;45(4):211-9.
4. Sangeorzan BJ, Ananthakrishnan D, Tencer AF. Contact characteristics of the subtalar joint after a simulated calcaneus fracture. J Orthop Trauma. 1995;9(3):251-8.
5. Borrelli Jr J, Torzilli PA, Grigiene R, Helfet DL. Effect of impact load on articular cartilage: development of an intra-articular fracture model. J Orthop Trauma. 1997;11(5):319-26.
6. Buckley R, Tough S, McCormack R, Pate G, Leighton R, Petrie D, et al. Operative compared with nonoperative treatment of displaced intra-articular calcaneal fractures: a prospective, randomized, controlled multicenter trial. J Bone Joint Surg Am. 2002;84(10):1733-44.
7. Folk JW, Starr AJ, Early JS. Early wound complications of operative treatment of calcaneus fractures: analysis of 190 fractures. J Orthop Trauma. 1999;13(5):369-72.
8. Ishikawa SN, Murphy GA, Richardson EG. The effect of cigarette smoking on hindfoot fusions. Foot Ankle Int. 2002;23(11):996-8.
9. Myerson M, Quill Jr GE. Late complications of fractures of the calcaneus. J Bone Joint Surg Am. 1993;75(3):331-41.
10. Saltzman CL, el-Khoury GY. The hindfoot alignment view. Foot Ankle Int. 1995;16(9):572-6.
11. Stephens HM, Sanders R. Calcaneal malunions: results of a prognostic computed tomography classification system. Foot Ankle Int. 1996;17(7):395-401.
12. Braly WG, Bishop JO, Tullos HS. Lateral decompression for malunited os calcis fractures. Foot Ankle. 1985;6(2):90-6.
13. Clare MP, Lee 3rd WE, Sanders RW. Intermediate to long-term results of a treatment protocol for calcaneal fracture malunions. J Bone Joint Surg Am. 2005;87(5):963-73.

14. Zwipp H, Rammelt S. Posttraumatic deformity correction at the foot. Zentralbl Chir. 2003;128(3):218-26.

15. Easley ME, Trnka HJ, Schon LC, Myerson MS. Isolated subtalar arthrodesis. J Bone Joint Surg Am. 2000;82(5):613-24.

16. Chandler JT, Bonar SK, Anderson RB, Davis WH. Results of in situ subtalar arthrodesis for late sequelae of calcaneus fractures. Foot Ankle Int. 1999;20(1):18-24.

17. Savva N, Saxby TS. In situ arthrodesis with lateral-wall ostectomy for the sequelae of fracture of the os calcis. J Bone Joint Surg Br. 2007;89(7):919-24.

18. Chahal J, Stephen DJ, Bulmer B, Daniels T, Kreder HJ. Factors associated with outcome after subtalar arthrodesis. J Orthop Trauma. 2006;20(8):555-61.

19. Carr JB, Hansen ST, Benirschke SK. Subtalar distraction bone block fusion for late complications of os calcis fractures. Foot Ankle. 1988;9(2):81-6.

20. Trnka HJ, Easley ME, Lam PW, Anderson CD, Schon LC, Myerson MS. Subtalar distraction bone block arthrodesis. J Bone Joint Surg Br. 2001;83(6):849-54.

21. Rammelt S, Grass R, Zawadski T, Biewener A, Zwipp H. Foot function after subtalar distraction bone-block arthrodesis. A prospective study. J Bone Joint Surg Br. 2004;86(5):659-68.

22. Pollard JD, Schuberth JM. Posterior bone block distraction arthrodesis of the subtalar joint: a review of 22 cases. J Foot Ankle Surg. 2008;47(3):191-8.

23. Huang PJ, Fu YC, Cheng YM, Lin SY. Subtalar arthrodesis for late sequelae of calcaneal fractures: fusion in situ versus fusion with sliding corrective osteotomy. Foot Ankle Int. 1999;20(3):166-70.

24. Romash MM. Reconstructive osteotomy of the calcaneus with subtalar arthrodesis for malunited calcaneal fractures. Clin Orthop Relat Res. 1993(290):157-67.

23

Arthroscopic Management of Late Complications of Calcaneal Fractures

Tun Hing Lui

"A man who has committed a mistake and doesn't correct it, is committing another mistake".

–Confucius

"I have made many mistakes myself; the best surgeon, like the best general, is he who makes the fewest mistakes".

–Astley Cooper

■ INTRODUCTION

Calcaneal fracture is one of the most common fractures of the foot and ankle region. Most of the calcaneal fractures consist of a primary fracture line that separates the sustentaculum fragment from the tuberosity fragment. The secondary fracture lines travel in the sagittal plane in any direction along the bone. These secondary fracture lines can split into the calcaneocuboid joint, the anterior calcaneal facet, or exit the calcaneal body medially or laterally. The posterior calcaneal facet can be shattered. Impaction of the talar body into the calcaneus can result in lateral cortical bulging.[1] The sustentaculum fragment generally remains attached to the talus by the interosseous ligament. The tuberosity fragment displaces superiorly and laterally, resulting in shortening and flattening of the calcaneus. It typically rests in a varus heel position. No single treatment is suitable for all calcaneal fractures. Treatment should be tailored to the individual fracture pathoanatomy, accompanying soft-tissue damage, associated injuries, functional demand, and comorbidities of the patient. If operative treatment is chosen, reconstruction of the overall shape of the calcaneum and joint surfaces is of utmost importance to obtain a good functional result. Despite meticulous reconstruction, primary cartilage damage due to the impact at the time of injury may lead to post-traumatic subtalar arthritis. Even if subtalar fusion becomes necessary, patients benefit from primary anatomical reconstruction of the hindfoot geometry because in situ fusion is easier to perform and associated with better results than corrective fusion for hindfoot deformities in malunited calcaneal fractures.[2] If the fracture lines are not reduced, late complications of calcaneal malunion such as

loss of height of the heel with concomitant dorsiflexion of the talus; widening of the heel with associated subfibular impingement causing peroneal stenosis, tendinitis, or dislocation; subtalar and/or calcaneofibular post-traumatic arthritis; altered gait secondary to hindfoot malalignment; and nerve impingement may occur. Clinical evidence of malunion is evident with complaints of inability to wear standard footwear and asymmetry when wearing shoes. However, pain may be felt and localized to the lateral aspect of the foot (with varus malunion) or at the lateral subfibular area (with valgus malunion). Varus malunions may occur with nonsurgical treatment or as a result of malpositioning the tuberosity fragment during surgery for fixation or arthrodesis. Weight-bearing is shifted to the lateral border of the foot, and the patient develops severe pain. Clinical examination may show a worn-out lateral shoe edge and deformed heel counter, an obvious varus deformity, a widened heel, callosities and sores over the lateral aspect of the foot, and a prominent fibula laterally. Radiologic evaluation of malunions includes obtaining lateral radiographs to document heel shortening and talar dorsiflexion and subtalar or calcaneocuboid arthritis.[3] A decreased heel height (decreased Böhler's angle) and relative dorsiflexion of the talus (loss of the talar declination angle) may lead to an anterior tibiotalar abutment and impingement. The trapezoidal shape of the talus facilitates normal ankle joint dorsiflexion and plantar flexion as well as normal rotational and translational movement. When the talus assumes a more horizontal position, the wider anterior aspect of the talar body may become wedged in the ankle mortise and possibly contribute to the development of ankle arthrosis.[1,4] Shortening of the heel may also cause a lower portion of the malleoli to the ground and shoewear impingement. Malunion of the posterior tuberosity also shortens the effective lever arm of the gastrosoleus complex, leading to secondary weakness of the foot and ankle plantar flexion.[3]

If conservative treatment fails to relieve the symptoms, different surgical options have been postulated, either trying to address all the deformities or concentrating on certain aspects that are most clinically pressing.[5] In case of severe calcaneal malunion deformities, calcanectomy, calcaneal allograft transplantation, vascularized autografts, and calcaneal prosthesis are the potential options.[6]

Techniques of reconstructive osteotomy with or without subtalar arthrodesis to correct all the deformities associated with the late complications have been reported.[7-11] The goals are to reestablish the calcaneal height, restore the talocalcaneal relationship, and create a stable, plantigrade foot.[6] The important concept is that the relative displacement of the fragments, especially the superior and lateral translation of the tuberosity fragment along shear fracture line, is the primary reason for the loss of height, widening of the heel, and lateral impingement.[7] The reconstructive osteotomy recreates the primary fracture. This permits repositioning of the tuberosity that narrows the heel, alleviates impingement, and returns height to the heel. The subtalar arthrodesis alleviates the symptoms of post-traumatic arthritis.[7] Recent advances in computer-assisted virtual surgical technology facilitate preoperative planning for the reconstruction of calcaneal fracture malunion.[12] However, these are technically demanding and sometimes they are overdone because not all the deformities are symptomatic at the same time.

Stephens and Sanders[13] have classified the calcaneal malunion into three types according to the computed tomography (CT) appearance and proposed treatment algorithms accordingly. Type 1 malunion is a lateral wall exostosis without subtalar arthrosis or with far-lateral arthrosis only. Treatment includes peroneal tenolysis and lateral exostectomy with a lateral joint resection. Type 2 malunion is a lateral wall exostosis with subtalar arthrosis. Treatment includes peroneal tenolysis, lateral exostectomy, and subtalar arthrodesis. Type 3 malunion is a lateral wall exostosis, subtalar arthrosis, and a varus malunion of >10°. Treatment includes peroneal tenolysis, lateral exostectomy, subtalar arthrodesis, and calcaneal osteotomy to correct varus and valgus malalignment and shortening of the hindfoot.

The majority of cases of symptomatic subtalar joint arthritis can be treated with in situ arthrodesis. However, significant depression of calcaneal height after a fracture of the calcaneus makes in situ arthrodesis of the subtalar joint

difficult in terms of hindfoot alignment. Subtalar distraction bone block arthrodesis using autografts, allografts, or titanium truss may be performed in restoring hindfoot alignment, calcaneal height, and talar declination.[11,14] Myerson and Quill[15] suggested that this procedure was indicated in case of loss of >8 mm of heel height and radiographic evidence of anterior tibiotalar impingement. Overall, the results of this technique have been favorable, with high rates of fusion and improvement in the talocalcaneal angle after surgery. However, Myerson and Quill[15] as well as Flemister et al.[16] cautioned against aggressive attempts to restore heel height as this may lead to hindfoot varus.

Others have argued that complete correction of the hindfoot at the time of subtalar arthrodesis is not necessary to obtain a successful clinical result. Distraction bone block fusion attempts to restore hindfoot alignment through correction of talocalcaneal height and talar inclination, but the need to fully correct these parameters is controversial. In a review of 19 in situ subtalar fusions performed for late sequelae of calcaneal fractures, Chandler et al.[17] reported that no significant correlation between patient outcome and talar declination or talar height was found. Similarly, Flemister et al.[16] noted that no correlation was found between postsubtalar arthrodesis talar declination angle and the American Orthopaedic Foot and Ankle Society (AOFAS) ankle-hindfoot score. They concluded that complete anatomic restoration of hindfoot, based on the talar declination angle, is not necessary for a satisfactory outcome. Therefore, in the absence of anterior ankle impingement, in situ fusions are recommended versus more complicated distraction bone block fusions.[16] Distraction arthrodesis was recommended only if anterior ankle impingement was present.[16,17]

■ ARTHROSCOPIC SURGERY

With the advancement of foot and ankle arthroscopy and endoscopy, many of the late complications of calcaneal fractures can be managed arthroscopically.[18-20] By means of different arthroscopic and endoscopic approaches, different facets of the calcaneal fractures can be accessed. The posterior subtalar joint can be approached through the standard lateral approach[21,22] or the posterior approach.[23,24] The lateral calcaneal wall can be approached with the extra-articular extension of the posterior subtalar arthroscopy.[25-27] The anterior/middle calcaneal facet can be approached with anterior (talocalcaneonavicular) subtalar arthroscopy[28,29] or medial subtalar arthroscopy.[30] The cuboid facet can be approached through calcaneocuboid arthroscopy.[21,31] The peroneal tendons can be approached by peroneal tendoscopy.[32-34] Finally, the posterosuperior process and the anterosuperior process can also be approached endoscopically.[24,35-37]

Arthroscopic management of late complications of calcaneal fracture is a symptom-focused surgical approach and does not focus on the correction of the talocalcaneal relationship or restoration of the height or length of the calcaneus. For the sake of a symptom-focused surgical approach, the late complications of calcaneal fractures can be classified according to a patient's symptoms into three groups.[19] Group 1 complications include different impingement syndromes and arthrosis leading to focal hindfoot or ankle pain, which can usually be managed arthroscopically and/or endoscopically. Group 2 complications cause functional deficit of the foot and ankle; only selected cases can be managed arthroscopically and/or endoscopically. Group 3 complications refer to those causing diffuse and poorly localized pain; surgical treatment is not indicated and may even drastically worsen the patient's condition.[19] For those patients with symptoms related to loss of height (dorsiflexed talus with anterior ankle impingement) or length (weakness of the ankle plantar flexion with easy fatigue of the calf muscle) of the bone, subtalar distraction bone block arthrodesis or corrective osteotomy is indicated. Arthroscopic surgery can be considered in management of different impingement syndromes, subtalar and/or calcaneocuboid arthrosis, arthrofibrosis, post-traumatic synovitis, and various peroneal tendon pathologies associated with calcaneal fracture.

Calcaneofibular Impingement

Lateral calcaneal cortical bulging frequently occurs in patients treated conservatively. This can cause calcaneofibular or peroneal impingement syndrome or footwear problems. Lateral ostectomy should be considered if conservative treatment fails to relieve the symptoms. According to Stephens and Sander,[13] this is an important component of surgery for different types of calcaneal malunion.

Endoscopic lateral exostectomy can be performed with two or three lateral subtalar portals[25,27] or two posterior ankle endoscopy portals.[38,39] Preoperative evaluation of calcaneal malunion with CT scan and coronal two-dimensional (2D) reconstructions is more useful not only to determine the type of malunion of the calcaneus but also to assess with accuracy the size and localization of the lateral calcaneal exostosis, its relations with the lateral malleolus as well as the extent of degenerative changes in the subtalar joint. These iconographic data will help the surgeon to precisely know the localization and amount of bone resection that will

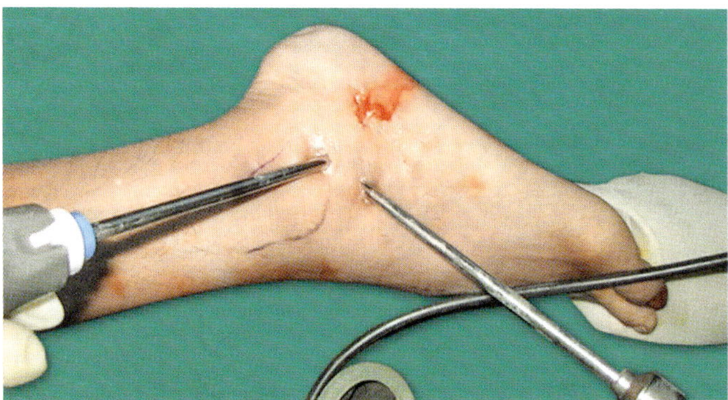

Fig. 1: Lateral calcaneal ostectomy with the anterolateral and middle subtalar portals. Ankle plantar flexion can relax the peroneal tendons and allow easier reach of the cortical bulge.

be necessary (particularly in the lateral part of the subtalar joint) and to adapt the portals.[25]

Intraoperatively, it is sometimes needed to locate the portals under fluoroscopy since the malunited calcaneus may distort the normal portal anatomy. The key of the procedure isstripping off the soft-tissue envelope from the lateral wall before bone shaving. Plantar flexion of the ankle can relax the peroneal tendons and allow easier reach of the cortical bulge **(Fig. 1)**.

Because of the integrity of the soft-tissue envelope, soft-tissue complication will be minimized. Moreover, the subtalar pathology can be examined and treated accordingly with the same approach.

This operation can also be performed through the peroneal tendoscopy (personal communication, Dr S Guillo, France). The apex of the cortical bulge can be reached after endoscopic resection of the deep part of the peroneal tendon sheath. It has the advantage of direct approach to the apex of the bulge and can deal with the associated pathology of the peroneal tendons.

Bauer et al.[25] have reported a case series of seven patients with calcaneofibular impingement treated by two-portal endoscopic exostectomy. Six out of the seven patients were "very satisfied" or "satisfied" about the results.

Posterior Ankle Impingement Syndrome Caused by Malunion of Joint Depressed-type Calcaneal Fracture

In cases of malunion of the joint depressed-type calcaneal fracture, the calcaneal bone spike immediately posterior to the depressed posterior calcaneal facet may cause posterior ankle impingement pain. The patient will complain of deep posterior ankle pain during activity with ankle plantar flexion, for example, walking downstairs. Operation should be considered if conservative management fails to relieve

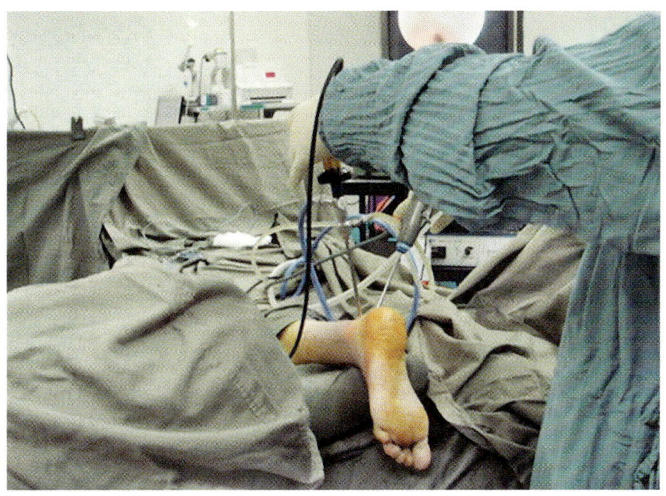

Fig. 2: Intraoperative fluoroscopy can help to identify the location of the bone spike.

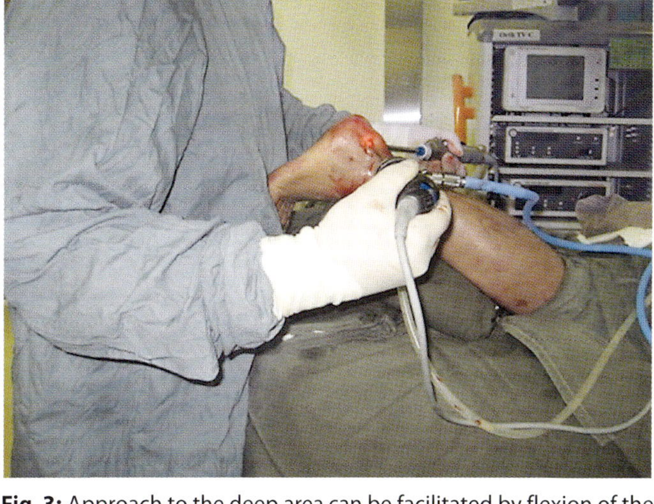

Fig. 3: Approach to the deep area can be facilitated by flexion of the knee and plantar flexion of the ankle during the procedure.

the pain. Similar to other causes of posterior ankle impingement, the bony impediment can be resected by means of a two-portal posterior ankle endoscopy.[24,39] Because of the malunion of the calcaneus, the portals should be modified to override the posterosuperior corner of the calcaneus in order to reach the posterior part of the subtalar joint. The posterior calcaneal facet is depressed and obscured by the calcaneal bone spike and scar tissue just posterior to it. The subtalar joint cannot be visualized easily. Intraoperative fluoroscopy **(Fig. 2)** is useful to identify the location of the bone spike and the posterior edge of the posterior calcaneal facet.[35]

Impingement to the Achilles Tendon by Malunited Tongue-type Calcaneal Process

Jung et al.[40] have reported two cases of secondary Haglund's deformity after malunion of tongue-type calcaneal fracture. The patients complained of posterosuperior heel pain due to a deformed bursal projection impinging on the Achilles tendon. They were treated by open excision of Haglund's deformity. With the technique of endoscopic calcaneoplasty,[41,42] this problem can be dealt with endoscopically. The resection of the posterosuperior process should be down to the insertion of the Achilles tendon since this is the site of impingement. The approach to the deep area can be facilitated by flexion of the knee and plantar flexion of the ankle during the procedure **(Fig. 3)**. Moreover, it is usually obscured by scar tissue between the bone and the Achilles tendon. This should be resected in order to gain adequate visualization of the Achilles insertion. Usually, the insertion can be left intact during the procedure. If it is detached accidentally, it can be repaired through the portal wounds by means of suture anchors.[43]

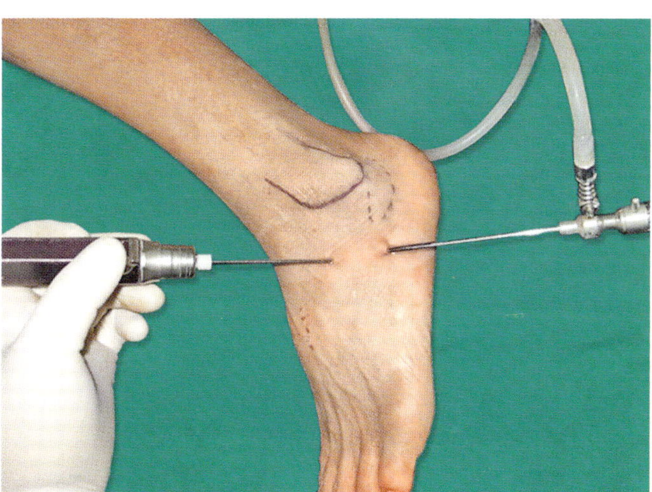

Fig. 4: Arthroscopic calcaneocuboid decompression.

Calcaneocuboid Impingement

Residual bone overhang from the displaced anterolateral calcaneal wall results in a loss of motion at the calcaneocuboid joint.[44] This will lead to pain over the calcaneocuboid joint and increased stress to the adjacent joints. Clare et al.[44] suggested that both the overhang and the lateral fourth of the distal aspect of the calcaneus should be removed as the articulation of this lateral portion with the cuboid is almost always arthritic. This can also be performed arthroscopically **(Fig. 4)**. The portals should be modified according to the location and span of the overhang. They should be placed at the dorsal and plantar ends of the overhang. After removal of the overhang, the joint can be examined for any synovitis or cartilage damage. The joint pathology can then be treated arthroscopically.

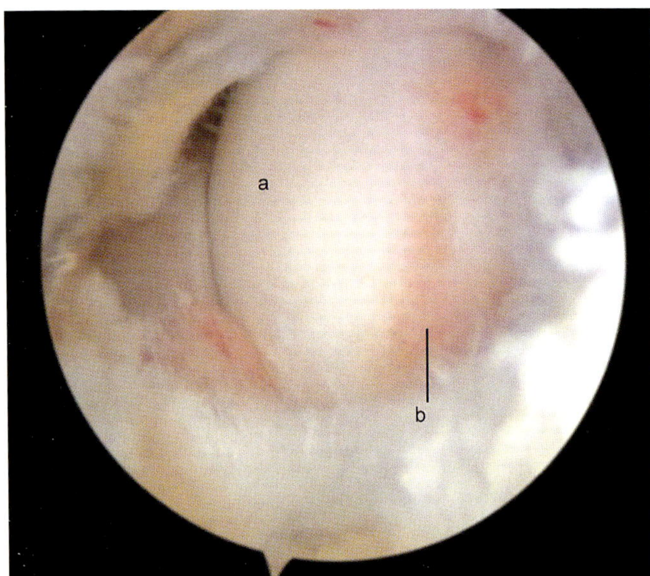

Fig. 5: Chondral lesion at the plantar lateral side of the talar head was seen after excision of the impinging anterosuperior calcaneal process. a: Talar head; b: Chondral lesion.

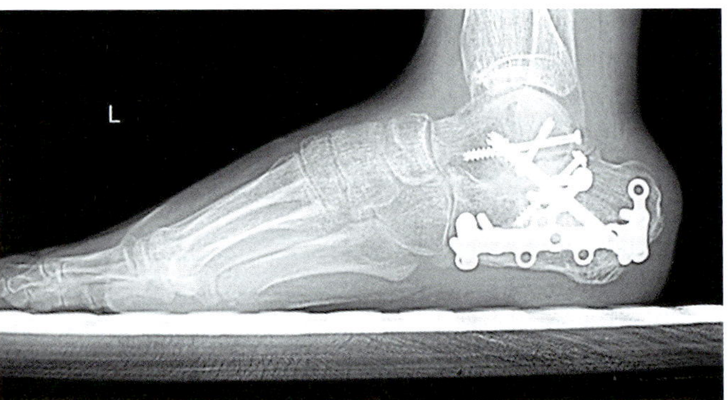

Fig. 6: Only those calcaneal screws that are blocking the insertion of the arthrodesis screw are needed to be removed.

Anterosuperior Impingement

Occasionally malunited anterosuperior process with elongation of the process or unhealed fragment at this region can impinge on the plantar lateral side of the talar head. The patient will complain of local swelling, deep pain and tenderness at that region, and limited foot inversion. A preoperative oblique radiograph of the foot is sufficient to confirm the diagnosis. A CT scan may be needed if the radiograph cannot reveal the lesion. Endoscopic excision of the anterosuperior calcaneal process[36,37] is indicative of conservative treatment that fails to relieve the symptoms. The working portal is at the junction between the talonavicular and calcaneocuboid joints. The visualization portal is either the anterolateral subtalar portal or the lateral midtarsal portal[21] depending on whether there is any associated subtalar or calcaneocuboid joint problem. If there is no associated subtalar or calcaneocuboid pathology, the lateral midtarsal portal is the preferred viewing portal. It is important to examine the plantar lateral part of the talar head after resection of the process. Cartilage lesion is frequently present at this part of the talar head due to previous impingement by the calcaneal process **(Fig. 5)**. Arthroscopic debridement and microfracture can be done if the lesion is present. This endoscopic technique provides a minimally invasive approach for excision of the symptomatic nonunion of the anterior calcaneal process. It can also allow detailed arthroscopic assessment of the adjacent sites for possible concomitant lesions. In our experience, the pain relief is good after the procedure, but the hindfoot motion may not be improved.

Subtalar and/or Calcaneocuboid Arthrosis

Subtalar joint arthrosis frequently occurs if the calcaneal fracture is managed conservatively because of the articular incongruity. Even in anatomically reduced fractures, however, arthritis can occur secondary to cartilage damage from the initial trauma.[1-3] Penetration of the joint by implants and residual incongruity of the posterior subtalar joint are other factors contributing to the development of post-traumatic subtalar arthrosis in operated cases. However, initial open reduction and internal fixation restore calcaneal shape, alignment, and height favoring in situ subtalar arthrodesis.[2,45] In situ subtalar arthrodesis is also indicated for symptomatic calcaneal malunion with minimal deformity but with significant subtalar arthritis (Stephens type II).[1,17] Patients who do not report anterior ankle pain and who have no pain anteriorly on forced passive ankle dorsiflexion or while squatting are candidates for this procedure.[1,17] Mi et al.[46] have reported good union rate and clinical results with the arthroscopic subtalar arthrodesis for malunion of calcaneal fracture.

Arthroscopic subtalar arthrodesis is best suited for patients requiring in situ fusion with minimal deformity or bony destruction. This can be performed with either the lateral portal or the posterior portal[23] technique. During the procedure, there is no need to remove all the calcaneal implant but only those screws that block the insertion of the arthrodesis screws **(Fig. 6)**. The posterior portal technique[23] provides better and safe access to the posteromedial corner, better control of the arthrodesis position, more thorough preparation of the fusion site, minimal bone removal, easier placement of the screws, and less chance of varus–valgus malunion.

In cases of Stephens type III malunion, calcaneal osteotomy is frequently performed in conjunction with the subtalar joint arthrodesis. Another approach is to correct the varus position through the subtalar joint level. This can be achieved by performing the "closing wedge procedure"[22] during the arthroscopic subtalar arthrodesis. However, further lateral impingement can occur if correction of the varus deformity by placing the subtalar joint into a valgus position. It is important to examine the lateral gutter again after the subtalar arthrodesis and decompress the lateral gutter further if needed.

Arthritic calcaneocuboid joint is frequently asymptomatic. If the subtalar joint is fused in plantigrade position, rotational motion across the calcaneocuboid joint only flexes or extends, and this motion is coupled with the motion of the lateral Lisfranc joint and stress across the midtarsal joint is minimized. Arthrodesis of the calcaneocuboid joint is only performed if the arthrosis is symptomatic.

Arthroscopic triple arthrodesis may be indicated when the hindfoot pathology involves the talonavicular joint and/or the calcaneocuboid joint. Triple arthrodesis also may be indicated in the patient with preexisting deformity in conjunction with calcaneal malunion. A patient with preexisting flatfoot deformity and symptomatic calcaneal malunion may benefit from triple arthrodesis to correct the deformity and address the malunion.[1]

Arthroscopic triple arthrodesis[21] includes arthroscopic arthrodesis of the subtalar joint, talonavicular joint, and calcaneocuboid joint. Subtalar arthroscopy is performed through the anterolateral and middle subtalar portals. The midtarsal arthroscopy is performed through the lateral, dorsolateral, dorsomedial, and medial portals. Lateral and dorsolateral portals are established for calcaneocuboid arthroscopy. The lateral portal is identified at the plantar-lateral corner of the calcaneocuboid joint. The dorsolateral portal is directly over the space between the talonavicular and calcaneocuboid joints.

It is the most important portal of this procedure because the medial aspect of the calcaneocuboid joint, the lateral and plantar aspects of the talonavicular joint, and the junction between the talus, calcaneum, navicular, and cuboid can be approached through this portal. The talonavicular joint is approached through the medial, dorsomedial, and dorsolateral portals. The medial portal is at the medial side of the talonavicular joint, just dorsal to the posterior tibial tendon. The dorsomedial portal is at the midpoint between the medial and dorsolateral portals. The hindfoot deformity can be corrected with the "closing wedge procedure"[22] after preparation of the fusion surfaces. Recently, the technique of three-portal arthroscopic triple arthrodesis has been developed, and preparation of fusion surfaces of all three joints can be achieved via the anterolateral subtalar, dorsolateral midtarsal, and medial midtarsal portals.[47]

Subtalar Arthrofibrosis

Subtalar arthrofibrosis with limited subtalar motion is common after calcaneal fracture, especially in operated patients. With a stiff subtalar joint, inversion eversion stresses are transferred to the ankle joint, especially the lateral ligamentous structures of the ankle. These compensatory stresses in the ankle joint, particularly in the coronal plane of motion, will result in residual pain on the lateral side of the ankle.[44] The patient may notice difficulty in walking on an uneven surface, and patient satisfaction will be impaired.

Open subtalar release is not a good choice as early vigorous mobilization exercise is prohibited by the extensive surgical scar. Arthroscopic subtalar release[26] has the advantage of smaller surgical wounds such that immediate vigorous mobilization is allowed. The tight lateral structure can be released in stages to minimize the risk of over-release resulting in subtalar instability.[26] The lateral ligaments are divided into deep, intermediate, and superficial layers and those contributing to the stability of the subtalar joint. We preserve most of the interosseous talocalcaneal ligament during arthroscopic subtalar release. In addition, we perform quite extensive soft-tissue release, even extending beyond the surgical scar **(Fig. 7)** in the patients with previous open reduction, according to the intraoperative subtalar inversion motion gained. Early peroneal strengthening exercise is incorporated into the rehabilitation program to improve the dynamic stability of the subtalar joint.

Synovitis

Post-traumatic synovitis of the subtalar and/or calcaneo-fibular joint is the common cause of lateral heel pain after calcaneal fracture. The anterior subtalar joint synovitis is a

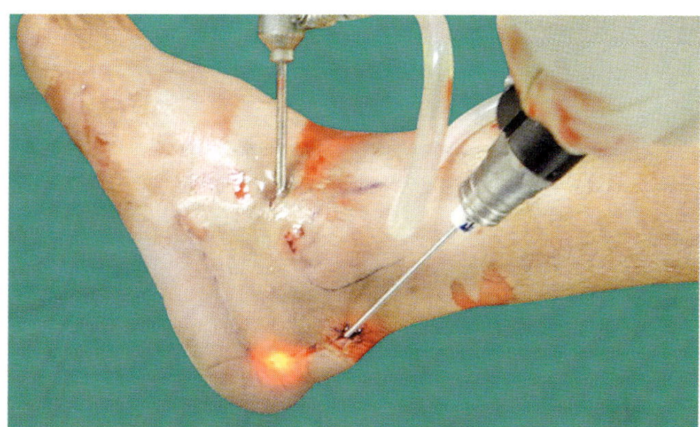

Fig. 7: Arthroscopic release of the subtalar joint should extend beyond the old surgical scar.

commonly missed diagnosis. The joint(s) involved can be determined by clinical localization of the site of tenderness. The posterior subtalar joint synovitis usually presents with tenderness at sinus tarsi and lateral subtalar gutter. The calcaneocuboid joint synovitis can be determined by local tenderness over the joint. Anterior subtalar synovitis usually presents with sinus tarsi pain and sometimes also medial heel pain around the sustentaculum tali. Tenderness is usually located at the junction between the talonavicular and the calcaneocuboid joints. The corresponding arthroscopy[21,28-31] and arthroscopic synovectomy can be performed to treat this problem.

Peroneal Tendon Pathologies

Various acute peroneal tendon abnormalities can occur with intra-articular calcaneal fractures, and these include lateral displacement, bony impingement, subluxation or dislocation, hematomas and scar tissue formation, and entrapment of tendons.[3] Peroneal tendonitis may occur secondarily by implant irritation when a lateral approach is used. It can present as pain over the lateral aspect of the heel. Buckling or giving way when walking also may suggest peroneal tendon dysfunction. Myerson and Quill[15] recommend confirming localization of the pain along the course of the peroneal tendon and eliciting pain with passive dorsiflexion and resistance to eversion of the hindfoot.

Nonoperative treatment options include the use of shoe inserts and massage and manipulation over the involved area in an attempt to break adhesions along the peroneal sheath.[3] Peroneal tendoscopy[32] can be considered if conservative treatment fails. Endoscopic peroneal tendon decompression, tendon repair, synovectomy, and retinaculum reconstruction can be performed.[33,34]

Combination of Pathologies

Symptomatic malunion often has multiple components, and combinations of different arthroscopic and endoscopic procedures are needed. Identification of the correct sources of symptoms is key to selecting the most appropriate surgical procedures and ensuring that the planned surgical procedures specifically address the underlying pathologies.[19]

For example, combined posterior impingement pain and lateral subfibular pain can be managed by posterior ankle endoscopy.[38,39] Through this endoscopic approach, the posterior ankle and lateral subfibular space can be accessed, and the impinging bones can be resected. The peroneal tendons can also be released via the same endoscopic approach **(Fig. 8)**.[38]

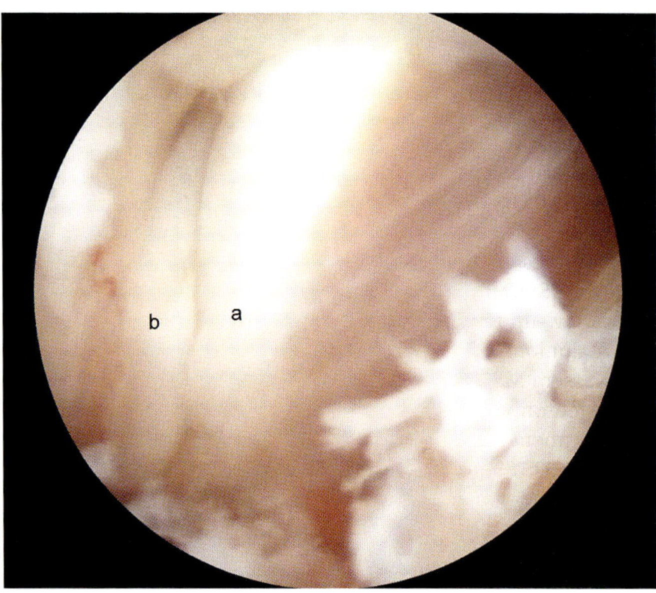

Fig. 8: Posterior ankle endoscopy with the posteromedial portal as the viewing portal and the posterolateral portal as the working portal. The peroneal tendons are released endoscopically. a: Peroneus brevis tendon; b: Lateral malleolus.

■ TAKE-HOME MESSAGE

Arthroscopic management of late complications after calcaneal fracture is symptom-focusing. Identification of the correct source of symptoms is the key in selecting the appropriate procedure. This may be challenging because symptomatic malunion often has multiple components.[1] Detailed history taking and clinical examination are the most important tools for surgical decision-making. Radiographic measures should not be the sole determinant for surgical decision-making.[1] Selective injections are sometimes helpful in determining the source of pathology.[15]

■ REFERENCES

1. Banerjee R, Saltzman C, Anderson RB, Nickisch F. Management of calcaneal malunion. J Am Acad Orthop Surg. 2011;19:27-36.
2. Rammelt S, Sangeorzan BJ, Swords MP. Calcaneal fractures—should we operate or should we not operate? Indian J Orthop. 2018;52:220-30.
3. Lim EVA, Leung JPF. Complications of intraarticular calcaneal fractures. Clin Orthop Relat Res. 2001;(391):7-16.
4. Rammelt S, Grass R, Zawadski T, Biewener A, Zwipp H. Foot function after subtalar distraction bone-block arthrodesis. A prospective study. J Bone Joint Surg Br. 2004;86:659-68.
5. Reddy V, Fukuda T, Ptaszek AJ. Calcaneus malunion and nonunion. Foot Ankle Clin. 2007;12:125-35.
6. Iceman KL, Magnus MK, Roukis TS. Salvaging the unsalvageable severe malunion deformity after displaced intra-articular calcaneal fractures: what options exist? Clin Podiatr Med Surg. 2019;36:339-47.

7. Romash MM. Reconstructive osteotomy of the calcaneus with subtalar arthrodesis for malunited calcaneal fractures. Clin Orthop Relat Res. 1993;(290):157-67.

8. Farouk A, Ibrahim A, Abd-Ella MM, El Ghazali S. Effect of subtalar fusion and calcaneal osteotomy on function, pain, and gait mechanics for calcaneal malunion. Foot Ankle Int. 2019;40:1094-103.

9. Clare MP, Crawford WS. Managing complications of calcaneus fractures. Foot Ankle Clin. 2017;22:105-16.

10. Lee HS, Kim WJ, Park ES, Kim JY, Kim YH, Lee YK. Mid-term follow-up results of calcaneal reconstruction for calcaneal malunion. BMC Musculoskelet Disord. 2019;20:43.

11. Kassem MS, Elgeidi A, Badran M, Farag F. Sagittal resection osteotomy with bone block distraction subtalar fusion for treatment of malunited calcaneal fractures. J Foot Ankle Surg. 2019;58:739-47.

12. Qiang M, Zhang K, Chen Y, Jia X, Wang X, Chen S, et al. Computer-assisted virtual surgical technology in pre-operative design for the reconstruction of calcaneal fracture malunion. Int Orthop. 2019;43:1669-77.

13. Stephens HM, Sanders R. Calcaneal malunions: results of a prognostic computed tomography classification system. Foot Ankle Int. 1996;17:395-401.

14. Persaud SJ, Catanzariti AR. Subtalar joint distraction arthrodesis utilizing a titanium truss: a case series. J Foot Ankle Surg. 2019;58:785-91.

15. Myerson M, Quill Jr GE. Late complications of fractures of the calcaneus. J Bone Joint Surg Am. 1993;75:331-41.

16. Flemister Jr AS, Infante AF, Sanders RW, Walling AK. Subtalar arthrodesis for complications of intra-articular calcaneal fractures. Foot Ankle Int. 2000;21:392-9.

17. Chandler JT, Bonar SK, Anderson RB, Davis WH. Results of in situ subtalar arthrodesis for late sequelae of calcaneus fractures. Foot Ankle Int. 1999;20:18-24.

18. Lui TH. Arthroscopy and endoscopy of the foot and ankle: indications for new techniques. Arthroscopy. 2007;23:889-902.

19. Lui TH, Pan XH, Pan Y. Arthroscopic and endoscopic management of common complications after displaced intra-articular calcaneal fractures. Clin Podiatr Med Surg. 2019;36:279-93.

20. Lui TH, Chan KB. Arthroscopic management of late complications of calcaneal fractures. Knee Surg Sports Traumatol Arthrosc. 2013;21:1293-9.

21. Lui TH. New technique of arthroscopic triple arthrodesis. Arthroscopy. 2006;22:464.e1-5.

22. Lui TH. Case report: correction of neglected club foot deformity by arthroscopic assisted triple arthrodesis. Arch Orthop Trauma Surg. 2010;130:1007-11.

23. Carro LP, Golanó P, Vega J. Arthroscopic subtalar arthrodesis: the posterior approach in the prone position. Arthroscopy. 2007;23:445.e1-4.

24. van Dijk CN, Scholten PE, Krips R. A 2-portal endoscopic approach for diagnosis and treatment of posterior ankle pathology. Arthroscopy. 2000;16:871-6.

25. Bauer T, Deranlot J, Hardy P. Endoscopic treatment of calcaneo-fibular impingement. Knee Surg Sports Traumatol Arthrosc. 2011;19:131-6.

26. Lui TH. Arthroscopic subtalar release of post-traumatic subtalar stiffness. Arthroscopy. 2006;22:1364.e1-4.

27. Lui TH. Endoscopic lateral calcaneal ostectomy for calcaneofibular impingement. Arch Orthop Trauma Surg. 2007;127:265-7.

28. Lui TH. Clinical tips: anterior subtalar (talocalcaneonavicular) arthroscopy. Foot Ankle Int. 2008;29:94-6.

29. Lui TH, Chan KB, Chan LK. Portal safety and efficacy of anterior subtalar arthroscopy: a cadaveric study. Knee Surg Sports Traumatol Arthrosc. 2010;18:233-7.

30. Mekhail AO, Heck BE, Ebraheim NA, Jackson WT. Arthroscopy of the subtalar joint: establishing a medial portal. Foot Ankle Int. 1995;16:427-32.

31. Oloff L, Schulhofer SD, Fanton G, Dillingham M. Arthroscopy of the calcaneocuboid and talonavicular joints. J Foot Ankle Surg. 1996;35:101-8.

32. van Dijk CN, Kort N. Tendoscopy of the peroneal tendons. Arthroscopy. 1998;14:471-8.

33. Lui TH. Endoscopic peroneal retinaculum reconstruction. Knee Surg Sports Traumatol Arthrosc. 2006;14:478-81.

34. Lui TH. Endoscopic management of recalcitrant retrofibular pain without peroneal tendon subluxation or dislocation. Arch Orthop Trauma Surg. 2012;132:357-61.

35. Lui TH. Posterior ankle impingement syndrome caused by malunion of joint depressed type calcaneal fracture. Knee Surg Sports Traumatol Arthrosc. 2008;16:687-9.

36. Lui TH. Endoscopic excision of symptomatic nonunion of anterior calcaneal process. J Foot Ankle Surg. 2011;50:476-9.

37. Lui TH. Arthroscopic resection of the calcaneonavicular coalition or the "too long" anterior process of the calcaneus. Arthroscopy. 2006;22:903.e1-4.

38. Chu KM, Lui TH. Endoscopic lateral calcaneal ostectomy and peroneal tendon decompression with the patient in the prone position as management of subfibular impingement after calcaneal fracture. Arthrosc Tech. 2019;8:e1069-73.

39. Lui TH, Siu YC, Ngai WK. Endoscopic management of calcaneofibular impingement and posterior ankle impingement syndrome caused by malunion of joint depressed-type calcaneal fracture. Arthrosc Tech. 2018;7:e71-6.

40. Jung HG, Yoo MJ, Kim MH. Late sequelae of secondary Haglund's deformity after malunion of tongue type calcaneal fracture: report of two cases. Foot Ankle Int. 2002;23:1014-7.

41. van Dijk CN, van Dyk GE, Scholten PE, Kort NP. Endoscopic calcaneoplasty. Am J Sports Med. 2001;29:185-9.

42. Lui TH. Endoscopic calcaneoplasty and Achilles tendoscopy with the patient in supine position. Arthrosc Tech. 2016;5:e1475-9.

43. Lui TH. Technique tip: reattachment of the Achilles tendon after endoscopic calcaneoplasty. Foot Ankle Int. 2007;28:742-5.

44. Clare MP, Lee III WE, Sanders RW. Intermediate to long-term results of a treatment protocol for calcaneal fracture malunions. J Bone Joint Surg. 2005;87:963-73.

45. Radnay CS, Clare MP, Sanders RW. Subtalar fusion after displaced intra-articular calcaneal fractures: does initial operative treatment matter? J Bone Joint Surg Am. 2009;91:541-6.

46. Mi K, Liu P, Liu W, Feng Z. Arthroscopical subtalar arthrodesis for malunion of calcaneal fractures. Zhongguo Xiu Fu Chong Jian Wai Ke Za Zhi. 2010;24:875-7.

47. Li HM, Lui TH. Correction of severe flatfoot deformity by 3-portal arthroscopic triple arthrodesis. Arthrosc Tech. 2019;9:e103-9.

Stress Fractures of the Calcaneus

Sidak Dhillon, Mandeep S Dhillon

"In my experience, stress is the cause of all injury and pain".

–Tobe Hanson

"It's not stress that kills us, it's our reaction to it".

–Hans Selye

■ INTRODUCTION AND HISTORY

Since the description of stress fractures in the mid-1800s by physicians in the Prussian Army, there has been significant documentation of this overuse injury.[1,2] Called by various names, these are basically fatigue fractures due to overloading of either normal bone or abnormal bone. In army recruits, they were called "*march fractures*" and when associated with diseases they were labeled "insufficiency fractures"; other synonyms such as "*pseudo fractures*", "*exhaustion fractures*", and "*creeping fractures*" are no longer used.[1,2] Much of the published literature focuses on other bones, with the tibia and metatarsals taking the bulk of the focus; the calcaneus stress fracture, although uncommon, would not fall into the rare variety **(Table 1)**.

A significant percentage of these cases have been documented as being bilateral; **Table 2** looks at the published series, and the reported incidence of bilaterality in calcaneus stress fractures ranges from 33 to 75% of cases.

■ CLINICAL PRESENTATION[13-15]

The clinical presentation is usually innocuous and can happen after strenuous activity in young adults (such as in army recruits) or in the elderly, where the bone is weakened, and more than usual stress is applied. Pain is the common initial presentation, and this may be vaguely localized in the initial phases; however, it becomes localized to the tuberosity over time. Swelling is unusual but may be associated with the pain. It is important to evaluate the patient clinically and order the appropriate investigations; otherwise, these fractures are frequently missed.

Elderly patients could present with these fractures which can occur in osteoporotic bones, where they may be labeled insufficiency fractures and are seen even with normal stresses of day-to-day life.

The heel pain is often mistaken for the more common presentations of plantar fasciitis and insertional tendinopathy as the symptoms may overlap with these conditions.

TABLE 1: Reported percentage of cases reported in major series of stress fractures.[3-8]

Author/year	Number of cases of stress fractures	Calcaneus cases
Hullinger, 1944	53	71 (some bilateral)
Yale, 1976	3,675 consecutive stress fractures	>2,000
Pester and Smith, 1992	1,338 stress fractures in 109,296 soldiers (0.96%)	• 20% calcaneus • 66% metatarsals
Greaney et al., 1983	250 marines, 839 abnormal sites on bone scan	95 abnormal signals

TABLE 2: Reported cases over the years and incidence of bilaterality.[3,9-12]

Author/year	Number of cases reported	Bilateral cases
Hullinger, 1944	53	33%
Winfield and Dennis, 1959	13	38%
Leabhart, 1959	113	73%
MacDonald, 1966	27	44%
Morris and Blickenstaff, 1967		50%
Hopson and Perry, 1977	12	75%

Proper evaluation of the site of tenderness will show that the tenderness is over the bone and not on the insertion of the tendo-Achilles or the plantar fascia; this may be difficult to determine in many cases.

Like in the other causes of heel pain, the pain in stress fractures is exacerbated by activity and could often be relieved by rest. Some cases have been documented where the pain is seen in the ipsilateral heel in elderly ladies who have undergone arthroplasty and have increased their activities after the arthroplasty.

■ DIAGNOSIS/IMAGING[16-18]

The most common investigation that is ordered is X-rays, and the standard protocol is to take X-rays in anteroposterior (AP) and lateral views. In the initial phases, these X-rays may not show any fracture, and other investigations may be required to confirm the diagnosis. Repeat X-rays at a later date will show the development of sclerotic lines, most commonly in the tuberosity; if adequately followed up, the healing of the fracture can be documented by X-rays also **(Figs. 1A to C)**.

Magnetic resonance imaging (MRI) is the gold standard investigation in the early phases, and it clearly defines the problem **(Figs. 2A and B)**; the signal change is the most common in the tuberosity. Initially, this could be a longitudinal line, but, in most cases, due to the delays in diagnosis, there is widespread bone edema involving the tuberosity **(Figs. 3A to J)**. Anterior process fractures have also been documented, but they are extremely rare.[18]

The signal change in the MRI may persist over long periods even after the pain has subsided; MRI is thus not a good follow-up tool to determine return to activity in young, aggressive individuals (such as army recruits) who have developed this overuse injury. Simple X-rays will be able to demonstrate appropriate healing **(Figs. 1A to C)**.

Other investigations such as bone scans have a role, but are rarely indicated; computed tomography (CT) scans have a negligible role.

Atypical situations:[11-15] Hyperparathyroidism, cerebral palsy, after arthroplasty, Charcot foot. Calcaneal stress fractures have been documented in abnormal situations, where the bone is affected indirectly. Stress fractures of the calcaneus in the elderly have been documented relatively frequently in recent years. Miki et al.[19] reported on five patients who developed a calcaneal stress fracture after a total knee or total hip arthroplasty; the average age of the patients reported was 78 years, and all had been diagnosed with osteoporosis. Most of the fractures were noted at about 10 weeks postsurgery and presented with heel-related pain. Initial X-rays did not show the fracture in two of five cases, but a sclerotic line appeared eventually in most of them. One fracture went on to displace, while four others healed with conservative treatment.

These stress fractures are not necessarily due to osteoporosis alone, and no clear explanation exists as to why they happen. One hypothesis is that these osteoporotic bones were inadequately loaded prior to surgery due to knee pain; they developed a stress reaction/fracture after cessation of knee pain by total knee replacement (TKR) and resumption of normal weight-bearing on the ipsilateral osteoporotic heel.

The message is to keep this possibility in mind in elderly females who have undergone ipsilateral knee replacement and develop heel pain without any obvious cause.

Kaya et al.[20] reported a rare case of bilateral stress fracture/reaction in a 41-year-old lady due to long-term antiepileptic

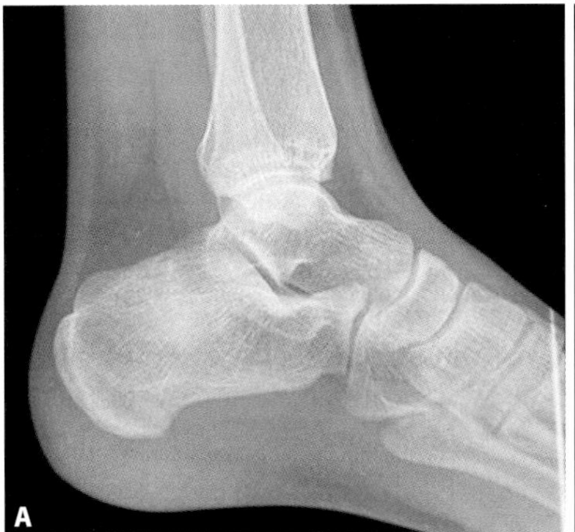
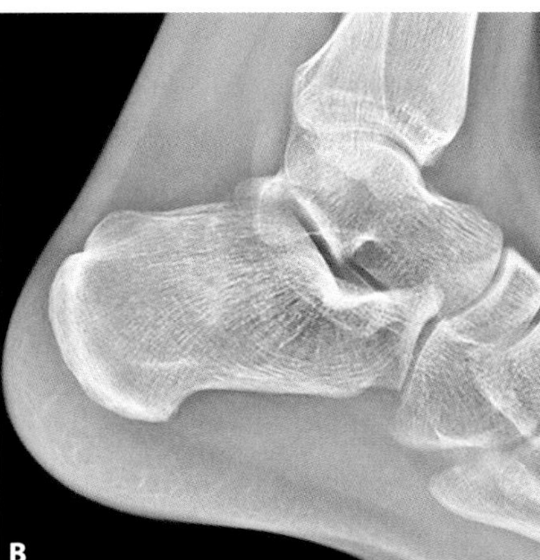
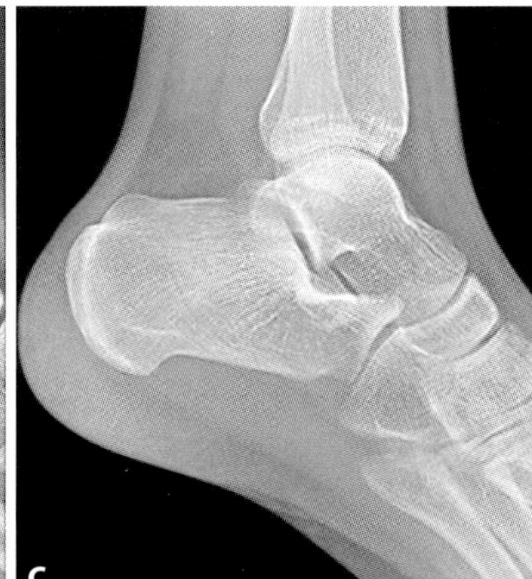

Figs. 1A to C: A 17-year-old male, military recruit; pain in heel after intensive training. Serial X-rays show stress reaction (A), developing into a fracture line (B), which ultimately is resolved with no symptoms (C) within 6 months of rest.

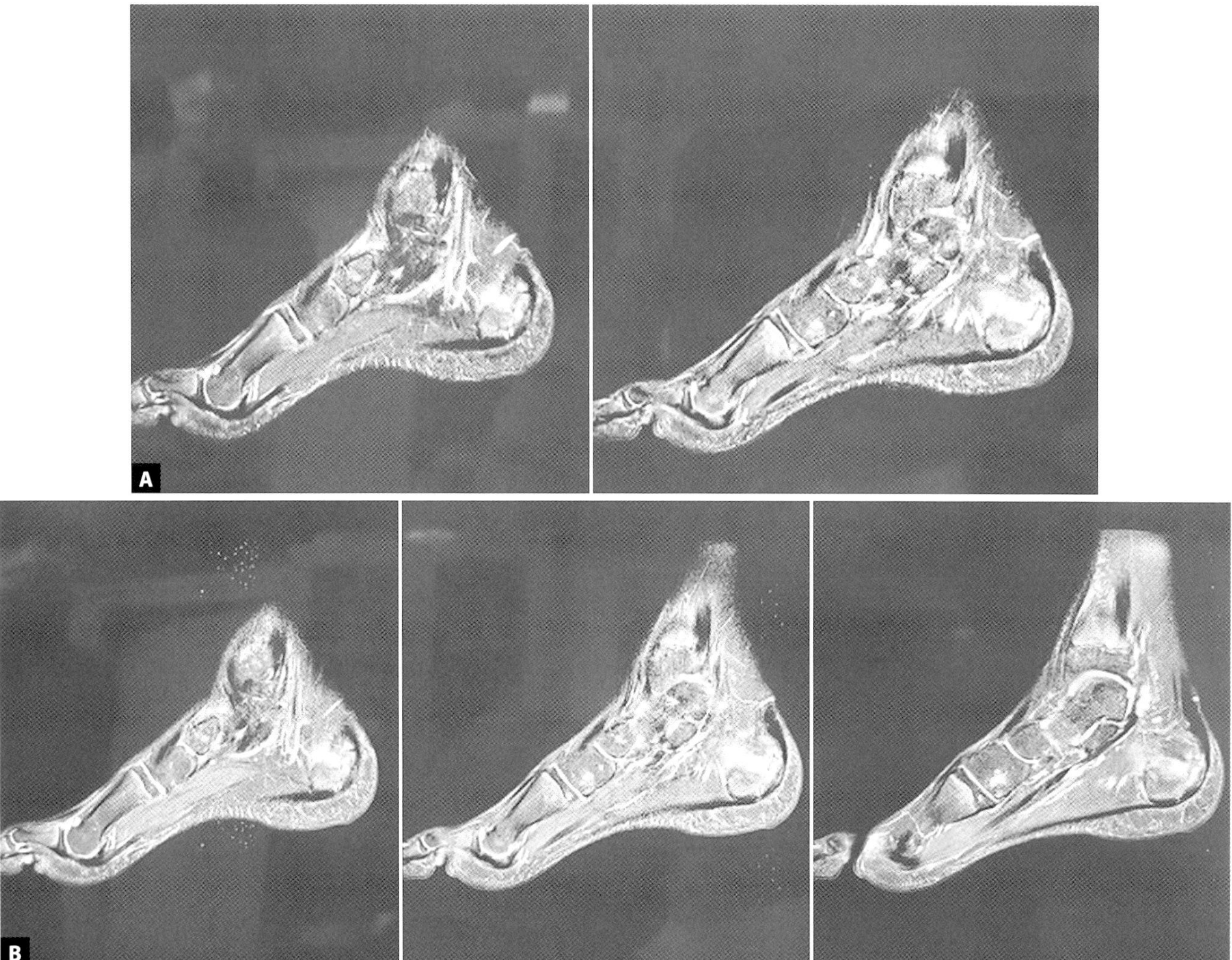

Figs. 2A and B: Magnetic resonance imaging (MRI) images showing a stress reaction in a 23-year-old cricket player which developed over 3 months. X-rays showed no evidence of fracture, but MRI revealed stress reaction in the posterior inferior part of the tuberosity.

drug use (carbamazepine), which was diagnosed after a long history of pain; MRI showed bilateral lesions.

Similarly, low bone density in other situations, such as celiac disease, has also shown this rare problem; Kose et al. reported a case which presented with planter pain, diagnosed as plantar fasciitis in a 33-year-old woman.[21]

Atypical heel pain masquerading as plantar fasciitis has also been reported in a patient who was subsequently diagnosed with hyperparathyroidism-induced stress fracture of the calcaneus.[22]

Lui[23] published a case of heel pain in a 75-year-old lady with previous history of back pain with radiation to the buttocks and was wheelchair-bound; the neurological issues were masked. She presented as a case of neglected insufficiency fracture with a preexisting neurological problem. The findings were presentation with a swollen foot without any history of trauma. Radiological presentation was

that of depression of the posterior facet of the calcaneus with malunion, which was confirmed by CT scans.

Similarly, Takai et al.[24] have reported on a 63-year-old male, with syphilis and Charcot's knee, who developed an avulsion fracture of the calcaneus after resuming walking after a knee arthroplasty. The cause of stress fracture was proposed to be decreased protective sensations in the limb, as the fracture could then occur unnoticed with minimal trauma.

Stein and Stelling documented this problem in a child with cerebral palsy,[25] while Pearce et al.[26] have shown that a stress fracture of the calcaneus developed in the anterior process in association with a calcaneonavicular coalition.

The above-mentioned conditions are documented to highlight the fact that these stress fractures can occur with systemic abnormalities leading to weakened bone or with altered biomechanics.

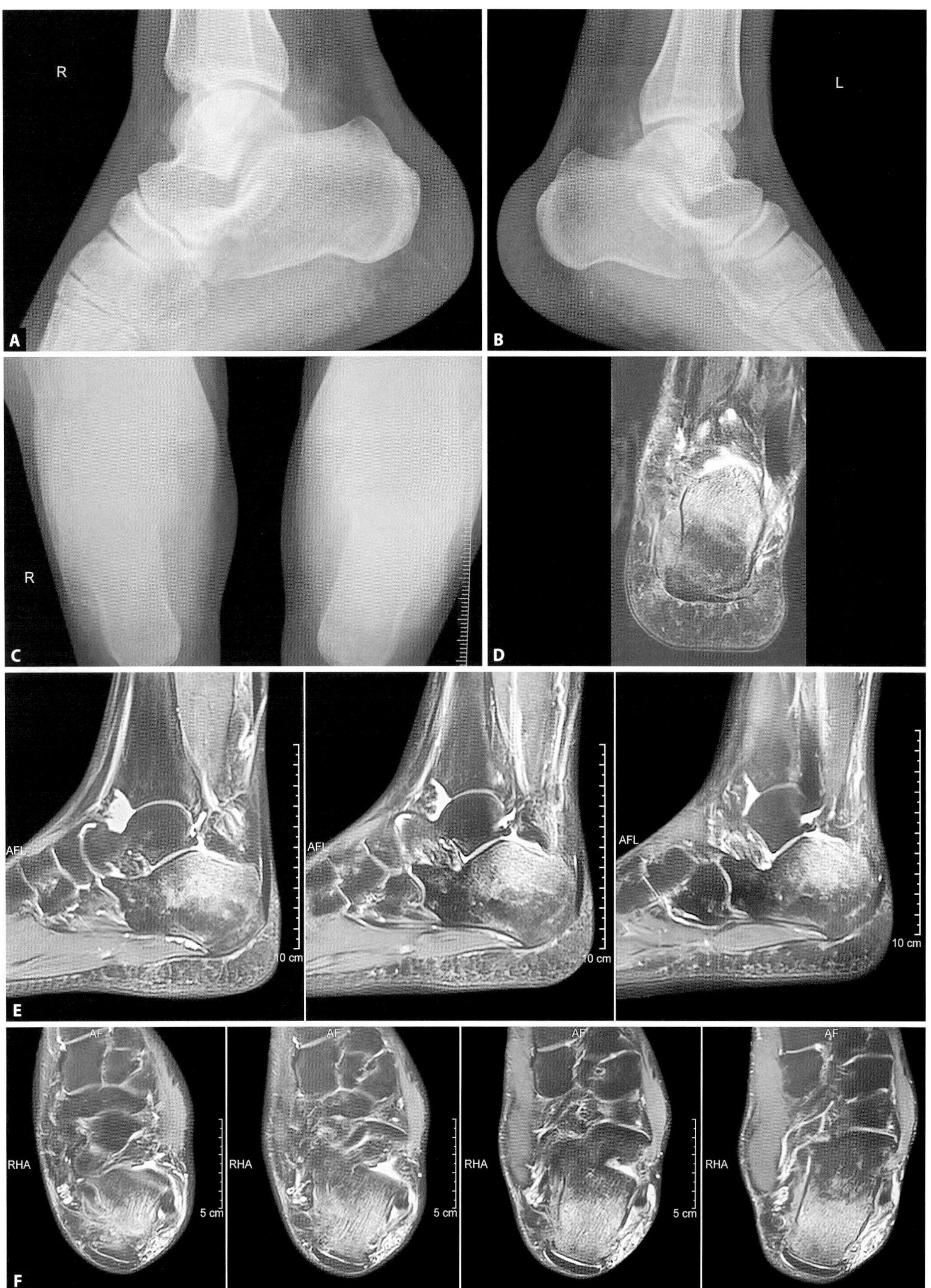

Figs. 3A to F

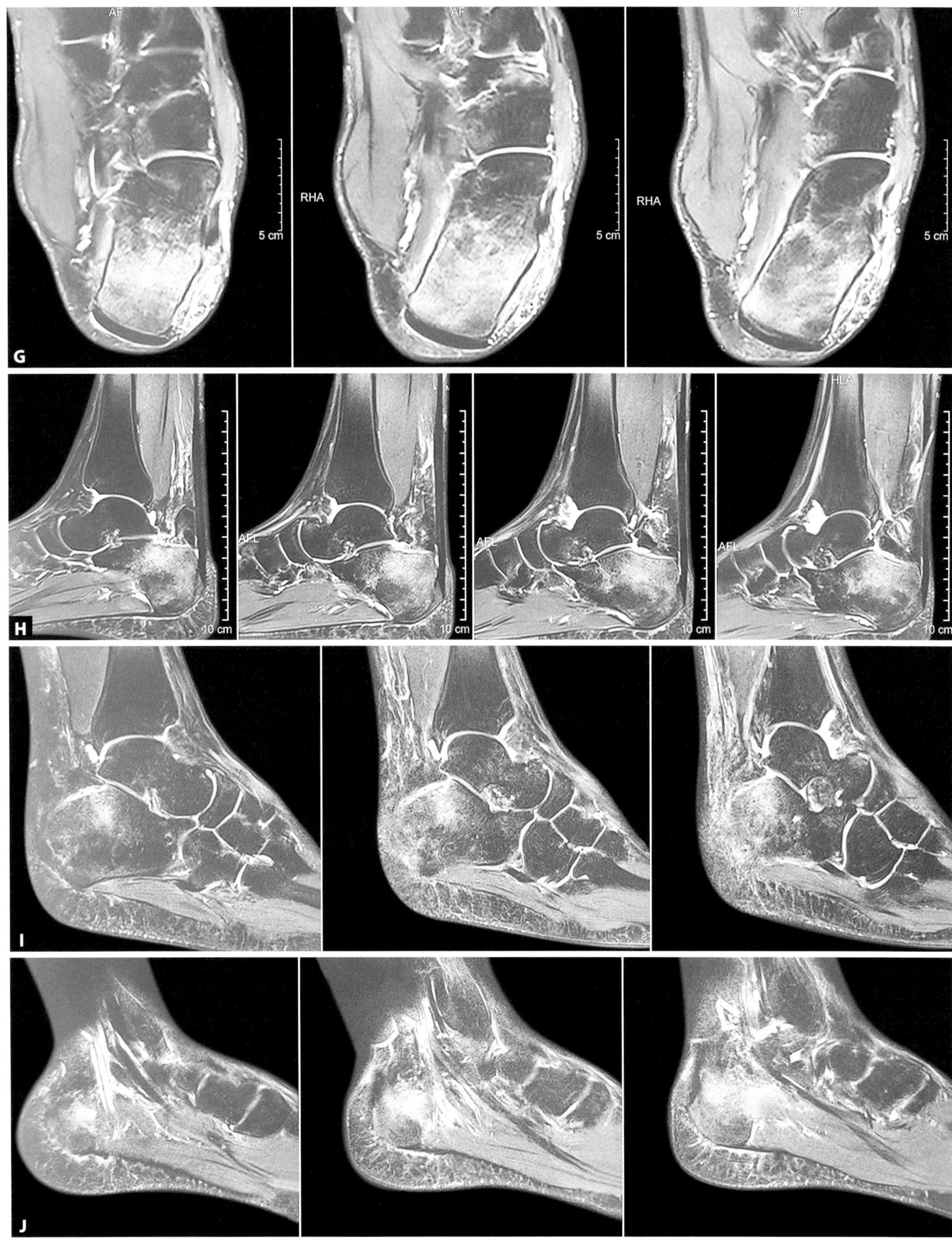

Figs. 3G to J

Figs. 3A to J: X-rays of a 28-year-old male surgeon in training who developed bilateral heel pain after playing badminton for over 4 weeks to lose weight. X-rays were noncommittal, but magnetic resonance imaging (MRI) showed a stress fracture in both heels, with signal change localized to the tuberosity. On one side, a fracture line extending to the subtalar joint was seen, but this was not clear on the other side.

MANAGEMENT OPTIONS

Calcaneal stress fractures usually heal on their own once the stress is removed and medical comorbidity is addressed. The basic treatment option in these cases is to limit weight-bearing till the fracture heals. Usually, there is no need for a protective cast, but a protective shoe or well-padded splint may be of benefit; the use of a walking aid is often beneficial in the elderly patients. A walking boot or cast in young active adults may be of benefit, but the key point is reduction of weight-bearing stress; the usual time to full healing is around 3 months, but weight-bearing could be started by 6–8 weeks.

Activity resumption has to be done gradually; if no immobilization has been done, then tibialis anterior (TA) stretches and leg press exercises should be allowed early. Swimming and stationary cycling are good options to restart the routine exercises in athletes.

In cases with significantly associated comorbidity, osteoporosis and any dietary deficiencies have to be addressed. Conditions such as celiac disease and hyperparathyroidism have to be looked at by the medical specialists and treated appropriately. Routine use of vitamin D and supplemental calcium has not been proven to give additional benefit unless a specific deficiency is documented. However, most physicians prescribe this in stress fractures.

REFERENCES

1. Weber JM, Vidt LG, Gehl RS, Montgomery T. Calcaneal stress fractures. Clin Podiatr Med Surg. 2005;22(1):45-54.
2. Pilgaard S. Stress fracture of the os calcis. Acta Orthop Scand. 1968;39(2):270-2.
3. Hullinger CW. Insufficiency fracture of the calcaneus similar to march fracture of metatarsal. J Bone Joint Surg Am. 1944;26:751-7.
4. Darby RE. Stress fractures of the os calcis. JAMA. 1967;200:1183-4.
5. Hopson CN, Perry DR. Stress fractures of the calcaneus in women marine recruits. Clin Orthop Relat Res. 1977;(128):159-62.
6. Yale J. A statistical analysis of 3,657 consecutive fatigue fractures of the distal lower extremities. J Am Podiatr Med Assoc. 1976;66:739-48.
7. Pester S, Smith PC. Stress fractures in the lower extremities of soldiers in basic training. Orthop Rev. 1992;21:297-303.
8. Greaney RB, Gerber FH, Laughlin RL, Kmet JP, Metz CD, Kilcheski TS, et al. Distribution and natural history of stress fractures in U.S. Marine recruits. Radiology. 1983;146:339-46.
9. Winfield AC, Dennis JM. Stress fractures of the calcaneus. Radiology. 1959;72:415.
10. Leabhart JW. Stress fractures of the calcaneus. J Bone Joint Surg Am. 1959;41-A:1285-90.
11. MacDonald RG. Early diagnosis and treatment of stress fractures of the calcaneus. J Am Podiatr Med Assoc. 1966;56:533-6.
12. Italiano J, Bitterman AD. Diagnosis and management of calcaneal stress fractures. Radiol Technol. 2021;93(2):177-94.
13. Giladi M, Alcalay J. Stress fracture of the calcaneus—still an enigma in the Israeli Army. JAMA. 1984;252(22):3128-9.
14. Morris JM, Blickenstaff LD. Etiology of fatigue fractures. Fatigue Fractures, A Clinical Study. Springfield, IL: Charles Thomas; 1967. pp. 7-10.
15. Voormolen N, Canete AN, Reijnierse M. Calcaneal stress fracture revisited. JBR-BTR. 2012;95(2):114-7.
16. Sormaala MJ, Niva MH, Kiuru MJ, Mattila VM, Pihlajamäki HK. Stress injuries of the calcaneus detected with magnetic resonance imaging in military recruits. J Bone Joint Surg Am. 2006;88(10):2237-42.
17. Bianchi S, Luong DH. Stress fractures of the calcaneus diagnosed by sonography: report of 8 cases. J Ultrasound Med. 2018;37(2):521-9.
18. Taketomi S, Uchiyama E, Iwaso H. Stress fracture of the anterior process of the calcaneus: a case report. Foot Ankle Spec. 2013;6(5):389-92.
19. Miki T, Miki T, Nishiyama A. Calcaneal stress fracture: an adverse event following total hip and total knee arthroplasty: a report of five cases. J Bone Joint Surg Am. 2014;96(2):e9.
20. Kaya O, Hurel C, Gumussuyu G, Kose O. Bilateral calcaneal insufficiency fractures due to chronic carbamazepine use for trigeminal neuralgia: a case report. Niger J Clin Pract. 2020;23(4):574-6.
21. Kose O, Kilicaslan OF, Ozyurek S, Ince A. Calcaneal insufficiency fracture secondary to celiac disease-induced osteomalacia: a rare cause of heel pain. Foot Ankle Spec. 2016;9(2):179-83.
22. Fishco WD, Stiles RG. Atypical heel pain. Hyperparathyroidism-induced stress fracture of the calcaneus. J Am Podiatr Med Assoc. 1999;89(8):413-8.
23. Lui TH. Insufficiency fracture of the body of the calcaneus. Foot (Edinb). 2013;23(2-3):93-5.
24. Takai H, Kiyota K, Nakane N, Takahashi T. Charcot fracture in the calcaneus after total knee arthroplasty: a case report. J Orthop Case Rep. 2016;6(5):92-5.
25. Stein RE, Stelling FH. Stress fracture of the calcaneus in a child with cerebral palsy. J Bone Joint Surg Am. 1977;59(1):131.
26. Pearce CJ, Zaw H, Calder JD. Stress fracture of the anterior process of the calcaneus associated with a calcaneonavicular coalition: a case report. Foot Ankle Int. 2011;32(1):85-8.

Outcome Evaluations of Calcaneal Fractures

Nikolaos Gougoulias, Donald McBride, Nicola Maffulli

"There are two possible outcomes: If the result confirms the hypothesis, then you've made a measurement. If the result is contrary to the hypothesis, then you've made a discovery".
–Enrico Fermi (1901–1954)

"The outcome of any serious research can only be to make two questions grow where only one grew before".
–Thorstein Veblen (1857–1929)

■ INTRODUCTION

"Ordinarily speaking, the man who breaks his heel bone is done, so far as his industrial future is concerned". The previous statement was made just over 100 years ago in a publication evaluating the results of fractures of the os calcis.[1] This "raw statement" is not necessarily based on "high quality scientific data", as we would say these days; it was based on observation of patients suffering these injuries.

How do we evaluate the outcome of these injuries today? Is our outcome assessment accurate? Has application of "temporary" management techniques improved outcomes? What do we define as a successful outcome? Is it important that the surgeon is satisfied, for example, with radiographic measurements revealing "anatomic reduction" or is it more important when the patients say how satisfied they are with the outcome of their management?

Orthopedic surgery has greatly evolved in the last two decades, while outcome evaluation of treatments tends to be based on documentation of "outcome scores". The quality of outcome scores depends on whether they are "scientifically validated". They can be disease specific (e.g., those evaluating foot and lower leg function) or assess general health and well-being. We also distinguish outcome evaluations between those based on physicians' assessment (e.g., radiographic measurements, range of motion clinical measurements) and those reported by patients (e.g., visual or verbal analog scales). Last but not least, one has to mention the sample size and the lack of bias and methodology issues in the published studies. A critical appraisal of the literature will show that evidence is often inadequate to make specific recommendations regarding calcaneal fractures management as either the study is "too small" in terms of number of patients included, and/or also maybe biased or not following robust methodology. Published research articles, systematic reviews, and meta-analyses have addressed these issues.[2-4]

Despite the advances in nonoperative and operative management, fractures of the calcaneus remain serious injuries that commonly affect young and active individuals, are often associated with long-term sequelae, permanent disability, and a considerable reduction in quality of life, and have a high socioeconomic cost.[4]

Nonoperative management of displaced intra-articular calcaneal fractures often results in marked deformity, bone loss, and post-traumatic arthrosis. The goal of operative management is to achieve anatomic joint reduction and restore the height, length, width, and axis of the calcaneus. Stable internal fixation should allow early motion to restore function. On the other hand, operative management can be associated with significant early complications, including infections and wound healing problems, which occasionally compromise the viability of the foot. Wound healing problems occur in 16–25% of patients after open reduction and internal fixation (ORIF) of calcaneal fractures and have been reported to be as high as 43%. Furthermore, it is not clear whether long-term outcome variables are significantly improved in patients undergoing surgery.[2-6]

The optimal management of calcaneal fractures remains controversial because of several unanswered questions on their outcome:[1-13]

- Are outcomes of surgery superior to those after nonoperative care?

- Do the benefits of operative management outweigh the risks?
- Do minimally invasive methods of fracture fixation provide any advantages over "traditional" open techniques?
- Are there any prognostic, patient-related factors associated with favorable or unfavorable outcomes?

To answer these key questions, we need to define objective, standardized outcome measures that can accurately describe the clinical situation at clearly defined time intervals after initiation of management.

Buckley et al.[5] conducted a large-scale multicenter trial randomizing patients with an intra-articular calcaneal fracture to receive ORIF or nonoperative care. One of their findings was that patients younger than 29 years, who did not receive worker's compensation and had a light workload, with a multifragmentary fracture and a low Böhler's angle (<14°), that was fixed optimally (with a step-off in the articular surface of <2°), had higher satisfaction rates if managed operatively than those managed nonoperatively.

The previous statement indicates how complex the issue of assessing the outcome of management of calcaneal fractures can be. Numerous factors affect the outcome. Therefore, the conclusions of any given study are unlikely to be definite. Several randomized studies and systematic reviews in the meantime (their main findings will be mentioned later) explored the question of superiority of surgical nanagement.

Nevertheless, the outcome of management has to be evaluated in relation to how bad the problem is. Therefore, appropriate evaluation should include assessment of the following:

- *The patient:* His/her physiological status before initiation of management, e.g., demographics, comorbidities, previous level of activities, work
- *The surgeon's expertise:* Special interest in these injuries, institution's workload
- *The fracture:* How bad was the injury?
- *The surgery* (if applicable): Was the technique appropriate? What was the radiographic outcome?
- *The clinical outcome:* Objective assessment by the physician according to validated outcome scores, complications, patient-derived outcome scores (describing foot function and quality of life).

Taking into account all the above and what has been published over the years, we present how the outcome of management of calcaneal fractures should be approached, based on the following categories:

- Demographics
- Radiographic variables
- Foot function outcome scores
- Pain scores

- Quality of life measuring scores
- Complications
- Need for unplanned operations/subsequent subtalar arthrodesis.

We will comment on the scientific validity of the outcome measures presently in use, identify which ones withstood the course of time, and propose outcome measures that should be used in everyday clinical practice and for scientific purposes.

We should not forget that evidence in favor or against a specific intervention/management option should be strong to be widely accepted by the scientific community.

GLOBAL UPDATE

Numerous case series have been published in peer-reviewed journals. Most studies present outcomes of surgical management of calcaneal fractures that were not evaluated by an independent assessor. In general, outcome reporting is inconsistent. The authors of most studies seem to prefer surgical management for displaced intra-articular calcaneal fractures. Mainly, the argument in favor of ORIF is the ability to restore the shape of the calcaneus and the integrity of the subtalar joint and, obviously, improve radiographic variables. The evidence provided by level IV studies is, however, not strong.

The traditional surgical approach to achieve ORIF is associated with extensive soft-tissue dissection within a zone of high-energy injury. The relatively high incidence of wound complications, and the fact that the soft-tissue condition is sometimes not suitable for open surgery, leads surgeons to apply minimally invasive methods for the management of at least certain types of calcaneal fractures. Again, looking at the quality of evidence, no definite answers can be given regarding the superiority of one operative management strategy over the other.

A systematic review of the literature, by the authors of this work,[2] included a large-scale trial, recruiting 424 calcaneal fractures. Of the 26 comparative studies initially identified, applying exclusion criteria, we were left with only five randomized controlled trials comparing operative versus nonoperative management. One trial examined the differences in the outcome of nonoperative management if impulse compression was used, and one study assessed the volume of the injured foot awaiting surgery when a foot pump was used. All these studies had methodological flaws, with their methodology scores ranging from 6 to 14 out of a possible total of 24. This, of course, limits the validity of their results, which will be discussed in the following sections. Similar conclusions were drawn from the latest Cochrane review published in 2013.[4]

The United Kingdom (UK) Heel Fracture trial,[6] a large multicenter study with scientifically robust methodology, included 151 patients with acute calcaneal fracture, randomized between nonoperative ($n = 78$) and operative ($n = 73$) management. The primary outcome functional score was the Kerr–Atkins scale,[14] while they also assessed complication rate, hindfoot pain, and function using the American Orthopaedic Foot and Ankle Society (AOFAS) score, general health [short form-36 (SF-36)], and quality of life [EuroQol-5 Dimensions (EQ-5D)]. Its results were published in 2014, showing no clinical benefit from operative management: Patients undergoing surgery had more often wound complications (19%) and required unplanned surgery.[6] Interestingly, the primary finding of this study ("surgery provides no benefits") was chosen to make the headline in the front page of the British Medical Journal. This, probably, irritated the orthopedic community in UK, and in combination with the fact that out of approximately 500 potential study participants, a large proportion was excluded (e.g., patients with fractures with lateral wall bulging, possibly at risk of peroneal tendons impingement, received surgical management), and the fact that many patients were treated according to their own (not the surgeon's) treatment preference, gave rise to criticism: Selection bias in the UK Heel Fracture trial may have influenced the results.[15] Furthermore, the results do not seem to have influenced indications for surgical management, as the rate of patients undergoing surgery for their calcaneal fracture in UK has remained stable and at around 7.35% of all calcaneal fractures seen at the UK hospitals, before and after publication of the trial results. On the other hand, minimally invasive calcaneal fracture fixation has raised from 7.3 to 13.5% of calcaneal fractures treated operatively, before and after publication of the UK Heel Fracture trial results in 2014.[16]

The latter also shows that data alone are not making the difference, as interpretation can be individualized, depending also on surgeons' preference, especially if the quality of evidence is flawed.

OUTCOME MEASURES FOR EVALUATION OF CALCANEAL FRACTURES MANAGEMENT

Demographic Data

Although not directly a measurement of outcome, presentation of demographic data is equally important as demographics provide variables that directly influence the outcome of management of calcaneal fractures.

A recent study by Gaskill et al.[17] emphasizes the effect of *age* on outcome. The authors found that patients over 50 years did at least as well as younger patients, with a similar complication rate. A patient's *physiological age* has to be taken into account, as his *level of activity* may play an important role in the outcome.

Similarly, patients' *occupation and workload* play an important role. Is it possible for a heavy laborer to return to his previous work after sustaining a calcaneal fracture? Evidence shows that 75% of patients will return to their previous job.[5]

Gender is another parameter. Barla et al.,[18] based on the data of the multicenter study by Buckley et al.,[5] showed that women did better after operative management, compared to those managed nonoperatively. However, was gender the independent variable that led to better outcomes? As the authors of the study clearly emphasized, women were more likely to sustain a low-energy fracture, producing less severe injuries, predisposing to better outcomes.

Patients' *ASA* (American Society of Anesthesiologists) score indicates the physiological status of the patient. It is related to age and to the level of activities. Higher ASA can possibly be related to higher complication rates after operative management, and a low demand (in terms of activity) patient may be safely managed nonoperatively.

Smoking adversely affects bone and soft-tissue healing, and evidence shows that it is related to unfavorable outcomes in patients with a calcaneal fracture managed operatively. Outcomes in smokers should be reported in comparison to the nonsmokers.

Sample size is very important. As the outcome of calcaneal fractures is multifactorial, one cannot draw valuable conclusions unless the assessment includes a large number of individuals. For prospective comparative studies, a power analysis should be performed before initiation of the study. Usually, a power of 90% and an alpha value of 0.05 are required.

Length of Follow-up

The management of calcaneal fractures requires an initial period of restrictions on weight bearing and activities in general, followed by a prolonged period of rehabilitation and gradual return to ordinary activities, work, sports, etc. Specialists in the field and published studies agree that a minimum of 2 years follow-up is required before valuable results should be published. Furthermore, the rate of *patients lost to follow-up* has to be clearly presented. Tracing trauma patients for follow-up is difficult; however, if >20% of patients are lost to follow-up, the presentation is likely biased toward more favorable outcomes.

Worker's Compensation Claim

Last but not least, when evaluating the outcome of a calcaneal fracture, one should take into account whether his patient is claiming compensation. This issue should also be a parameter in relevant scientific studies. There is strong evidence, derived from a large-scale multicenter randomized trial,[5] that surgical results are not as good in the subgroup of patients claiming worker's compensation.

FRACTURE CHARACTERISTICS AND CLASSIFICATION

To evaluate the outcome of an injury, its characteristics have to be defined first. How bad is the fracture? Common sense and scientific evidence indicate that the worse the problem is, the less favorable the outcome is likely to be. Is the fracture the result of high- or low-energy trauma? Is it open? Is it an isolated injury? These issues should be addressed in everyday clinical practice as well as in scientific publications.

Open fractures require special care, lead, logically, to worse outcomes, and should be evaluated as a separate category.

Unilateral versus Bilateral Fractures

Are outcomes of patients with bilateral calcaneal fractures (approximately 5–15% of all calcaneal fractures) directly comparable to those with a unilateral fracture? Can we define which fracture causes disability and to what degree? Probably not, and we would suggest that those patients should be assessed in a different category.

Concomitant injuries are also important to be assessed and presented. Spinal injuries or other musculoskeletal injuries can accompany approximately 10% of calcaneal fractures and may affect outcome. In other words, if disability is present or health-related quality of life is affected, it cannot be attributed to the calcaneal fracture alone if other injuries were present at the same time.

Classification of the fracture itself is essential to evaluate the outcome in relation to "how bad the problem was". The most widely accepted modern classification is *Sanders classification*,[19] based on the degrees of articular surface comminution (number of fracture lines through the posterior facet) as shown on a *computed tomography (CT) scan* and *is prognostic*. However, the amount of depression of the posterior facet of the subtalar joint may be underestimated based on CT alone,[20] and therefore, lateral radiographs remain of paramount importance. Several parameters measured on *plain radiographs* are used to assess not only the severity of the fracture but also the outcome of management.

RADIOGRAPHIC PARAMETERS

Plain radiographs' evaluation allows assessment not only of the severity of the fracture but also of the accuracy of fracture reduction and restoration of normal anatomy. Both a lateral **(Figs. 1A and B)** and an axial **(Figs. 2A and B)** view are needed.

Böhler's angle (B): The angle formed by the intersection of line drawn from the most cephalic point of the tuberosity to the highest point of the posterior facet with a line from

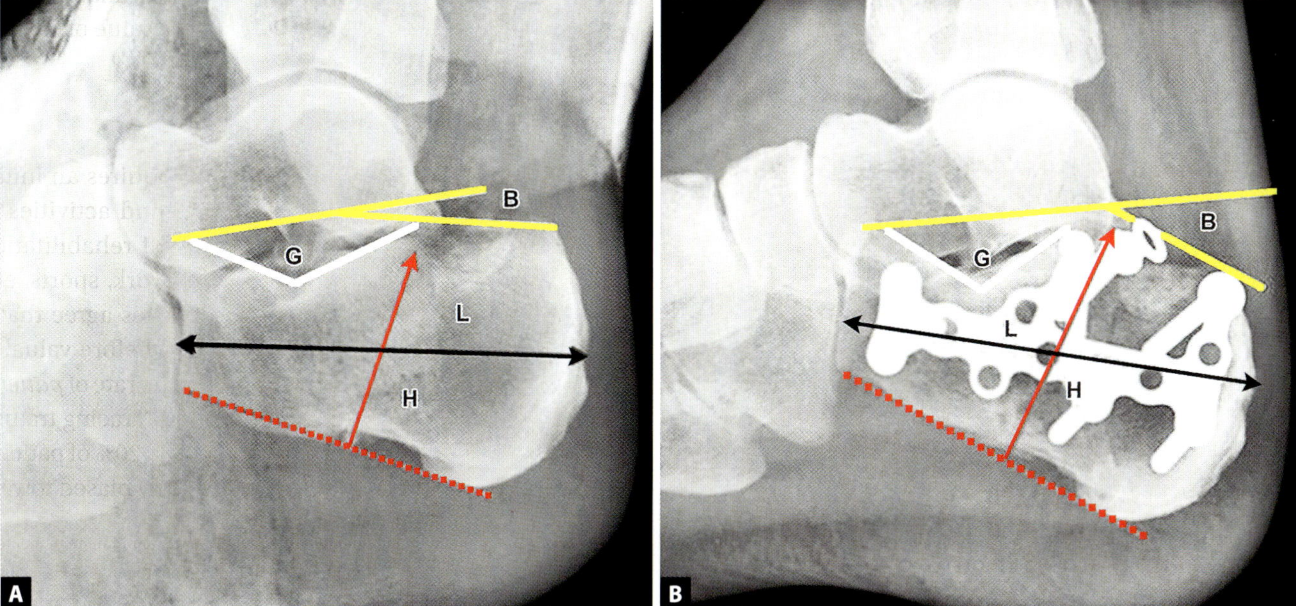

Figs. 1A and B: Lateral view of the heel, (A) pre- and (B) postoperatively after open reduction and internal fixation (ORIF). (B: Böhler's angle; G: Gissane angle; L: length; H: height)

the latter to the most cephalic part of the posterior process of calcaneus (**Figs. 1A and B**, yellow lines) measures the height of the posterior facet. The normal range is 20–40°. In most cases, a decreased *Böhler's* angle implies fracture and disrupted posterior facet. Persistent, severe decreases (<0°) have been associated with poor long-term results.

Gissane angle (G): In 1947, Gissane described his "critical angle" or "crucial angle". It reveals the angular relationship of the calcaneal facets (**Figs. 1A and B**, white lines) and should appear identical when taken bilaterally. The angular measurements vary from 130° to 145°, with an average of 130°, on a lateral radiographic view.

Calcaneal height and length: Measurement of these parameters after surgical reduction of the fracture, in comparison to the "healthy side" on a lateral radiographic view (**Figs. 1A and B**, red and black lines), indicates accuracy of restoration of calcaneal shape. Care should be taken that radiographs of both feet should be taken in the same fashion.

Calcaneal width/subfibular impingement: An axial view of the os calcis is needed (**Figs. 2A and B**). Comparison to the "healthy" side is needed to assess normalization of the width of the calcaneus. On that view (which is difficult to standardize), subfibular impingement (the distance between the distal fibula and the lateral wall of the calcaneus) can be detected.

Subtalar joint congruity: It can be evaluated on the lateral radiographic view. The posterior facet is checked for the presence of "step-off" bigger than 2 mm. Its validity is debatable as plain radiography projections (two-dimensional imaging of a three-dimensional structure) may lead to mistakes. Brodén's view is useful in assessing congruity of the posterior facet of the subtalar joint (**Fig. 3A**). However, a CT scan is more accurate than plain radiographs in order to assess joint congruity (**Fig. 3B**).[21] Routine use of CT scan postoperatively is not always used in clinical practice as it involves radiation for patients and cost for health care systems. It is essential for symptomatic patients and useful for research purposes.

New technologies allowing weight-bearing CT scanning with low radiation exposure are available and widely used in North America and some countries in Central Europe. They provide a useful diagnostic tool in foot and ankle surgery and allow accurate assessment of calcaneus shape, subtalar joint congruity, and hindfoot alignment.[22]

■ FOOT FUNCTION ASSESSMENT

In general, it involves assessment of pain, range of movement, walking ability, physical activity, and ability to work.

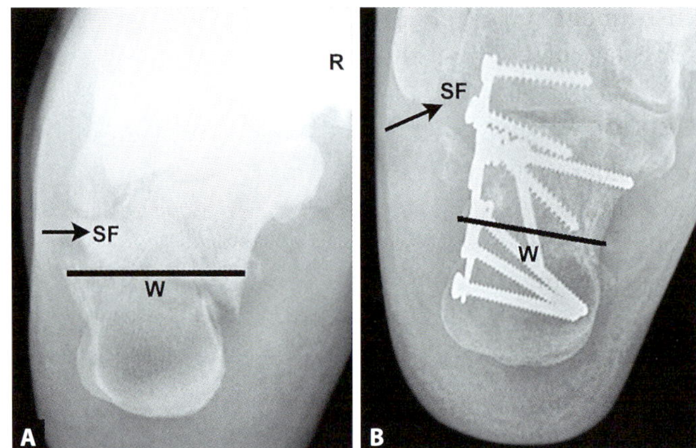

Figs. 2A and B: Axial view of the heel (A) pre- and (B) postoperatively after open reduction and internal fixation (ORIF). (W: width of calcaneus; SF: subfibular space)

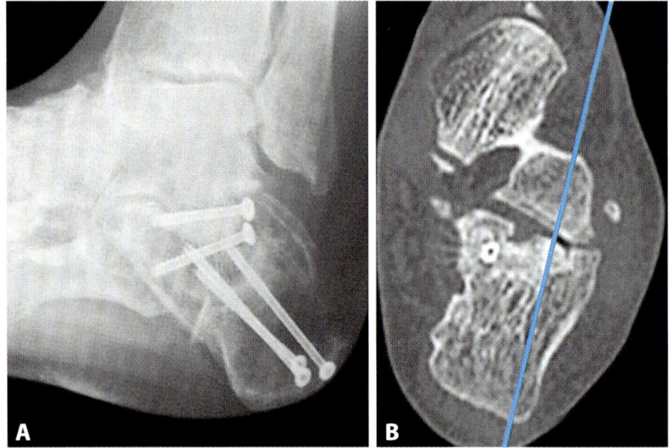

Figs. 3A and B: (A) Brodén's view is useful in evaluating subtalar joint congruity. However, (B) computed tomography (CT) scan is more accurate.

Unspecified Pain Scores

Many of the older studies do not clearly define or quantify pain. Thus, presentation of "painful" or "painless" heel or description of pain level as "severe" or "moderate" does not appear to be based on an accurate outcome measure. We will present hereinafter the "newer developments" on how to quantify pain, namely the use of visual analog scale (VAS) scores.

Range of Movement

Studies mention the mobility of the subtalar and ankle joints. We doubt whether small differences in the range of movement can really indicate superior or inferior outcomes of fracture management. Furthermore, usually, the technique of movement measurement is not mentioned and not standardized. However, several outcome measurement "instrument" use the parameter "range of motion" as a percentage of the "healthy" side.

Walking Ability

Some older studies report on how many "blocks" the patient can walk or whether he is able to walk a certain distance (e.g., 1 mile). The validity of this measure can be criticized as it can vary depending on the patients' general health status.

Return to Work

This is an objective end point, reported in many studies. Scientific studies should explicitly mention the proportion of patients who are heavy labor workers.

Shoe Wear

Malalignment of the hindfoot (e.g., excessive valgus) can be restrictive regarding the type of shoe wear the patient has to use (e.g., "orthopedic" custom-made shoes).

Pedobarography

Some studies have used pedobarography to assess the outcome of calcaneal fractures management. Pedobarography reveals differences in pressures in certain parts of the foot and differences in the overall center of pressure in the foot. A systematic review found no certain correlation of specific pressure changes with the functional outcome. Hence, pedobarography may not be useful, at least not yet, in outcome prediction, but may help in further management of patients, requiring custom-made insoles.[23]

Mortality (Long-term)

Mortality is not one of the direct outcome measures of calcaneal fractures management. However, one retrospective study showed that male patients undergoing ORIF of their calcaneal fracture have an increased risk for long-term morality compared to an age- and gender-matched population. The reasons are unclear and need to be explored to possibly tackle the reasons leading to an increased mortality rate.[24]

Visual Analog Scale Scores

Newer studies (since the mid-1990s) are using this "tool" for patients' assessment. This is an outcome measure based on the patient's perspective. The patient quantifies the degree of pain. We would suggest that, in general, this is an "easy" and reliable way to quantify the degree of success of a patient's management in orthopedics. Even when not involved in a scientific study, it would be worth asking our patients how they would describe their pain on a scale from 0 to 10 (verbal scale). It is, of course, more reliable if the patient is asked to draw an arrow on a 10 cm-long line without the physician's physical presence.

Example:

Does your foot limit your ability to run?

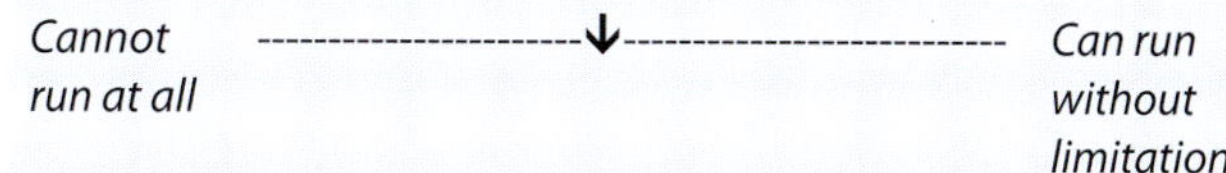

We would like to emphasize the use of function scores containing *VAS* in order to quantify pain, physical activity, satisfaction, etc., in the last decade. This enables patients to "express" their views regarding the outcome of their orthopedic problem without the physical presence of a physician or another accessor. This obviously applies in the assessment of outcomes of calcaneal fractures as we will present in the next section. The description of the commonly used scores will highlight the importance of the development of VAS and show their application in clinical practice and research.

■ FOOT FUNCTION SCORES

American Orthopaedic Foot Ankle Society Ankle-hindfoot Score[25]

The AOFAS score includes pain, function, and alignment evaluation and allows a maximum total of 100 points, with higher scores indicating better outcomes. In the past, it was considered the "gold standard" score for the assessment of outcomes of hindfoot surgery. Currently, the AOFAS score seems to be "out of date", as it is not validated. However, it is often used for research purposes even today, mainly because it allows direct comparison of recent and "historic" studies.

Pain (40 points)
- None — 40
- Mid, occasional — 30
- Moderate, daily — 20
- Severe, almost always present — 0

Function (50 points)
- *Activity limitations, support requirement*
  - No limitations, no support — 10
  - No limitations of daily activities, limitations of recreational activities, no support — 7
  - Limited daily and recreational activities, cane — 4
  - Severe daily and recreational activities, walker, crutches, wheelchair, brace — 0
- *Maximum walking distance (blocks)*
  - >6 — 5
  - 4–6 — 4
  - 1–3 — 2
  - <1 — 0

Contd...

Contd...

- *Walking surfaces*
  - No difficulty with any surface — 5
  - Some difficulty on uneven terrain, stairs, inclines, ladders — 3
  - Severe difficulty on uneven terrain, stairs, inclines, ladders — 0
- *Gait abnormality*
  - None slight — 8
  - Obvious — 4
  - Marked — 0
- *Sagittal motion (flexion plus extension)*
  - Normal or mild restriction (30° or more) — 8
  - Moderate restriction (15–29°) — 4
  - Severe restriction (<15°) — 0
- *Hindfoot motion (inversion plus eversion)*
  - Normal or mild restriction (75–100% of normal) — 6
  - Moderate restriction (25–74% of normal) — 3
  - Marked restriction (<24% of normal) — 0
- *Ankle-hindfoot stability (anteroposterior, varus–valgus)*
  - Stable — 8
  - Definitely unstable — 0

Alignment (10 points)
- Good, plantigrade foot, midfoot well aligned — 15
- Fair, plantigrade foot, some degree of midfoot malalignment observed, no symptoms — 8
- Poor, nonplantigrade foot, severe malalignment, symptoms — 0

Total — 100

Source: Kitaoka et al. (1994).[25]

Foot Function Index[26]

This validated score is subdivided into assessment of pain, disability, and activity limitation. Each of the three categories has subcategories which are scored individually, with a possible range from 0 to 10 points, with lower values indicating better outcomes. A VAS is used.

See below:

Pain subscale: How severe is your foot pain?	*No pain*	*Worst pain imaginable*
Foot pain at its worst?		1 2 3 4 5 6 7 8 9 10
Foot pain in morning?		1 2 3 4 5 6 7 8 9 10
Pain walking barefoot?		1 2 3 4 5 6 7 8 9 10
Pain standing barefoot?		1 2 3 4 5 6 7 8 9 10
Pain walking with shoes?		1 2 3 4 5 6 7 8 9 10
Pain standing with shoes?		1 2 3 4 5 6 7 8 9 10
Pain walking with orthotics?		1 2 3 4 5 6 7 8 9 10
Pain standing with orthotics?		1 2 3 4 5 6 7 8 9 10
Foot pain at end of day?		1 2 3 4 5 6 7 8 9 10

Contd...

Contd...

Disability subscale: How much difficulty did you have?	*No difficulty*	*Unable*
Difficulty walking in house?		1 2 3 4 5 6 7 8 9 10
Difficulty walking outside?		1 2 3 4 5 6 7 8 9 10
Difficulty walking 4 blocks?		1 2 3 4 5 6 7 8 9 10
Difficulty climbing stairs?		1 2 3 4 5 6 7 8 9 10
Difficulty descending stairs?		1 2 3 4 5 6 7 8 9 10
Difficulty standing tiptoe?		1 2 3 4 5 6 7 8 9 10
Difficulty getting up from chair?		1 2 3 4 5 6 7 8 9 10
Difficulty climbing curbs?		1 2 3 4 5 6 7 8 9 10
Difficulty walking fast?		1 2 3 4 5 6 7 8 9 10

Activity limitation subscale: How much of the time do you:	*None of the time*	*All of the time*
Stay inside all day because of feet?		1 2 3 4 5 6 7 8 9 10
Stay in bed all day because of feet?		1 2 3 4 5 6 7 8 9 10
Limit activities because of feet?		1 2 3 4 5 6 7 8 9 10
Use assistive device indoors?		1 2 3 4 5 6 7 8 9 10
Use assistive device outdoors?		1 2 3 4 5 6 7 8 9 10

Source: SooHoo et al. (2006).[26]

Calcaneal Fracture Scoring System

The calcaneal fracture scoring system was developed by Kerr et al. in 1996.[14] A maximum of 100 points in total can be achieved. A higher score indicates a better outcome. It is subdivided into assessment of pain, ability to work, ability to walk, and the need to use walking aids.

Maximum of 100 points	*Score*	
Assessment of pain (36 points)	*At rest*	*On activity*
None	18	18
Slight	12	12
Moderate	6	6
Severe	0	0
Assessment of work (25 points)		
No change in job	25	
Modification of job	16	
Enforced change of job	8	
Unable to work	0	
Assessment of walking (25 points)		
No change in walking ability	25	
Minimal restriction	16	
Moderate restriction	8	
Severe restriction	0	
Assessment of walking aids (14 points)		
None	14	
Occasional stick	10	
Constant stick	6	
1 stick	3	
Crutches	0	

Source: Kerr et al. (1996).[14]

Maryland Foot Score[27]

The Maryland Foot Score was designed to evaluate the outcome of foot injuries. Pain, function (gait and activities), and cosmesis (deformity) are evaluated and scored to a possible total of 100 points.

1. *Pain:*
   a. None including with sports — 45
   b. Slight, no change in ADLs or work ability — 40
   c. Mild, minimal change in ADL or work — 30
   d. Moderate, significant change in ADLs taken ASA — 20
   e. Marked. During minimal ADLs, e.g., bathroom, simple housework. Stronger, more frequent analgesics — 10
   f. Disabled, unable to work or shop — 0

2. *Function:*
   a. *Gait*
      1. Distance walked
         - Unlimited — 10
         - Slight limitation — 8
         - Moderate limitation (2–3 blocks) — 5
         - Severe limitation (1 block) — 2
         - Indoors only — 0
      2. Stability
         - Normal — 4
         - Weak feeling—no true giving way — 3
         - Occasional giving way (1–2 months) — 2
         - Frequent giving way — 1
         - Orthotic device used — 0
      3. Support
         - None — 4
         - Cane — 3
         - Crutches — 1
         - Wheelchair — 0
      4. Limp
         - None — 4
         - Slight — 3
         - Moderate — 2
         - Severe — 1
         - Unable to walk — 0

   b. *Functional activities*
      1. Shoes
         - Any type — 10
         - Minor concessions — 9
         - Flat, laced — 7
         - With orthotics — 5
         - Space shoes — 2
         - Unable to wear shoes — 0
      2. Stairs
         - Normally — 4
         - With banister — 3
         - Any method — 2
         - Unable — 0
      3. Terrain
         - Any surface — 4
         - Problems on hills, uneven surfaces — 2
         - Problems on flat surfaces — 0
      4. Motion

Points	5	4	2	0
Ankle dorsal flexion	Normal	Slight	Marked	Ankylosed
Ankle plantar flexion				
Subtalar inversion				
Subtalar eversion				
Midfoot abduction				
Midfoot adduction				
Metatarsophalangeal (MTP) dorsal flexion				
MTP plantar flexion				

3. *Cosmesis:*
   a. Normal — 10
   b. Mild deformity — 8
   c. Moderate — 5
   d. Severe — 0
   e. Multiple deformities — 0

Source: Sanders et al. (1993).[27]

Modified Rowe Score

The original Rowe score was developed in 1963 and modified by Buckley and Meek in 1992.[28] It is used by physicians for clinical evaluation, assessing pain, range of motion, gait, activities, and working ability as shown in the table below.

Level of	Score
Pain:	
• None	30
• Exercise induced	25
• Mild on daily activity	20
• Pain with weight-bearing	10
• Pain at rest	0
Range of motion:	
• 100–75%	20
• 74–50%	10
• 49–25%	5
• 24–0%	0
Gait:	
• Normal	15
• Mild limp (exercise)	10
• Moderate limp	5
• Severe limp	0
Activities:	
• Normal	20
• Restricted on rough ground	15
• Moderate daily restrictions	10
• Able to walk short distances only	5
• Unable to walk	0
Work:	
• No restrictions	15
• Some restrictions on usual occupation	10
• Change of job or substantial restrictions	5
• Unable to work	0
Total	100

Source: Buckley and Meek (1992).[28]

"Calgary" Score[29]

Based on the previously presented Rowe score modified by Buckley and Meek in 1992[28] and the SF-36 score, the Calgary team developed a VAS score.[29] It is based on both patients' and physicians' perspective, assessing pain, physical function, and overall impression regarding the outcome.

Patient Visual Analog Scale Form

Assessment of pain:

1. How often does your heel hurt?
   Always--Never

2. How bad is the pain in your heel foot?
   As bad as it could be--No pain

3. I have heel/foot pain at night, making it difficult for me to sleep
   Always--Never

Contd...

Contd...

4. I have stiffness/discomfort in my heel/foot first thing in the morning when I wake up
   Always--Never

5. I have aching in my heel/foot at the end of the day
   Always--Never

Assessment of physical function:

6. I have difficulty walking on level ground
   Extreme difficulty--No difficulty

7. I have difficulty walking on rough or uneven ground
   Extreme difficulty--No difficulty

8. I have difficulty walking up or down hills or inclines
   Extreme difficulty--No difficulty

9. I have difficulty walking long distances
   Extreme difficulty--No difficulty

10. I have difficulty standing for prolonged periods of time
    Extreme difficulty--No difficulty

11. I have difficulty running
    Extreme difficulty--No difficulty

12. I limp when I walk
    Always--Never
    Taking everything into consideration, rate your overall result from your heel at this point of time on the following line
    The worst possible--Perfect

Surgeon and independent assessor visual analog scale form:

1. The treating surgeon will rate each patient on the following scales

   The first scale refers to the amount of pain that the patient is having

   As bad as it could be--No pain

2. The second scale refers to gait and related activities

   Extreme difficulty--No difficulty

3. Rate the overall result of this fractured calcaneus at this point of time

   The worst possible--Perfect

Source: Hildebrand et al. (1996).[29]

"Hannover" Calcaneal Fracture Score[30]

This is one of the most recently developed outcome scores. The producers of this score took into consideration the flaws of the existing scores at the time. They validated their score toward SF-36 (another validated score), originally in the German language. It is based on a VAS form (see below), filled in by the patient after reading essential instructions.

How much do foot problems
affect your gait?

Strong   --   *No changes,*
limping   *normal gait*

Contd...

Contd...

How often do you have foot pain in physical rest?

Constantly always -- Never, very rarely

How intense is your foot pain in physical rest?

Extreme pain -- No pain

How often do you have foot pain during physical activity?

Constantly always -- Never, very rarely

Do you have the impression that one leg is weaker than the other?

The weakness restricts me substantially -- Same strength as in the healthy leg

Do you have callous at the foot/feet?

Widespread, painful callous -- No callous

Do you have a limitation of ankle/foot range of motion?

My foot/ankle is constantly rigid -- No limitation of range of motion at any time

Do you have problems when climbing stairs?

Climbing stairs impossible -- Climbing stairs without limitation possible

How much do foot problems affect your occupation?

Occupation cannot be practiced anymore -- No limitation

How much do foot problems affect you driving a car (operating clutch, accelerator, brake pedals)?

Driving a car not possible -- Driving a car without limitation possible

How long can you stand without foot problems?

Only briefly and with crutches/stick -- For hours, without limitation

Contd...

Contd...

How much do foot problems affect your ability to stand on one leg?

Standing on one leg impossible -- No limitation

How long can you walk without foot problems?

Only briefly and with crutches/stick -- For hours, without limitation

Do foot problems stop you from running (e.g., jogging/on soft or uneven ground)?

Even short jogging is impossible -- Jogging for extended periods possible

How much do foot problems affect your daily activities (e.g., getting dressed, eating, washing)?

Impossible on my own, need constant help -- No limitation

How much do foot problems restrict traveling (e.g., traveling with trains, buses, aircraft)?

Even short jogging is impossible -- No limitation

Do you have problems finding good footwear?

Can only wear orthopedic shoes -- Can wear any type of shoe

How much do foot problems restrict walking on uneven ground?

On uneven ground, walking is impossible -- No limitations on uneven ground

How much is sensation on your feet reduced?

No sensation -- Normal sensation

Source: Richter et al. (2006).[30]

European Foot and Ankle Society Score[31]

A newly developed foot and ankle disease-specific score by the European Foot and Ankle Society (EFAS), consisting of only six questions (and four supplementary questions for those who participate in sports), is a useful tool for assessing patient-reported outcomes of the management of foot and ankle chronic problems and trauma. It has already been translated and validated in various languages and could be used for the assessment of outcomes of calcaneal fractures.

See below the questions as presented to patients in the English language.

Below you will find six questions relating to your foot and/or ankle problem.

Please answer each question by selecting the answer that best describes your situation in the last week. Each question can be answered on a 5-point scale, with descriptions given for the two end points of the scale.

If a question does not apply to you, please indicate this by checking the N/A box on the left.

Question no.	Question	Answer
1	Do you have pain in your foot and/or ankle when you are at rest?	Always Never 0 1 2 3 4
2	How far can you walk before you get pain in your foot and/or ankle	Impossible No limitation 0 1 2 3 4
3	How much has your gait (i.e., the way you walk) changed because of your foot and/or ankle problem?	Extreme gait change No change 0 1 2 3 4
4	Do you have difficulty walking on uneven surfaces?	Always Never 0 1 2 3 4
5	Do you have pain in your foot and/or ankle when you are walking?	Always Never 0 1 2 3 4
6	How often do you have pain in your foot and/or ankle during physical activity?	Always Never 0 1 2 3

■ SPORTS QUESTIONS

Please only answer these questions if you regularly engage in sports activities; if a specific question does not apply to your chosen sport, please check the N/A box number.

	Question	Answer
S1	Can you run?	Impossible No limitation 0 1 2 3 4

Contd...

Contd...

S2	Can you jog?	Impossible No limitation 0 1 2 3 4
S3	Do you have problems landing after jumping?	Impossible No limitation 0 1 2 3 4
S4	Are you able to perform your sports with your usual technique?	Impossible No limitation

■ QUALITY OF LIFE MEASURING SCORES

Short Form Health Survey (SF-36)[32]

The SF-36 was developed from work performed by the RAND Corporation and the Medical Outcomes Study (MOS), based on the measurement strategy of the RAND Health Insurance Study in the 1980s. SF-36 is a multipurpose, short-form health survey with only 36 questions. It yields an 8-scale profile of functional health and well-being scores as well as psychometrically based physical and mental health summary measures and a preference-based health utility index.

The SF-36 can be either self-administered or administered by a trained interviewer, either in person or by telephone. Over the years, the SF-36 has been used in surveys of general and specific populations, for comparing the relative burden of diseases across different subgroups and in differentiating the health benefits produced by health care treatments.

The *SF-36* is a validated, contemporary, widely accepted assessment tool and used set of generic, coherent, and easily administered quality-of-life measures. These measures rely upon patient self-reporting and are now widely utilized by managed care organizations and by physicians and researchers for routine monitoring and assessment of care outcomes in adult patients.

Short SF-36 questionnaire:

1. In general, would you say your health is:

Excellent	1
Very good	2
Good	3
Fair	4
Poor	5

2. *Compared to 1 year ago*, how would your rate your health in general *now*?

Much better now than 1 year ago	1
Somewhat better now than 1 year ago	2
About the same	3
Somewhat worse now than 1 year ago	4
Much worse now than 1 year ago	5

The following items are about activities you might do during a typical day. Does *your health now limit you* in these activities? If so, how much? *(Circle one number on each line)*

	Yes, limited a lot	Yes, limited a little	No, not limited at all
3. *Vigorous activities*, such as running, lifting heavy objects, participating in strenuous sports	1	2	3
4. *Moderate activities*, such as moving a table, pushing a vacuum cleaner, bowling, or playing golf	1	2	3
5. Lifting or carrying groceries	1	2	3
6. Climbing *several* flights of stairs	1	2	3
7. Climbing *one* flight of stairs	1	2	3
8. Bending, kneeling, or stooping	1	2	3
9. Walking *more than a* mile	1	2	3
10. Walking *several blocks*	1	2	3
11. Walking *one block*	1	2	3
12. Bathing or dressing yourself	1	2	3

During the *past 4 weeks*, have you had any of the following problems with your work or other regular daily activities *as a result of your physical health*? *(Circle one number on each line)*

	Yes	No
13. Cut down the amount of time you spent on work or other activities	1	2
14. *Accomplished less* than you would like	1	2
15. Were limited in the *kind* of work or other activities	1	2
16. Had *difficulty* performing the work or other activities (e.g., it took extra effort)	1	2

During the *past 4 weeks,* have you had any of the following problems with your work or other regular daily activities *as a result of any emotional problems* (such as feeling depressed or anxious)? *(Circle one number on each line)*

	Yes	No
17. Cut down the *amount of time* you spent on work or other activities	1	2
18. *Accomplished less* than you would like	1	2
19. Did not do work or other activities as *carefully* as usual	1	2

20. During the *past 4 weeks,* to what extent has your physical health or emotional problems interfered with your normal social activities with family, friends, neighbors, or groups? *(Circle one number)*

Not at all	1
Slightly	2
Moderately	3
Quite a bit	4
Extremely	5

21. How much *bodily* pain have you had during the *past 4 weeks*? *(Circle one number)*

None	1
Very mild	2
Mild	3
Moderate	4
Severe	5
Very severe	6

22. During the *past 4 weeks*, how much did *pain* interfere with your normal work (including both work outside the home and housework)? *(Circle one number)*

Not at all	1
Slightly	2
Moderately	3
Quite a bit	4
Extremely	5

These questions are about how you feel and how things have been with you *during the past 4 weeks.* For each question, please give the one answer that comes closest to the way you have been feeling.

How much of the time during the *past 4 weeks*? *(Circle one number on each line)*

	All of the time	Most of the time	A good bit of the time	Some of the time	A little of the time	None of the time
23. Did you feel full of pep?	1	2	3	4	5	6
24. Have you been a very nervous person?	1	2	3	4	5	6
25. Have you felt so down in the dumps that nothing could cheer you up?	1	2	3	4	5	6
26. Have you felt calm and peaceful?	1	2	3	4	5	6
27. Did you have a lot of energy?	1	2	3	4	5	6
28. Have you felt downhearted and blue?	1	2	3	4	5	6
29. Did you feel worn out?	1	2	3	4	5	6
30. Have you been a happy person?	1	2	3	4	5	6
31. Did you feel tired?	1	2	3	4	5	6

32. During the *past 4 weeks,* how much of the time has your *physical health or emotional problems* interfered with your social activities (such as visiting with friends, relatives)? *(Circle one number)*

All of the time	1
Most of the time	2
Some of the time	3
A little of the time	4
None of the time	5

How *true* or *false* is each of the following statements for you? *(Circle one number on each line)*

	Definitely true	Mostly true	Do not know	Mostly false	Definitely false
33. I seem to get sick a little easier than other people	1	2	3	4	5
34. I am as healthy as anybody I know	1	2	3	4	5
35. I expect my health to get worse	1	2	3	4	5
36. My health is excellent	1	2	3	4	5

A newer version of the SF-36, the SF-36v2, was designed to improve on the original instrument. Refinements in item wording and format and an increase in the range of scores covered were achieved without increasing respondent burden. Norms and guidelines are available for maintaining backward comparability with studies published with the first version of the SF-36, providing standardization between the two versions of the instrument and allowing for comparison of data sets for trend analyses. It can be accessed online at https://www.rand.org/health-care/surveys_tools/mos/36-item-short-form/survey-instrument.html.[32]

■ EQ-5D

Another "tool" to assess the general health status, most commonly used in the European community, is the EQ-5D. This method has been advanced by a collaborative group from Western Europe known as the EuroQol group (originally formed in 1987). It comprises a network of international, multidisciplinary researchers originally from seven centers in England, Finland, the Netherlands, Norway, and Sweden. More recently, researchers from Spain as well as researchers from Germany, Greece, Canada, the United States, and Japan have joined the group. The intention of this effort is to develop a generic currency for health that could be used commonly across Europe. The original version of the EuroQol had 14 health states in six different domains. More recent versions of the EuroQol, known as the EQ-5D, are now in use in a substantial number of clinical and population studies. The questionnaire can be accessed online via https://euroqol.org/eq-5d-instruments.[33]

■ COMPLICATIONS

There are key issues in assessing the outcome of calcaneal fracture management. These include:

- Wound healing problems/skin necrosis, which are the most worrying complications
- Infections (deep and superficial) are, probably, synonymous to wound healing complications. However, in the vast majority of published studies, wound healing problems and infections are presented distinctively
- Thromboembolic events (deep vein thrombosis and pulmonary embolism) should always be reported

- Malunion/malalignment. One should define what exactly the exact nature of the problem is (e.g., hindfoot valgus or varus, malunited lateral wall causing peroneal tendons and subfibular impingement, congruity of the subtalar articular surfaces, reduction of Böhler's and Gissane's angles)
- Nonunion.

NEED FOR UNPLANNED OPERATIONS

This is an objective end point. Common unplanned procedures that are performed subsequent to operative management are given as follows:
- Removal of metal
- Wound debridement for infection ± soft-tissue coverage (e.g., using skin graft, flaps)
- Reoperation for malalignment of the fracture
- Reoperation of debridement of the lateral calcaneal wall (possibly for subfibular impingement)
- Subtalar arthrodesis for post-traumatic joint degeneration. This is a key issue because it clearly defines an end point.

SUMMARY

- *Patient-related factors* (socio-economic factors, general health issues, occupation, worker's compensation) strongly influence outcome and should be evaluated.
- *Fractures* should be classified (Sanders classification) and measurements on plain radiographs should be carried out.
- Several scientific instruments are available for outcome evaluation. Contemporary studies should include the following:
  - *Radiographic evaluations* of the outcome (measurement of Böhler's and Gissane's angles, calcaneal height and width, before initiation of management and at follow-up). CT scans are more accurate, compared to plane radiographs, in assessing fracture reduction
  - *General health status* assessment (SF-36 questionnaire)
  - *Foot function* evaluations (e.g., AOFAS score, foot function index, calcaneal fracture score)
  - Use questionnaires containing *visual analog scales* for quantification of outcomes from the patients' perspective
  - Presentation of the rate of *complications, unplanned procedures*, patients undergoing *subtalar arthrodesis.*

REFERENCES

1. Cotton F, Henderson F. Results of fracture of the os calcis. J Bone Joint Surg Am. 1916;s2-14:290-8.
2. Gougoulias N, Khanna A, McBride DJ, Maffulli N. Management of calcaneal fractures: systematic review of randomized trials. Br Med Bull. 2009;92:153-67.
3. Bajammal S, Tornetta 3rd P, Sanders D, Bhandari M. Displaced intra-articular calcaneal fractures. J Orthop Trauma. 2005;19(5):360-4.
4. Bruce J, Sutherland A. Surgical versus conservative interventions for displaced intra-articular calcaneal fractures. Cochrane Database Syst Rev. 2013;(1):CD008628.
5. Buckley R, Tough S, McCormack R, Pate G, Leighton R, Petrie D, et al. Operative compared with nonoperative treatment of displaced intra-articular calcaneal fractures: a prospective, randomized, controlled multicenter trial. J Bone Joint Surg Am. 2002;84:1733-44.
6. Griffin D, Parsons N, Shaw E, Kulikov Y, Hutchinson C, Thorogood M, et al. Operative versus non-operative treatment for closed, displaced, intra-articular fractures of the calcaneus: randomised controlled trial. BMJ. 2014;349:g4483.
7. Ibrahim T, Rowsell M, Rennie W, Brown AR, Taylor GJ, Gregg PJ. Displaced intra-articular calcaneal fractures: 15-year follow-up of a randomised controlled trial of conservative versus operative treatment. Injury. 2007;38(7):848-55.
8. McBride DJ, Ramamurthy C, Laing P. The hindfoot: calcaneal and talar fractures and dislocations—part I: fractures of the calcaneum. Current Orthopaedics. 2005;19:94-100.
9. Sangeorzan BJ, Benirschke SK, Sanders R, Carr JB, Thordarson DB. The literature on calcaneal fractures is highly controversial. Foot Ankle Int. 2001;22(10):844-5.
10. Schepers T, Ginai AZ, Mulder PGH, Patka P. Radiographic evaluation of calcaneal fractures: to measure or not to measure. Skeletal Radiol. 2007;36:847-52.
11. Thordarson DB, Krieger LE. Operative vs. nonoperative treatment of intra-articular fractures of the calcaneus: a prospective randomized trial. Foot Ankle Int. 1996;17:2-9.
12. Zwipp H, Rammelt S, Barthel S. Calcaneal fractures—open reduction and internal fixation (ORIF). Injury. 2004;35:SB46-54.
13. Buckley RE, Tough S. Displaced intra-articular calcaneal fractures. J Am Acad Orthop Surg. 2004;12(3):172-8.
14. Kerr PS, Prothero DL, Atkins RM. Assessing outcome following calcaneal fracture: a rational scoring system. Injury. 1996;27(1):35-8.
15. Pearce CJ, Wong KL, Calder JD. Calcaneal fractures: selection bias is key. Bone Joint J. 2015;97-B(7):880-2.
16. Humphrey JA, Woods A, Robinson AHN. The epidemiology and trends in the surgical management of calcaneal fractures in England between 2000 and 2017. Bone Joint J. 2019;101-B(2):140-6.
17. Gaskill T, Schweitzer K, Nunley J. Comparison of surgical outcomes of intra-articular calcaneal fractures by age. J Bone Joint Surg Am. 2010;92(18):2884-9.

18. Barla J, Buckley R, McCormack R, Pate G, Leighton R, Petrie D, et al. Displaced intraarticular calcaneal fractures: long-term outcome in women. Foot Ankle Int. 2004;25(12):853-6.

19. Sanders R. Displaced intra-articular fractures of the calcaneus. J Bone Joint Surg Am. 2000;82:225-50.

20. Ogawa BK, Charlton TP, Thordarson DB. Radiography versus computed tomography for displacement assessment in calcaneal fractures. Foot Ankle Int. 2009;30(10):1005-10.

21. Looijen RC, Misselyn D, Backes M, Dingemans SA, Halm JA, Schepers T. Identification of postoperative step-offs and gaps with Brodén's view following open reduction and internal fixation of calcaneal fractures. Foot Ankle Int. 2019;40(7):797-802.

22. Ha AS, Cunningham SX, Leung AS, Favinger JL, Hippe DS. Weightbearing digital tomosynthesis of foot and ankle arthritis: comparison with radiography and simulated weightbearing CT in a prospective study. AJR Am J Roentgenol. 2019;212(1):173-9.

23. Sanders FRK, Peters JJ, Schallig W, Mittlmeier T, Schepers T. What is the added value of pedobarography for assessing functional outcome of displaced intra-articular calcaneal fractures? A systematic review of existing literature. Clin Biomech (Bristol, Avon). 2020;72:8-15.

24. Brewster O, Clement ND, Duckworth AD, McQueen MM, Court-Brown CM. Long-term mortality after internal fixation of calcaneal fractures: a retrospective study. Eur J Orthop Surg Traumatol. 2020;30(1):157-62.

25. Kitaoka HB, Alexander IJ, Adelaar RS, Nunley JA, Myerson MS, Sanders M. Clinical rating systems for the ankle-hindfoot, midfoot, hallux, and lesser toes. Foot Ankle Int. 1994;15(7):349-53.

26. SooHoo NF, Samimi DB, Vyas RM, Botzler T. Evaluation of the validity of the foot function index in measuring outcomes in patients with foot and ankle disorders. Foot Ankle Int. 2006;27:38-42.

27. Sanders R, Fortin P, DiPasquale T, Walling A. Operative treatment in 120 displaced intraarticular calcaneal fractures. Results using a prognostic computed tomography scan classification. Clin Orthop Relat Res. 1993;(290):87-95.

28. Buckley RE, Meek RN. Comparison of open versus closed reduction of intraarticular calcaneal fractures: a matched cohort in workmen. J Orthop Trauma. 1992;6:216-22.

29. Hildebrand KA, Buckley RE, Mohtadi NG, Faris P. Functional outcome measures after displaced intra-articular calcaneal fractures. J Bone Joint Surg Br. 1996;78(1):119-23.

30. Richter M, Zech M, Geerling J, Frink M, Knobloch K, Krettek C. A new foot and ankle outcome score: questionnaire based, subjective, visual-analogue-scale, validated and computerized. Foot Ankle Surgery. 2006;12:191-9.

31. Richter M, Agren PH, Besse JL, Cöster M, Kofoed H, Maffulli N, et al. EFAS score - multilingual development and validation of a patient-reported outcome measure (PROM) by the score committee of the European Foot and Ankle Society (EFAS). Foot Ankle Surg. 2018;24(3):185-204.

32. RAND Corporation. 36-Item Short Form Survey Instrument (SF-36). [online] Available from: https://www.rand.org/health-care/surveys_tools/mos/36-item-short-form/survey-instrument.html. [Last accessed March, 2023].

33. EQ-5D. Explaining the EQ-5D in about two-and-a-half-minutes. [online] Available from: https://euroqol.org/eq-5d-instruments/. [Last accessed March, 2023].

26

Rehabilitation Protocols after Calcaneal Fractures

Bibek Adhya, Himmat S Dhillon, Sidak Dhillon

"Everyone has a doctor in him or her; we just have to help it in its work. The natural healing force within each one of us is the greatest force in getting well".

–Hippocrates (460–377 BC)

◼ INTRODUCTION

The calcaneus is responsible for transferring weight-bearing forces from the ankle to the ground during standing, walking, and running activities. The fractures of calcaneus are potentially so variable and complex that it has taken a long time to classify them and understand the complex injury patterns, which in turn determines what is the best treatment for each particular type. The most common trauma mechanisms are fall from height, motor vehicle accidents, or industrial accidents. When the fracture occurs, the patient is immediately aware of significant pain and is unable to bear weight on the foot or feet involved. Pain is often severe and unpleasant with significant swelling of the heel and ankle area of the foot. Whatever the initial treatment protocol, inherent in any good management method is a focus on rehabilitation of the injured foot. The physiotherapist has to focus on early ambulation to minimize stiffness and prevent complications such as reflex sympathetic dystrophy.

Rehabilitation concerns generally are multiple; undisplaced calcaneal fractures are usually managed with rest and protection until the fracture has healed, and in this scenario, the rehabilitation specialist comes into play almost immediately. Undisplaced fractures may be treated by casting in a short leg walking cast for 6 weeks; here the local area is protected, but the rest of the body has to be mobilized, and patient ambulation without straining the part or increasing edema has to be planned. The course of rehabilitation following this period of immobilization is generally the same as for ankle sprains.[1]

Displaced fractures are more frequently being treated with open reduction and internal fixation (ORIF). This is especially recommended in calcaneal fractures, which present with significant displacement of articular or lateral wall segments, impinged peroneal tendons, or entrapped structures in the medial compartment. The rehabilitation protocols here are different, and adequate planning and interaction with the treating surgeon are mandatory for all physiotherapists.

As has been mentioned in previous chapters, the treatment protocols are dependent on the fracture type, and most commonly, fractures of calcaneus may be:

- Extra-articular, 25–40% (not affecting the joint, mostly avulsion type: anterior process, sustentaculum tali, calcaneal tuberosity)[2]
- Intra-articular (involving the talocalcaneal and calcaneal cuboid joints) types

Various classification systems have been described, and their role in the rehabilitation process only becomes significant along with the proposed treatment.

- *Rowe classification:* Types I–III do not involve the subtalar joint. In type I (20%), the fracture line may be through the tuberosity, the sustentaculum tali, or the anterior process of the calcaneus. Type II or beak fractures are uncommon. Type III (20%) are oblique fractures. Types IV and V (60%) involve the subtalar joint. Type V fractures are comminuted fractures with a centrally depressed fragment.[2,3]
- *Essex-Lopresti classification:* There are two fracture lines in this classification, and based on the location of the secondary fracture line, there are two types of fracture. (1) Tongue-type fracture: The secondary fracture line extends directly posteriorly, producing a large superior, posterior, and lateral fragment, with the rest of the body forming the inferior fragment. (2) Joint depression fracture: The secondary fracture line begins at the crucial angle, extends posteriorly, and exits the bone just posterior to the posterior articular facet.[4]

Two other classification systems are most widely recognized and utilized in the evaluation of calcaneal fractures. Sanders, utilizing computed tomography (CT) scanning, divides calcaneal fractures into four categories.

Crosby–Fitzgibbons also using CT scans divide calcaneal fractures into three categories:

- *Type I:* Small fracture segments which are slightly displaced or undisplaced.
- *Type II:* Fracture segments which are displaced by 2 mm or more.
- *Type III:* Comminuted fracture.[2]

In addition to the above types, modern sports and overuse of the limb in different situations have led to more frequent occurrence of stress fractures.[5]

The role of the physiotherapist thus becomes multidimensional, and the rehabilitation protocol should include a detailed clinical examination as given in the following text.

OBSERVATION AND PHYSICAL EXAMINATION

Observation of the foot may reveal deformity of the foot, heel, or plantar arch. Deformity of the hindfoot, such as shortening, widening, or angulation, is common. Swelling (edema) and/or a pattern of ecchymosis that tracks along the outside (distal) of the foot to the sole may be present. An open wound may be present, especially if the injury was sustained during a motor vehicle accident. Holding the heel and gently squeezing it (palpation) **(Fig. 1)** elicits pain over the calcaneal tuberosities or the hindfoot. A thorough neurovascular examination is also essential. Ankle range of motion is often diminished, with pain at the extremes of motion. The individual may have difficulty in plantar flexion, especially with fractures of the posterior tuberosity, or avulsion injuries. With impaction fractures, there may be deformity in the Achilles tendon area and ecchymosis

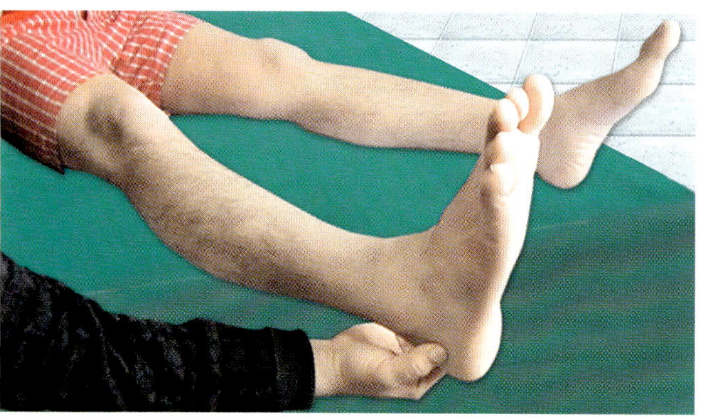

Fig. 1: Squeeze test of calcaneus.

along the sole of the foot. Examination of both feet, ankles, and knees, as well as the spine, is necessary to rule out any associated injuries.

A thorough physical examination, including subtalar and ankle range of motion, ankle and hindfoot stability, and gait, is essential and should be documented prior to starting rehabilitation.

AIMS OF REHABILITATION AND PROGNOSIS

Whatever may be the fracture type, there is always some stiffness in the subtalar joint following calcaneal fracture. Although some patients make an excellent recovery, some people find returning to a very active lifestyle difficult after these fractures, and this is dependent upon the initial fracture type, treatment protocols employed, and more importantly the rehabilitation process. Employment involving walking and climbing, industrial labor, or even prolonged standing may be difficult to return in the preinjury capacity. Appropriate rehabilitation helps to minimize the complications and ensures early return to normal function.

Most patients with a fractured calcaneus usually make a full recovery with appropriate management (whether surgical or conservative). Return to activity or sport (in case of sports person) can usually take place in a number of weeks to many months and should be guided by the treating physiotherapist and specialist. In patients with severe injuries involving damage to other bones, soft tissue, nerves, or blood vessels, recovery time may be significantly prolonged.

NONOPERATIVE TREATMENT

Nonoperative treatment of calcaneus fractures requires a multidisciplinary team involving a physiotherapist, an orthotist, and an occupational therapist, all familiar with the pattern of injury and the treatment protocol employed.

Many extra-articular calcaneus fractures are managed nonoperatively, provided that the injury does not change the weight-bearing surface of the foot and provided it does not alter hindfoot biomechanics.[6] Nonoperative treatment may be opted when there is no impingement on peroneal tendons and the fracture segments are undisplaced; if displaced, it should be <2 mm. Nonoperative care is also recommended when articulating surfaces are not disturbed. Older patients or who have preexisting health conditions, such as diabetes, severe osteoporosis, or peripheral vascular disease, are also commonly treated using nonoperative techniques.[7]

Severely comminuted intra-articular fractures may be managed nonoperatively, particularly in the elderly or when reconstruction is likely to be unsuccessful.[8] Many authors recommend short leg casting and no weight-bearing for 2 weeks, followed by range-of-motion exercises. Progressive weight-bearing should begin at 8 weeks, with full weight-bearing (FWB) by 12 weeks.

Surgical Procedure

Protocols for managing surgically treated patients may be somewhat different, although rehabilitation and physiotherapy techniques are similarly applicable. Regular interaction with the surgeon is mandatory as the surgical problems, degree of stability achieved, and associated injury and its management would dictate most aspects of the rehabilitation protocol.[9,10]

■ PREOPERATIVE REHABILITATION

Preoperative rehabilitation involves care of the patients who are awaiting surgery and the surgeon is waiting for the swelling to subside. This usually takes 7–14 days, and the physiotherapist should be aware of the time frames, the aims of waiting, and should observe the foot serially. Foot elevation, toe exercises, ipsilateral limb exercises, and, if possible, general body exercises should be done. Ambulation is minimized as the aim is to reduce edema prior to surgery, and compression along with medical interventions may be of benefit. The surgeon is informed when wrinkling of the skin sets in, and the patient is then taken up for surgery.

■ POSTOPERATIVE DETAILS

A small suction drain is frequently used after ORIF. This drain is typically removed when <10 mL of drainage fluid is collected over 8 hours.[11] Postoperatively, the foot is elevated with the ankle in the standard neutral position of a 90° angle between the foot and the tibia. This position is maintained for up to 72 hours to reduce postoperative swelling.[11]

Early range-of-motion exercises are encouraged after the surgical incision has begun healing, usually 10–12 days after surgery. A well-fitting orthosis is provided for comfort and to prevent gastrocnemius–soleus contracture. Sutures are removed at 3–4 weeks, but weight-bearing is delayed for up to 12 weeks, depending on the original fracture comminution and the subsequent rigidity of the fixation.

The progression of both nonoperative and postoperative rehabilitation management of calcaneal fractures includes traditional immobilization and early motion rehabilitation protocols. Much debate remains on the preferable management of calcaneal fractures after operative management. Böhler, Palmer, and Parmer recommend traditional immobilization after surgical repair, while Essex-Lopresti, Paley, and Wei advocate early mobilization

beginning within 24–72 hours of surgical repair.[4,12-17] Debate also exists on the preferable management of calcaneal fractures with nonoperative management. Barnard proposes the use of traditional immobilization in the form of a short leg cast, while Lance, Paley, and Parmer recommend early mobilization with nonoperative management.[18]

■ REHABILITATION PROTOCOL FOR CALCANEAL FRACTURE (NONOPERATIVE AND POSTOPERATIVE)[19]

Godges and Klingman

Phase-I		
Weeks	**Goals**	**Intervention**
1–4	• Control edema and pain • Prevent extension of fracture or loss of surgical stabilization • Minimize loss of function and cardiovascular endurance	• Cast with ankle in neutral and sometimes slight eversion • Elevation of involved extremity with ankle maintained at 90° angle in relation to the lower leg (or tibia) • Ice combined with compression wrap • After 24–72 hours, active range-of-motion exercises in small amounts of movement begin at all joints of the foot and ankle, including tibiotalar, subtalar, midtarsal, and toe joints, and are completed every hour **(Figs. 2 and 3)** • After 2–4 days, instruct in nonweight-bearing (NWB) ambulation utilizing crutches or walker • After 14 days, instruct in proper fitting and usage of prescribed surgical shoe or orthosis to prevent contracture • Instruct in wheelchair: use of wheelchair, appropriate way of sitting and limit the time of gravity assisted position of the affected extremity • Instruct in comprehensive exercise and cardiovascular program utilizing upper extremities and uninvolved lower extremity
Phase-II		
Weeks	**Goals**	**Intervention**
5–8	• Control remaining or residual edema and pain	• Continued elevation, icing, and compression as needed for involved lower extremity

Contd...

Contd...

- Prevent reinjury or complication of fracture by progressing weight-bearing safely
- Prevent contracture and regain motion at ankle/foot joints
- Minimize loss of function and cardiovascular endurance

- After 6–8 weeks, instruct in partial weight-bearing ambulation utilizing crutches or walker
- Initiate vigorous exercise and range of motion to regain and maintain motion at all joints: Tibiotalar, subtalar, midtarsal, and toe joints, including active range of motion in large amounts of movement and progressive isometric or resisted exercises **(Figs. 4 to 6)**
- Progress and monitor comprehensive upper extremity and cardiovascular program

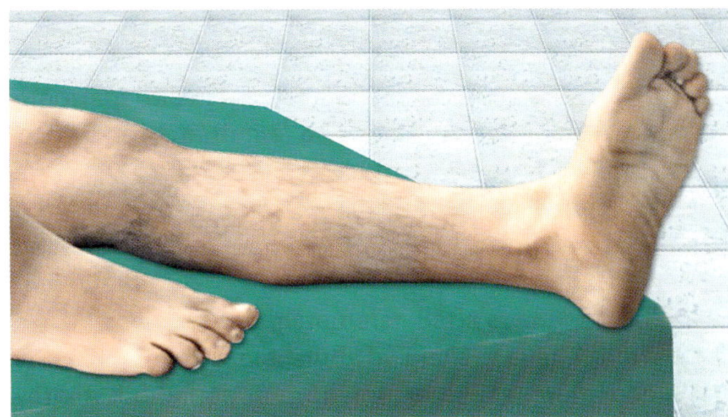

Fig. 2: Inversion exercise.

Phase-III		
Weeks	**Goals**	**Intervention**
9–12	• Progress weight-bearing status • Normal gait on all surfaces • Restore full range of motion Restore full strength • Allow return to previous work status	• After 9–12 weeks, instruct in normal FWB ambulation with appropriate assistive device as needed • Progress and monitor the subtalar joint's ability to adapt for ambulation on all surfaces, including graded and uneven surfaces • Joint mobilization to all hypomobile joints including tibiotalar, subtalar, midtarsal, and two toe joints **(Figs. 7 and 8)** • Soft-tissue mobilization to hypomobile tissues of the gastrocnemius complex, plantar fascia, or other appropriate tissues • Progressive resisted strengthening of gastrocnemius complex through use of pulleys, weighted exercise, toe walking ambulation, ascending/descending stairs, skipping or other plyometric exercise, pool exercises, and other climbing activities • Work hardening program or activities to allow return to work between 13 and 52 weeks

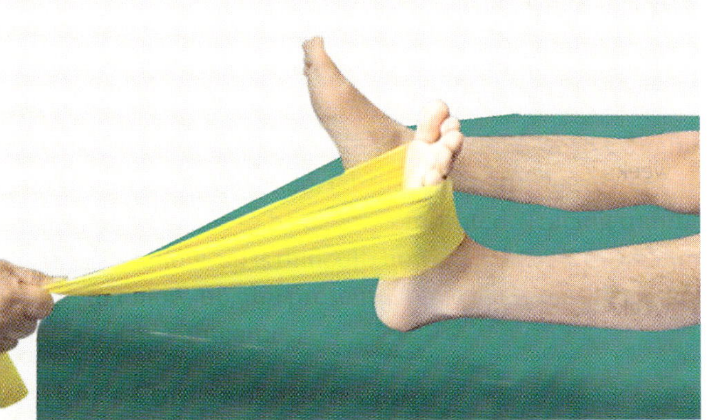

Fig. 3: Eversion exercise.

Fig. 4: Resisted strengthening of dorsiflexors.

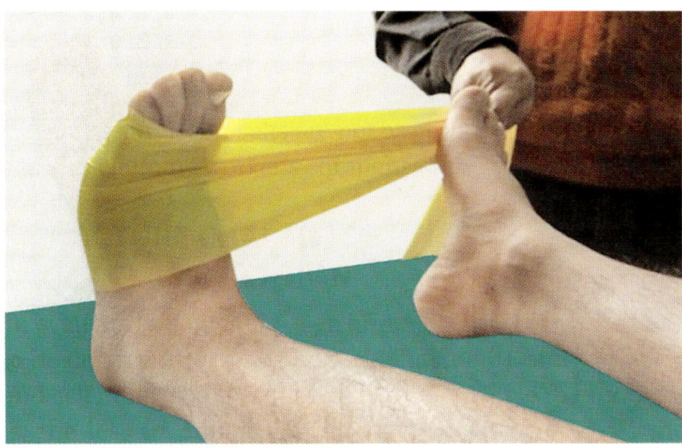

Fig. 5: Resisted strengthening of evertors.

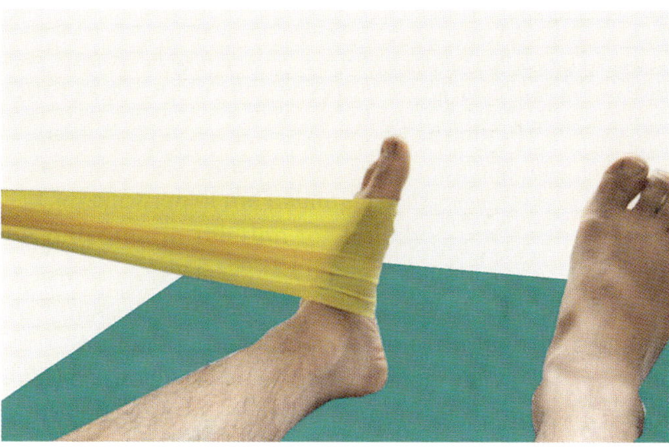

Fig. 6: Resisted strengthening of invertors.

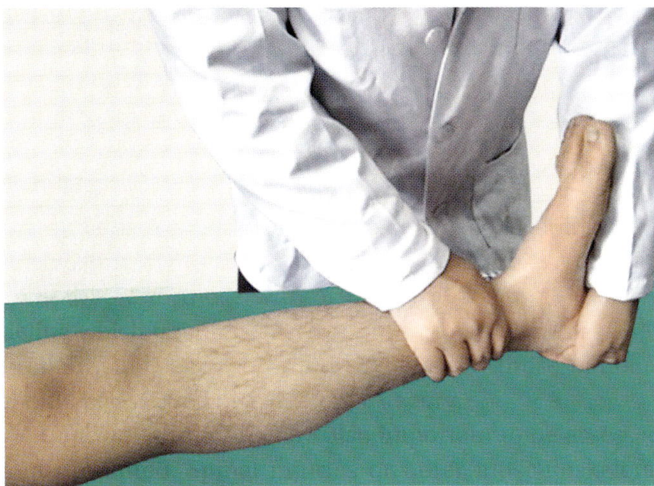

Fig. 7: Joint mobilization techniques.

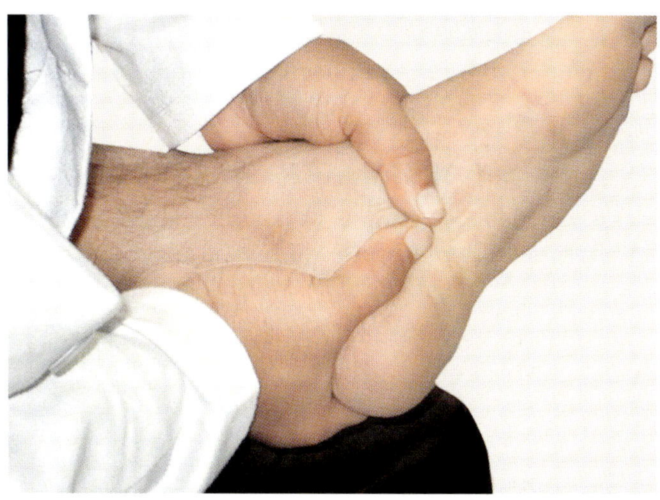

Fig. 8: Subtalar mobilization.

CALCANEUS FRACTURE POSTOPERATIVE PROTOCOL[20]

Sussex Foot and Ankle Center

Time	Interventions
Day 1	• Foot is wrapped in bulky bandage and splint. Elevate leg, take pain medication • Expect numbness in foot for 12–24 hours. Bloody drainage through bandage is expected. Do not bear any weight
1 week	• Use crutches, walker, wheelchair, or roll-a-bout. Do not change dressing/splint • Do not get the leg wet • Important to elevate the leg in the first 2 weeks
2 weeks	• First follow-up in outpatient department. Dressing changed • Sutures may be removed • A removable boot is applied

Contd...

Contd...

Time	Interventions
	• Start motion out of the boot as instructed • Can shower, provided the incision is clean and dry. Do not soak the foot until the incision is completely dry • Can soak in bath when the incision is completely dry, usually about 3 weeks
3 weeks	• Start swimming in a pool using a flipper to help movement of the ankle • Patient can bear some weight in the pool if there is no discomfort or pain • Start physiotherapy
8 weeks	Start exercise bicycle **(Fig. 9)**. No resistance. Begin partial weight-bearing
10–12 weeks	• Full weight-bearing without boot. Continue physiotherapy • X-rays taken in the outpatient department

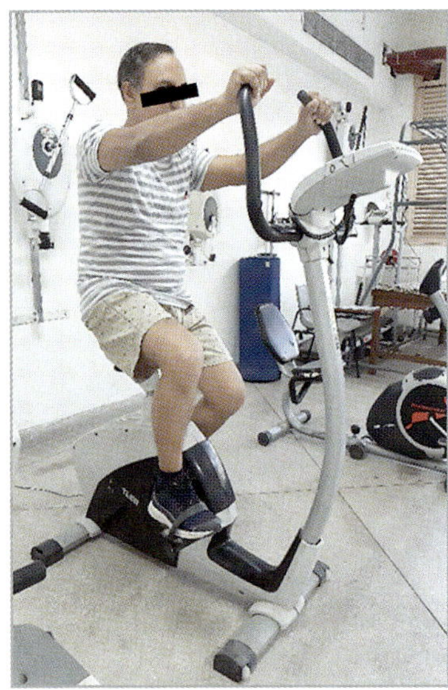

Fig. 9: Exercise bicycle.

REHABILITATION PROTOCOL FOR CALCANEAL FRACTURE[21]

Preoperative	Upper extremity (UE) strengthening; uninvolved extremity strengthening involved extremity hip, knee isometrics; crutch training for short distance (primary elevation of extremity)

Postoperative	
Time	**Intervention**
Day 1	UE strengthening; uninvolved extremity active range of movement (AROM) strengthening
Days 2–3	Crutch training, nonweight-bearing (NWB) involved extremity (limited time in dependent position)
Days 4–7	Early ankle, subtalar AROM when surgical incision is sealed
Week 1 to month 3	Continue early AROM ankle, subtalar, toes; gentle passive range of movement (PROM) toe dorsiflexion and plantar flexion; progress involved extremity; hip-knee conditioning. NWB ambulation
Advanced stage	
Month 3	Gradually increase weight-bearing starting at 20% to full weight-bearing over 1 month; gradually wean from assistive device as patient tolerates; pool therapy if available; gait training, reeducation; desensitization techniques as needed; ankle, subtalar active assisted range of movement (AAROM); isometrics; low impact endurance training

Contd...

Contd...

Months 4–6	Gait progression, advanced balance, and proprioceptive activities; ankle, subtalar isometric, isotonic strengthening with tubing/theraband; no free weights; soft-tissue immobilization
Month 6	Ankle, subtalar PROM; joint mobilization; isokinetic assessment, strength-endurance training; advanced balance, gait training as indicated

REHABILITATION FOR A CALCANEAL STRESS FRACTURE

Treatment for a stress fracture of the calcaneus typically involves an initial period of rest, usually involving reduced weight-bearing activity. This may include the use of crutches or a protective boot. This initial period of reduced weight-bearing may occur for approximately 6 weeks. Following this, a gradual increase in weight-bearing activity and exercise can usually take place, provided symptoms do not increase. This should occur over a period of weeks to months with direction from the treating physiotherapist and will vary depending on the severity of the injury.

Alternative exercises placing minimal weight-bearing forces through the affected bone should be performed to maintain fitness such as swimming, cycling, and water running. Exercises to restore flexibility, strength, balance, and function should also be performed to ensure that the foot and ankle are functioning correctly. The treating physiotherapist can advise which exercises are most appropriate and when they should be commenced.

Physiotherapy Techniques for a Calcaneus Stress Fracture

Physiotherapy treatment is vital in all patients with a calcaneus fracture to hasten healing and ensure an optimal outcome **(Table 1)**.

TABLE 1: Physiotherapy interventions in different stages of calcaneal stress fracture.	
Stage	**Interventions**
Early rehabilitation (0–6 weeks)	• NWB–PWB with crutches and protective boot/bracing. Cryotherapy to reduce edema and swelling • Gradual ROM exercise (e.g., foot and ankle up and down as far as possible and comfortable without pain). Repeat 10–20 times, provided there is no increase in symptoms. Move foot and ankle in and out as far as possible and comfortable without pain. Repeat 10–20 times, provided there is no increase in symptoms.

Contd...

Contd...

Stage	Interventions
	Move foot and ankle in a circle as large as possible and comfortable without pain. Repeat 10 times in each direction, provided there is no increase in symptoms. Hydrotherapy, patient education, activity modification
Advanced rehabilitation phase (6 weeks and above)	Gradual increase in weight-bearing to FWB, wear ankle support **(Fig. 10)**, contrast bath, paraffin wax bath, ultrasonic therapy, soft-tissue massage, hydrotherapy, strengthening exercise for foot and ankle muscles (theraband/elastic band, springs may be used) **(Figs. 11 and 12)**, stretching exercise **(Figs. 13 to 15)**, balance and proprioception exercises (e.g., mini trampoline and balance board) **(Figs. 16 and 17)**. Return to normal lifestyle

(FWB: full weight-bearing; NWB: nonweight-bearing; PWB: progressive weight-bearing; ROM: range of motion)

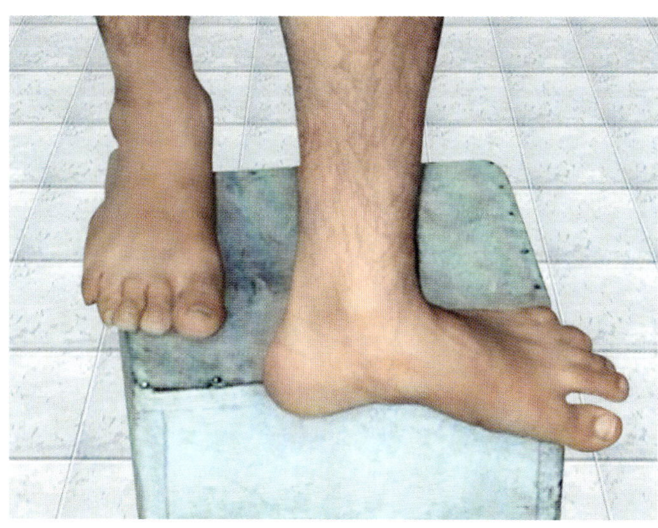

Fig. 12: Eccentric exercise for inverters.

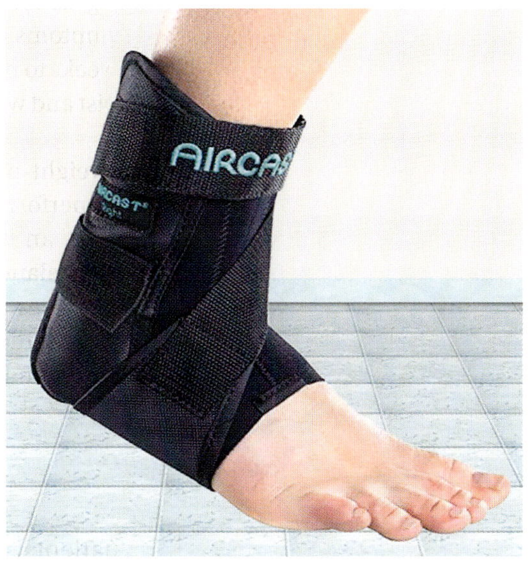

Fig. 10: Ankle support.

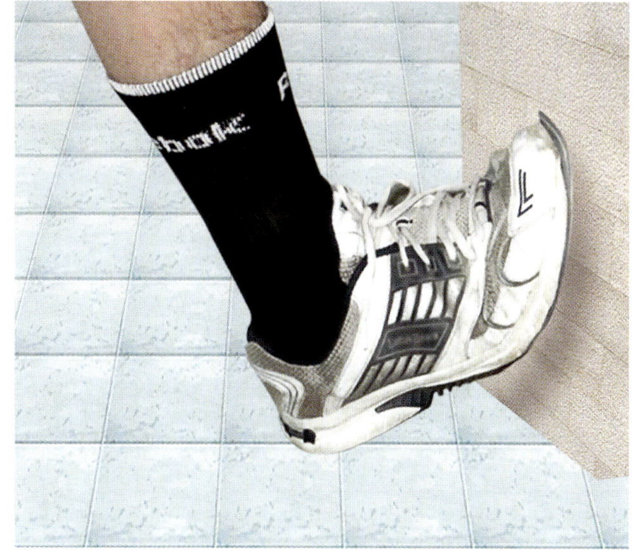

Fig. 13: Plantar fascia stretching.

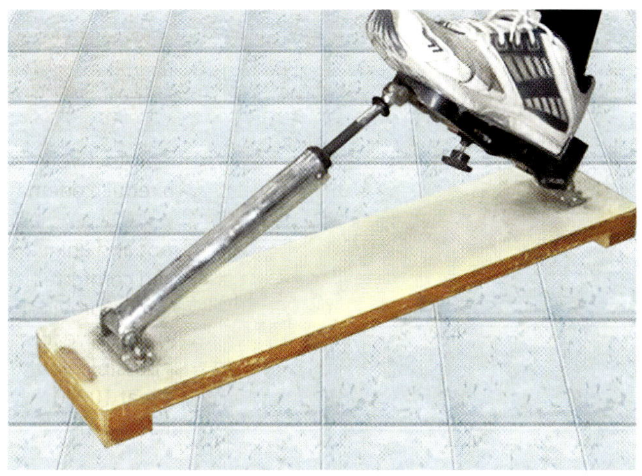

Fig. 11: Spring exercise.

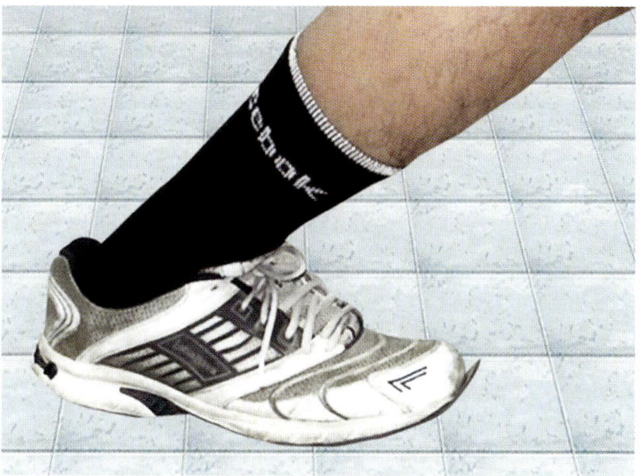

Fig. 14: Stretching of plantar flexors.

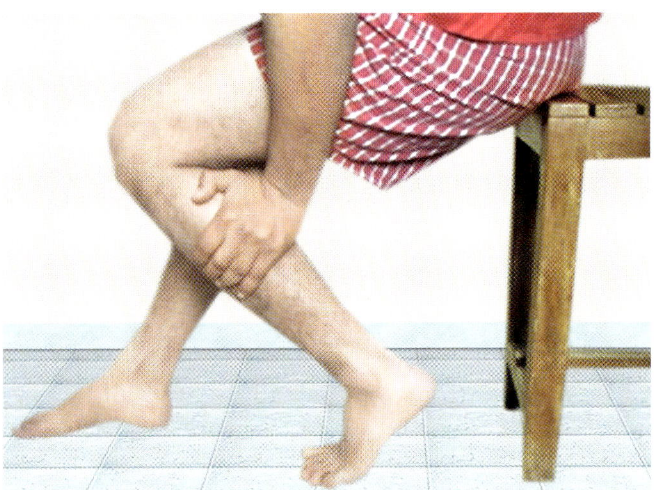

Fig. 15: Seated plantar fascia stretch.

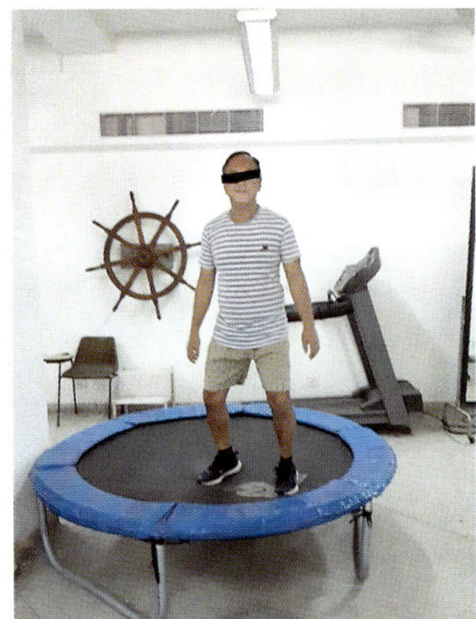

Fig. 16: Proprioceptive training (mini trampoline).

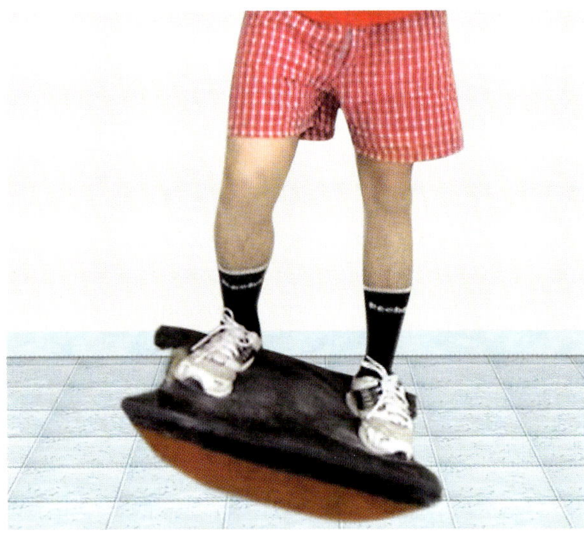

Fig. 17: Proprioceptive training (balance board).

■ REFERENCES

1. Prentice WE. Rehabilitation Techniques for Sports Medicine and Athletic Training, 4th edition. New York: McGraw Hill; 2004.
2. Schepers T, Ginai AZ, Van Lieshout EMM, Patka P. Demographics of extra-articular calcaneal fractures: including a review of the literature on treatment and outcome. Archives of Orthopaedic and Trauma Surgery. Arch Orthop Trauma Surg. 2008;128(10):1099-1106.
3. Rowe CR, Sakellarides HT, Freeman PA, Sorbie C. Fractures of the os calcis: a long-term follow-up study of 146 patients. JAMA. 1963;184:920-3.
4. Essex-Lopresti P. The mechanism, reduction technique, and results in fractures of the os calcis. Br J Surg. 1951;39:395-419.
5. Brukner P, Khan K. Clinical Sports Medicine, 3rd edition. North Ryde, NSW: McGraw Hill; 2005.
6. Degan TJ, Morrey BF, Braun DP. Surgical excision for anterior-process fractures of the calcaneus. J Bone Joint Surg Am. 1982;64(4):519-24.
7. Rammelt S, Sangeorzan BJ, Swords MP. Calcaneal fractures—should we or should we not operate? Indian J Orthop. 2018;52:220-30.
8. Pozo JL, Kirwan EO, Jackson AM. The long-term results of conservative management of severely displaced fractures of the calcaneus. J Bone Joint Surg Br. 1984;66(3):386-90.
9. Dhillon MS, Prabhakar S. Treatment of displaced intra-articular calcaneus fractures: a current concepts review. SICOT J. 2017;3:59.
10. Dhillon M, Khurana A, Prabhakar S, Sharma S. Crush fractures of the anterior end of calcaneum. Indian J Orthop. 2018;52:244-52.
11. Nicklebur S, Dixon TB, Probe R. Calcaneal fractures. EMedicine; 2004.
12. Lorenz B. Diagnosis, pathology, and treatment of fractures of the os calcis. J Bone Joint Surg. 1931;13:75-89.
13. Burdeaux Jr BD. The medical approach for calcaneal fractures. Clin Orthop Relat Res. 1993;(290):96-107.
14. Palmer I. The mechanism and treatment of fractures of the calcaneus; open reduction with the use of cancellous grafts. J Bone Joint Surg Am. 1948;30A(1):2-8.
15. Parmar HV, Triffitt PD, Gregg PJ. Intra-articular fractures of the calcaneum treated operatively or conservatively. A prospective study. J Bone Joint Surg Br. 1993;75(6):932-7.
16. Paley D, Hall H. Calcaneal fracture controversies—can we put Humpty Dumpty together again? Orthop Clin North Am. 1989;20:665-77.
17. Wei SY, Okereke E, Esmail AN, Born CT, DeLong Jr WG. Operatively treated calcaneus fractures: to mobilize or not to mobilize. Univ of Penn Orthop J. 2001;14:71-3.
18. Barnard L, Odegard JK. Conservative approach in the treatment of fractures of the calcaneus. J Bone Joint Surg Am. 1955;37-A(6):1231-6.
19. Godges J, Klingman R. Calcaneal fracture and rehabilitation surgical indications and considerations anatomic considerations. Loma Linda U DPT Program KPSoCal Ortho PT Residency 1. [online] Available from: http://xnet.kp.org/socal_rehabspecialists/ptr_library/09footregion/31foot-calcanealfracture.pdf. [Last accessed March, 2023].
20. Redfern DJ, Bendall SP. (2009). Fracture of the Calcaneus: Open Reduction and Internal Fixation. Sussex: Sussex Foot and Ankle Centre.
21. SIU School of Medicine [homepage on the Internet]. Division of Orthopaedics: Fracture Treatment Protocols; c2009-2011 [updated 26 Jan 2011]. Available from: http:// www.siumed.edu.

27

Evidence-based Orthopedics: What is Optimal for Calcaneus Fracture Today

Marianne Comeau-Gauthier, Harman Chaudhry, Raman Mundi, Mohit Bhandari

"The most savage controversies are those about matters as to which there is no good evidence either way".

"The fact that an opinion has been widely held is no evidence whatever that it is not utterly absurd; indeed in view of the silliness of the majority of mankind, a widespread belief is more likely to be foolish than sensible".

–Bertrand Russell (1872–1970)

■ INTRODUCTION

Although calcaneal fractures represent only 2% of all fractures, they are fraught with complications and patient morbidity. Calcaneal fractures are typically high-energy injuries which occur predominantly in working-age males, with a mean age of incidence between the 30s and 40s.[1,2] The vast majority of these injuries—between 65 and 75%— are intra-articular and therefore have the capacity to alter hindfoot biomechanics and function.[1,2] Although the poor prognosis associated with calcaneal fractures has been duly acknowledged for over a century,[3] there has been a long-standing controversy as to whether operative or non-operative management of these fractures is optimal.[4-7]

As scientific thinking has advanced, the advent of evidence-based medicine (EBM) in the 1980s finally provided a powerful tool to put such long-standing controversies to rest. As summarized by Guyatt and Busse,[8] EBM is defined by two important principles. The first is that evidence alone is never enough. Any clinical decision must represent an optimal intersection of patient values, clinical resources, and the best available evidence. The second principle attempts to elucidate what the best available evidence refers to by providing a systematic hierarchy of different study designs. In the hierarchy of evidence, the importance of a control group cannot be overstated. A control group provides a direct comparator against which an intervention can be evaluated. In this way, an intervention can be definitively shown to be superior to current practice (represented by the control group). Hence in the hierarchy of evidence, study designs that employ a control group rank higher than those that do not. Within study designs that utilize a control group, study designs are ranked based on the ability to minimize bias, with experimental designs being higher than observational designs. **Table 1** provides a simplified model of the hierarchy of evidence.[9] It is important to understand that high-quality trials ranked lower on the hierarchy may offer more valid conclusions than lower-quality trials ranked higher on the hierarchy. Therefore, it is important to conduct a thorough critical appraisal of any study to determine both the internal and external validity of its conclusions.

This chapter will provide a panoramic survey of the current best evidence regarding optimal management of displaced intra-articular calcaneal fractures (DIACFs). Subsequently, an outline of currently ongoing research trials will be provided. Finally, the chapter will conclude with recommendations for future research. As mentioned above, the best evidence regarding optimal management requires a control group. Therefore, this chapter will focus its content predominantly on studies that employ a control group in order to summarize only the best available evidence and identify where gaps in that evidence exist.

■ NONOPERATIVE MANAGEMENT

Clinical consensus and years of case series have collectively established nonoperative management as the treatment of choice for extra-articular fractures. The notable exception to this has been fractures of the calcaneal tuberosity (typically secondary to an avulsion mechanism) because of the ability of this injury to alter heel height, hindfoot biomechanics, and associated devastating risk of posterior heel skin compromise.[2] Most series and studies have indicated that nonoperative intervention consists of immobilization,

TABLE 1: A simplified model of the levels of evidence for therapeutic studies.[6]

Level	Study design	Control	Features
1	Systematic review	Yes	Systematic identification, data abstraction, data synthesis, and subsequent reporting of results of all studies pertaining to a specific clinical question. May include a meta-analysis of outcomes
2	Randomized controlled trial	Yes	Experimental clinical studies that randomly assign two or more groups to different treatment arms and follow these groups prospectively over time
3	Observational cohort study	Yes	Clinical studies that identify two or more groups of patients, one or more of which have received the intervention of interest over a period of time
4[*]	Case-control	Yes	• Clinical studies that identify patients having undergone a certain intervention and identify similar patients that did not undergo the intervention • These groups are retrospectively compared
	Case series	No	Clinical studies that follow a single patient or group of patients that have received an intervention over a period of time
5	Mechanism-based reasoning	No	Nonclinical studies that identify physiological or pathophysiological mechanisms that are used to suggest possible clinical outcomes

[*]Both study designs are categorized under level 4. Note that one employs a control group and one does not.

ice, rest, and elevation, with subsequent mobilization and physiotherapy. There have been no major high-level, high-quality studies comparing different nonoperative management options, timelines to mobilization, physiotherapy protocols, or other nonoperative parameters.

In terms of intra-articular fractures, various studies have attempted to outline indications for nonoperative management, including nondisplaced intra-articular fractures, local or systemic contraindications to surgical intervention, and severely comminuted fractures. However, because much of this is still controversial, this issue will be discussed in the following section.

OPERATIVE VERSUS NONOPERATIVE MANAGEMENT

There has been a long-standing controversy as to whether operative or nonoperative management is ideal for DIACF. Operative intervention has typically been undertaken by orthopedic surgeons to restore the articular surface between the calcaneus and talus, restore hindfoot biomechanics, and restore heel height and length. Although operative intervention is certainly the best way to achieve these goals in the short term, whether this restoration has any long-term implications is not certain. More importantly, whether achieving a stringent anatomical reduction has any impact on patient-important outcomes in either the short term or the long term is controversial. This section will review the pertinent observational cohort studies, randomized controlled trials (RCTs), and systematic reviews pertaining to these questions.

Observational Cohort Studies

Two observational cohort studies that have investigated operative compared to nonoperative management of calcaneal fractures have two specific patient populations. The first study looked at older patients, which represent a group of patients who are less likely than average to experience a calcaneal fracture but more likely to be treated nonoperatively due to a perception of lower physical demands. Basile[10] retrospectively followed a group of 33 patients, ages ranging between 65 and 75 years, treated at one of two different hospitals. One of the hospitals followed an open reduction and internal fixation (ORIF) protocol, while the other treated these patients nonoperatively. They assessed the patients after a minimum of 4 years for outcomes based on the American Orthopaedic Foot and Ankle Society (AOFAS) scoring system, pain as determined by a 100-mm visual analog scale (VAS), and radiographically. The authors determined that operatively managed patients had better outcomes in all domains. Interestingly, and importantly, among the 18 patients that underwent ORIF, those with anatomical reductions had significantly better AOFAS and VAS scores compared to those in which reductions were nearly, but not completely, anatomic. The study therefore provides objective level 3 evidence that anatomic reduction during surgery results in improved functional, patient-important outcomes.

The second study focused on outcomes in children—an age group in which fractures of the calcaneus are relatively rare.[11] Ceccarelli et al.[12] reported a retrospective cohort study of 46 calcaneal fractures in children between the ages of 3 and 17 years who underwent either operative or nonoperative intervention. They concluded that children aged 14 years and below (labeled "skeletally immature" patients) achieved similar results with operative or nonoperative management. In the age group above 14 years (labeled "skeletally mature" patients), operative management achieved superior results.

The third pertinent relevant retrospective cohort study compared three treatment modalities: (1) nonoperative (n = 18), (2) ORIF (n = 27), and (3) percutaneous fixation (n = 33).[13] Greatest disability, as measured by the foot function index (FFI), was found in the nonoperative control group, while other functional outcome measures [AOFAS, short-form 36-item questionnaire (SF-36), EuroQol-5 dimension (EQ-5D)] in patients treated nonoperatively were not significantly different from those in operative management. It remains unclear if ORIF and percutaneous fixation differed in regard to functional and clinical outcome as it was not explicitly mentioned.

Randomized Controlled Trials

The largest trial on calcaneal fracture management to date was conducted by Richard Buckley and his research team at the University of Calgary in Canada.[14] This was a multicenter RCT, which randomized patients to receive one of two interventions: (1) ORIF through an extensile lateral approach (ELA) and rigid fixation with plates, screws, or wires (bone graft use was not standardized and left to the discretion of each individual surgeon) or (2) nonoperative management consisting of ice, rest, and elevation only (no closed reduction). A total of 424 patients were randomized and followed up for a minimum of 2 years and up to a maximum of 8 years. Outcome measures included a validated VAS designed specifically for evaluating functional outcomes following calcaneal fractures[15] and the SF-36 general health survey. This study came to a number of important conclusions. Firstly, it was noted that overall, without group stratification, there was no difference between the outcomes of operatively and nonoperatively managed patients. However, if patients involved in a worker's insurance claim were excluded from the analysis, then a significant benefit of operative intervention over nonoperative management emerged. A patient who received workers' compensation had unfavorable clinical outcomes regardless of treatment modality. The reasoning for this was not entirely clear. It could be postulated that insurance claim patients were involved in heavier labor resulting in either more severe injuries preoperatively or increased physical demands postoperatively. Finally, several prognostic factors were associated with higher postoperative satisfaction such

as higher Böhler's angle at presentation (>15°), a nonwork-related injury, and a unilateral injury.

The research team went on to conduct a post hoc analysis and delineate which subgroups of patients respond favorably to operative intervention; these subgroups included Women, young adults (ages 20–29 years), patients with a light-to-moderate workload, patients with a Böhler's angle between 0° and 14°, and fractures classified as type II under the Sanders classification (i.e., less comminution).

A second publication by the same research group attempted to elucidate both major and minor complications which occurred during their RCT.[16] Major complications represent the more important outcome reported in this study and included wound infections, thromboembolic events, and major reoperations such as secondary arthrodesis. In the patient subgroup in which ORIF was shown to be superior (i.e., noninsurance claim patients), ORIF was also more likely to result in a major complication (31 vs. 12% of patients, $p < 0.001$). Insurance claim patients were found to have a higher rate of complications regardless of management option. Interestingly, patients with severely comminuted fractures (Sanders type IV) were also more likely to develop a major complication regardless of management option.

A number of subsequent studies were conducted from the database produced from the Buckley research group's RCT. These studies served to further clarify any differences between operative and nonoperative management. One study found that patient satisfaction with their own gait was no different between operative and nonoperative groups, except in patients younger than 30 years.[17] A subsequent study determined that outcomes in patients with bilateral calcaneal fractures were no different than in those with unilateral fractures.[18] Another secondary analysis found several prognostic determinants of subsequent secondary subtalar fusion: Lower Böhler's angle at presentation (<0°) (10 times more likely), Sanders type IV (5.5 times more likely), nonoperative management, and patients receiving workers' compensation.[19] Finally, one study looked specifically at women and quantified how much more favorable their prognosis was with operative intervention. They determined that women who underwent ORIF for calcaneal fractures had greater SF-36 scores at follow-up than women who underwent nonoperative management (relative risk of approximately 3, $p < 0.05$). The authors attributed this to the observed lower energy traumas and less severe injuries sustained by women. They concluded that operative intervention in women is certainly warranted.[20]

More recently, the UK Heel Fracture trial (HeFt) by Griffin et al.[21] reported no added clinical benefits, as reported by the Kerr–Atkins score, from operative management by ORIF (n = 73) compared with nonoperative management (n = 78) for treatment of DIACFs at 2 years after injury. Based on their results, they recommended against operative treatment by ORIF. Similarly, Agren et al.[22] did not find any significant clinical improvement based on the VAS for pain and function, SF-36, and AOFAS scale from operative management at 8–12 years post injury. However, a major limitation to these more recent RCTs is the absence of group stratification. Modern medicine includes tailoring of a medical treatment to the individual characteristics of each patient. This is supported by the largest clinical trial to date, which found several subgroups or patient's characteristics to be associated with better outcomes following operative management.[14,20,23]

Brauer et al.[24] conducted an economic analysis on the RCT data at the Harvard Center for Risk Analysis. They retrospectively evaluated both direct and indirect health care costs over a 4-year follow-up period. Their detailed analysis found that CAD$19,000 were saved per patient undergoing operative management. However, the predominance of these savings was attributable to the indirect costs of missed time from employment. When costs associated with missed employment were excluded from the analysis, ORIF costs the system CAD$2,800. In other words, although surgery is initially more costly, patients return to employment faster, resulting in several thousands of dollars in savings for the economy. These results are supported by a more recent study who found operative treatment to be cost-effective, regardless of whether or not lost wages were included in the analysis.[25] In this study, they found savings of approximately $4,700 per patient initially managed operatively.[25]

Ibrahim et al.[26] have recently published the 15-year follow-up of an RCT originally published in 1993.[27] The original trial utilized a pseudo-randomization process to place 66 patients in one of two groups: (1) ORIF through a lateral approach and fixation with Kirschner wires or (2) nonoperative management with ice and elevation. The outcomes measured were both clinical (AOFAS score, FFI, and calcaneal fracture score) and radiological (Böhler's angle and calcaneal height). The 15-year follow-up study also measured radiological grade of arthritis as an outcome. Only 26 patients were available for long-term follow-up. They found absolutely no statistical difference between the operatively and nonoperatively managed groups for any of the outcomes. However, one must take into account the high lost to follow-up rate (>60%) which poses a serious risk of bias.

Overall, the most recent RCTs reporting data on functional outcomes did not find a significant difference between operative and nonoperative management.[7,14,18,21,22,26,28,29] More specifically, no difference was reported in regard to VAS score,[14,18,22,28] SF-36,[14,18,21,22] FFI questionnaire, Kerr–Atkins score,[21,28] AOFAS ankle-hindfoot scale,[21,22,26,29] and calcaneal fracture scoring systems.[26] As mentioned by Dhillon and Prabhakar,[30] while some authors may support operative intervention under selected circumstances,[14,18,31,32] other reported equivocal findings[22,26-28] or recommended against any surgical intervention.[21] Several other RCTs were published in the 1990s; however, all were relatively small trials and their conclusions are summarized in the following systematic reviews.

Systematic Reviews

Several up-to-date systematic reviews and meta-analyses have been published on the topic of operative versus nonoperative management of DIACFs.[4,5,7,33,34] Although most have concluded that there is still insufficient evidence supporting operative management over nonoperative treatment, there is a general consensus that operative treatment leads to a higher complication rate.[4,5,7,33,34] Although three recent RCTs implied no difference in the rate of subsequent arthrodesis whether surgery was performed or not,[21,22,26] the largest clinical trial to date completed by Buckley et al.[14] reported a higher rate of subsequent arthrodesis with the nonoperatively managed group. This is supported by pooled results from meta-analyses reporting a lesser risk of subsequent arthrodesis with operative management.[4,7,33] Operative treatment was associated with significantly better restoration of Böhler's angle,[5,7] and better walking ability and show wear,[33,34] although the latter remains an inconsistent finding.[4,5,7] Functional outcomes, as reported from pooled results of AOFAS, SF-36, or VAS scores, did not demonstrate added benefits from operative management,[4,5,7,33,34] while others reported reduced time to return to work.[4,5,33] Operative management may lead to less chronic pain,[7] but this finding was inconsistent.[4] All systematic reviews and meta-analyses reviews have come to essentially the same conclusion: There are not enough high-quality studies to make a definitive decision on the issue. Nevertheless, the majority of the systematic reviews make clinical suggestions that are fairly consistent with the conclusions made by Buckley and colleagues. This is hardly surprising, as this was by far the largest trial included in either review. Furthermore, as Schepers noted,[35] they all compared the so-called gold standard ELA and ORIF to nonoperative management. Perhaps, with the avenue of new minimally invasive approaches (MIA) (i.e., extended or limited sinus tarsi, arthroscopic) and new constructs (i.e., percutaneous pinning), practice may change toward operative management to prevent the devastating clinical outcomes associated with DIACFs.

OPERATIVE MANAGEMENT: TECHNIQUES AND PARAMETERS

Whereas the controversy between operative and nonoperative management has been explored and continues to be addressed in ongoing research trials **(Table 2)**, data on which operative strategies produce superior outcomes has not been well reported. There have been no level 1 or 2 studies comparing different operative exposures, techniques, instrumentation, or other parameters. Several controlled cohort studies, RCTs, and meta-analyses addressing this issue have been published in the last 10 years. We will outline the most determinant studies in this section. As no universal theme has emerged from these studies, it is difficult to conclude that there is a well-concerted effort to determine the best approach to operative care at this time.

Observational Cohort Studies

Gaskill and his research team[36] retrospectively identified two groups of patients at a tertiary care center: All patients above the age of 50 years who had undergone ORIF for calcaneal fractures and all patients below the age of 50 years meeting the same criteria. A total of 158 patients were followed up for an average of 9 years, and injury-specific outcomes were determined for each patient; specifically, the calcaneal fracture scoring system, the AOFAS ankle-hindfoot scale, and the FFI were used. The group of patients older than 50 years reported a significantly better AOFAS and calcaneal fracture score, while the group of patients under 50 years reported a significantly better FFI score. Furthermore, complications between the two groups of patients were

TABLE 2: Currently registered randomized controlled trials involving calcaneal fractures.

Trial	Location	Intervention	Control	Primary outcomes	Secondary outcomes	Target sample size	Estimated primary completion date
ORIF of calcaneal fractures with or without bone graft[38]	University of Alabama, Birmingham, USA	ORIF with tricortical iliac crest bone graft	ORIF without bone graft	Union and healing	Not available	49	Completed
External fixation versus splinting of acute calcaneus fractures prior to definitive surgery[39]	University of California, CA, USA	External fixation	Splinting	Time from injury to definitive surgery, soft tissue complications	Union, radiological, FFI-R, FAAM ADL, FAAM Sport, VAS	100	August 29, 2021
Osteosynthesis of intraarticular calcaneal fractures: Arthroscopically assisted percutaneous technique versus sinus tarsi approach[40]	Oslo University Hospital, Oslo, Norway	Arthroscopically assisted percutaneous technique	Sinus tarsi approach (STA)	MOxFQ	AOFAS ankle-hindfoot score, CFSS, SEFAS, complications, radiological	70	December, 2030
Sinus tarsi versus extensile lateral approach for ORIF of intra-articular calcaneus fractures[41]	Erlanger Health System, Chattanooga, Tennessee, USA	Sinus tarsi approach	Extensile lateral approach	Wound complication rate	Union and healing, sural nerve injury, peroneal tendon injury, operative time, secondary surgery, VAS, AOFAS, FFI, SF-36	110	December, 2019

(ADL: activities of daily living; AOFAS: American Orthopaedic Foot and Ankle Society; CFSS: Calcaneal Fractures Scoring System; FAAM: Foot and Ankle Ability Measure; FFI-R: foot function index-revised; MOxFQ: Manchester–Oxford Foot Questionnaire; ORIF: open reduction and internal fixation; SEFAS: Self-reported Foot and Ankle Score; SF-36: short-form 36-item questionnaire; VAS: visual analog scale)

not significantly different, even though the older group of patients had a higher perioperative risk as per the American Society of Anesthesiologists (ASA) score. In attempting to explain their findings, the authors did suggest that the similar outcomes following ORIF were likely attributable to more severe injuries and increased physical demands in the group of younger patients, as opposed to better-than-expected function in the older patients. Nevertheless, the study ultimately determined that age, per se, was not a contraindication to operative intervention.[37]

Weber et al.[42] performed a retrospective cohort study comparing 50 patients who had experienced calcaneal fractures classified as either Sanders II or Sanders III. The patients had undergone either an ORIF with an ELA or an ORIF with limited lateral incision and percutaneous fixation (i.e., a limited-exposure ORIF). Although no significant differences were detected in patient function or radiological assessment of anatomical outcomes, the limited-exposure ORIF had a significantly shorter operating time—approximately 52 minutes shorter. However, the limited-exposure approach also required more minor surgical procedures, such as pin removal, secondary to pain and irritation.

Grala et al.[43] reported the results of a prospective cohort study using a historical control group, which compares the use of a large bone distractor versus standard technique during ORIF of DIACFs. A total of 42 patients were analyzed. The large bone distractor is described as an instrument used to assist the orthopedic surgeon with both retraction and reduction. One end of the large bone distractor acts in place of K-wires in the standard technique, which among other things, assists with retraction of lateral soft tissue. The other end of the large bone distractor replaces the S-pin in the standard technique as a "joystick" for bony manipulation. The study demonstrated a reduced time to posterior articular surface fixation (22.6 minutes compared to 28.2 minutes for the standard technique, $p < 0.05$). The study did not detect any significant difference in functional outcomes (as measured by the Creighton-Nebraska Health Foundation Assessment score) or radiological outcomes.

Besch et al.[44] reported a prospective cohort study which attempted to elucidate the utility of a hinged external fixator for calcaneal fractures. Two groups of patients were prospectively followed and assessed both radiologically and functionally based on the AOFAS ankle-hindfoot scale. Twenty-four patients were treated definitively with hinged external fixation, while 13 patients were initially treated with hinged external fixation and later converted to ORIF if certain indications were met. Such indications included no necrosis, fracture blisters or infection, and minimal soft-tissue swelling. No significant differences in outcomes were seen between groups. In assessing the results of this study, it is important to note that there was no comparison of a hinged external fixator to ORIF alone (without a hinged external fixator). Therefore, it cannot be concluded that the hinged external fixator is a beneficial addition. However, the authors do outline various numerical outcome measures of the hinged external fixator which certainly adds to the utility of the study as a case series. However, the effectiveness of the hinged external fixator as an intervention warrants further study.

When comparing nonoperative treatment ($n = 18$) with ORIF ($n = 27$) and percutaneous fixation ($n = 33$), de Boer et al. found no difference in the infection rate between percutaneous fixation and ORIF. Furthermore, the percutaneous group was found to have a higher hardware removal rate and a higher number of secondary arthrodesis procedures compared with ORIF.[13]

Randomized Controlled Trials and Systematic Reviews

In recent years, there has been a surge of MIA in order to circumvent the high rate of postoperative wound complications following the conventional ELA. MIA refers to various types of limited incision approaches [limited or extended sinus tarsi approach (STA)] or percutaneous fixation (cannulated screws, K-wires, percutaneous plating positioning) relying on direct image intensifier arthroscopy-assisted techniques.[45-49] Several RCTs,[50-58] observational studies,[13,42,59-67] and meta-analyses[68-73] compared the STA to the conventional ELA. Only the most recent and up-to-date studies will be discussed.

Studies across meta-analyses were generally compared based on reported VAS score,[53,55,56,58] AOFAS ankle-hindfoot score,[51-53,55-58] Maryland score,[54,57] wound complications,[50-58] length of surgery,[50,52-57] restoration of Böhler's angle,[51-58] restoration of the angle of Gissane,[51,54,56-58] and final calcaneal width,[52,54,56,57] length,[52,54,56] and height.[54,56] A large and significantly reduced postoperative wound complications rate is found with MIA (2.3–4.9%) compared with ELA (18.7–24.9%),[68,69,71-73] with minimal heterogeneity throughout the studies. Pooled results from meta-analyses report less overall infection rate in favor of STA,[68,71] shorter duration of surgery,[68-70,73] and decreased length of stay.[72] These benefits are obtained without apparent significant compromise in reduction, as demonstrated by nonsignificant difference in Böhler's angle,[68,70,72] angle of Gissane,[68,72] recovery of calcaneus length,[72] height,[68] and width,[68,72] and reduction as assessed by computed tomography (CT) scan.[73] However, significant heterogeneity remains in regard to radiological outcomes and these results must be interpreted cautiously.[73] Some showed a significant difference in some subcomponents of selected functional outcome scales favoring the less invasive procedure.[57,70,72] However, this remains largely inconsistent.[53,68,74] Furthermore, a cost-effectiveness analysis found the STA to be the least expensive ($23,329), followed by nonoperative management ($24,530) and traditional ORIF using ELA ($27,530) ($p < 0.001$) for Sanders II and III intra-articular calcaneus fractures.[75] This was attributed mostly to lost time of work.

Three systematic reviews and meta-analyses pooling results from case-controlled series and RCTs have compared percutaneous reduction with K-wire versus ORIF.[76-78] There is a general consensus on reduction of wound complication rate with percutaneous techniques, while pooled results in regard to functional outcomes are contradicting.

One meta-analysis compared MIA, percutaneous reduction, and screw osteosynthesis with external fixation.[79] MIA and percutaneous techniques were significantly better than external fixation in regard to outcomes (AOFAS) and improvement in the Böhler's angle. When comparing MIA and percutaneous techniques, there seems to be no difference in outcomes, infection, or restoration of the Böhler's angle, although not specifically mentioned.

EVIDENCE FOR BONE GRAFTS AND SUBSTITUTES

Given the paucity of evidence and the use of bone grafts and substitutes in the operative management of DIACFs, their use has historically been a matter of surgeon's preference. Proponents reason that bone graft provides mechanical strength to prevent collapse and maintain reduction,[80,81] whereas opponents argue that the calcaneal fractures can heal fairly quickly without bone graft supplementation owing to its strong vascular supply.[81] In an attempt to transition this clinical decision into one that is evidence-based, two notable studies have directly investigated the outcomes associated with bone graft and bone graft substitute in the operative management of these fractures.

In a 2001 cohort study conducted by Longino and Buckley,[81] 20 patients treated with ORIF plus bone graft were matched to 20 patients treated with only ORIF. The majority of fractures were Sanders types II and III classifications. The results of the study showed no significant differences between the groups with respect to anatomic reduction as measured by postoperative CT, the improvement in Böhler's angle immediately postoperatively, or the decrease in Böhler's angle measured at 3 months postoperatively. There were also no significant differences found between the groups for functional outcomes, as measured by the SF-36

and a VAS assessing patients' perceptions of outcomes. It was concluded, "the efficacy of bone graft supplementation in the operative treatment of DIACFs (displaced intra-articular calcaneal fractures) is of no value and demands further study".[81]

In a more recently published RCT led by Johal et al.,[82] the efficacy of bioresorbable calcium phosphate paste was evaluated for its ability to maintain postoperative reduction of DIACFs. This trial was composed of 52 cases, with 24 fractures randomized to treatment with ORIF plus bone substitute material (α-BSM) and 28 randomized to ORIF alone. Fractures treated with ORIF plus α-BSM had significantly less collapse of Böhler's angle compared to treatment with ORIF alone, at both 6 months (5.6 vs. 9.1, $p = 0.03$) and after 1 year postoperatively (6.2 vs. 10.4, $p = 0.05$). However, there was no significant difference between the groups in regard to secondary outcome measures, including general health (SF-36) at 1 year, limb-specific function (lower extremity measure) at 1 year, and pain (oral analog scale) at 2 years. Given the significant radiographic findings, the authors endorsed the use of bioresorbable calcium phosphate paste to fill the bone void during the operative management of these fractures.[82]

In a recent RCT of 57 cases published in 2018, Cao et al.[83] did not find any added clinical or radiological benefits from adding bone graft during ORIF for Sanders type III. The only difference between the two groups was the increased occurrence of postoperative pain in the group who had undergone bone grafting. Therefore, they recommend against the use of bone grafts.

A meta-analysis combining the results from three retrospective studies[84-86] and six RCTs[57,81-83,87,88] could not find a significant difference in restoration of Böhler's angle, restoration of the angle of Gissane, and calcaneal height between groups with or without bone graft, despite low heterogeneity.[89] Application of local bone graft was not associated with a significant increase of local complication rates, wound edge necrosis, or wound infection. However, pooled results from three studies reporting AOFAS scores[83,84,88] showed a significantly higher score in the bone graft group at the last follow-up.[89] More RCTs are needed to elucidate the necessity of bone grafts in setting of acute calcaneal fractures.

EVIDENCE FOR COMPLICATIONS

Irrespective of operative or nonoperative initial management, DIACFs are prone to post-traumatic subtalar arthritis.[19] Although the optimal management of this complication with subtalar arthrodesis appears to be well accepted, there remains an interest in understanding which factors influence the risk of requiring arthrodesis as well as the expected outcomes of arthrodesis. It is known that the surgeon can expect a high union rate of 96% following any arthrodesis procedures, however, accompanied by a higher complication rate of up to 38%.[90-92]

In a retrospective cohort study, 44 patients with DIACFs (originally from the randomized trial by Buckley et al.[14]) were assessed as a cohort after requiring subtalar arthrodesis for unrelenting pain. Of these 44 patients, seven were initially managed with ORIF and the remaining 37 nonoperatively. All underwent a subtalar distraction autograft bone-block-screw arthrodesis with a tricortical bone graft. They were compared to the remaining patients in the Buckley trial[14] not requiring arthrodesis for analysis of factors predicting fusion. The analysis found that a Böhler's angle <0°, Sanders type IV classification, nonoperative initial treatment, and Workers' Compensation Board patients were all significantly more likely to require subtalar arthrodesis. Given the functional improvements associated with fusion, the authors concluded that late subtalar arthrodesis was able to adequately salvage a poor initial outcome.[19] The same group conducted an RCT comparing functional outcomes for Sanders IV treated by either standard ELA with ORIF or standard ELA with ORIF plus primary subtalar arthrodesis (PSTA).[93] They were unable to demonstrate a significant difference between treating Sanders type IV fractures with either ORIF or ORIF + PSTA. However, they suggest that a PSTA may reduce health care costs on a long-term basis as well as reduce lost time from work by preventing the need for late secondary subtalar fusion. In a systematic review by Schepers, it was demonstrated that PSTA provides overall with good outcomes; return to work was reported in ranges of 75–100% and wound complication rates around 19%. However, more high-quality evidence is required to make definitive recommendations.[91]

In a recently published retrospective cohort study, the outcomes of late subtalar arthrodesis were compared in patients who were initially managed with ORIF (36 fractures) for DIACFs to those managed initially nonoperatively (39 fractures). The indications for arthrodesis included pain, poor function, and radiological evidence of post-traumatic arthritis. At a minimum follow-up of 4 years, the group treated initially with ORIF displayed significantly better outcomes as measured by the Maryland Foot Score and the AOFAS ankle-hindfoot score. The results of this study suggest that, when indicated, ORIF should be the preferred method of management as it provides for better long-term functional results with subsequent arthrodesis.[94] This was corroborated with a recent review pooling results from most recent RCTs, which found a significant risk 4.4 times higher in the nonsurgical group as compared to the surgical group for subsequent subtalar arthrodesis.[95]

The cost-effectiveness and indications of PSTA need to be demonstrated with more studies harboring better and more rigorous methodology, as most of the evidence pertaining to complications management following DIACFs are graded as level IV on the EBM scale.

■ INSTITUTIONAL FACTORS

One of the factors influencing patient outcomes often overlooked is the effect of factors outside the control of the individual orthopedic surgeon. Poeze et al.[96] performed a systematic review to determine whether institutional fracture volume had any impact on complications following surgery for calcaneal fracture. They systematically retrieved 236 studies (including case series with no control group), but only included only in their final analysis. Reasons for exclusion reasonably included unreported data on endpoints. They extracted outcome data on rates of deep wound infection and secondary subtalar arthrodesis alongside data on institutional fracture load. Their findings were impressive. Inverse relationships between number of subtalar arthrodesis and institutional fracture load ($r^2 = -0.7$, $p < 0.01$) and deep infection rate and institutional fracture load ($r^2 = -0.5$, $p < 0.05$) were detected. As an added strength to their study, the authors performed a methodological assessment of all included studies and determined that methodological quality did not confound any of their conclusions. The authors' findings are consistent with other evidence that has posited case volume is related to patient outcomes and that high-volume centers typically have better outcomes than lower-volume centers.[97,98]

■ RECOMMENDATIONS FOR FUTURE RESEARCH

In evaluating the evidence in the management of calcaneal fractures, we have found that the available evidence remains far from definitive. Despite the availability of a large RCT, the controversy between operative and nonoperative intervention remains ongoing. Although the single large trial found no difference with nonoperative management, subsequent analyses and other related publications have pushed the pendulum toward the surgical option, especially for select subgroups of patients.

The solution to this question ultimately requires more high-quality, high-level research. Ideally, more RCTs will be needed. Such trials have the ability to generate sufficient power to detect clinically important differences. Furthermore, employing larger and more diverse patient populations allows more representation of diversity, thereby improving the external validity (i.e., generalizability) of the findings. Fortunately, a couple of such trials are currently underway **(Table 2)**.

Secondly, although much of the attention has been directed toward operative versus nonoperative management of calcaneal fractures, more high-level research is needed toward determining exactly which operative exposures, techniques, instrumentations, and other parameters are ideal. In other words, research is needed to determine how to optimize the surgical treatment of calcaneal fractures.

Finally, all researchers must continue to bear in mind the goal of any research endeavor: To produce evidence that will positively impact patient care. The best and most valid evidence is ultimately produced by a systematic review of high-quality RCTs. Ideally, this also demands the integration of data from various trials by means of a meta-analysis. To that end, researchers need to come to a consensus as to the most important outcome measures. There has already been a move in that direction with recent research focusing on patient-important functional outcomes, such as the AOFAS ankle-hindfoot scale. We suggest a continuation of this trend and employment of at least one common fracture-specific outcome tool in future studies. Furthermore, the added value of pedobarography has been called into question; we suggest refraining from spending more resources on gait analysis and focus other measures of clinical outcomes until sufficient evidence supports a relation between pedobarography and functional outcomes.[99] Consistent reporting of these outcomes will enable data synthesis, thereby allowing the research community to come to clinically meaningful conclusions that will ultimately improve patient care.

■ REFERENCES

1. Atkins RM, Allen PE, Livingstone JA. Demographic features of intra-articular fractures of the calcaneum. Foot Ankle Surg. 2001;7(2):77-84.
2. Schepers T, Ginai AZ, Van Lieshout EMM, Patka P. Demographics of extra-articular calcaneal fractures: including a review of the literature on treatment and outcome. Arch Orthop Trauma Surg. 2008;128(10):1099-106.
3. Cotton FJ, Henderson FF. Results of fracture of the os calcis. J Bone Joint Surg. 1916;2(5):290-8.
4. Bruce J, Sutherland A. Surgical versus conservative interventions for displaced intra-articular calcaneal fractures. Cochrane Database Syst Rev. 2013;(1):CD008628.
5. Wei N, Yuwen P, Liu W, Zhu Y, Chang W, Feng C, et al. Operative versus nonoperative treatment of displaced intra-articular calcaneal fractures: a meta-analysis of current evidence base. Medicine (Baltimore). 2017;96(49):e9027.
6. Monaco SJ, Calderone M, Fleming JJ. Paradigm shift for the surgical management of calcaneal fractures? Clin Podiatr Med Surg. 2018;35(2):175-82.
7. Luo X, Li Q, He S. Operative versus nonoperative treatment for displaced intra-articular calcaneal fractures: a meta-analysis of randomized controlled trials. J Foot Ankle Surg. 2016;55(4):821-8.
8. Guyatt GH, Busse JW. The philosophy of evidence-based medicine. Evidence-based Endocrinology. Berlin: Springer; 2006. pp. 25-33.
9. OCEBM Levels of Evidence Working Group. The 2011 Oxford CEBM Levels of Evidence. Oxford: Oxford Centre for Evidence-Based Medicine; 2011.
10. Basile A. Operative versus nonoperative treatment of displaced intra-articular calcaneal fractures in elderly patients. J Foot Ankle Surg. 2010;49(1):25-32.
11. Petit CJ, Lee BM, Kasser JR, Kocher MS. Operative treatment of intraarticular calcaneal fractures in the pediatric population. J Pediatr Orthop. 2007;27(8):856-62.
12. Ceccarelli F, Faldini C, Piras F, Giannini S. Surgical versus non-surgical treatment of calcaneal fractures in children: a long-term results comparative study. Foot Ankle Int. 2000;21(10):825-32.
13. De Boer AS, Van Lieshout EMM, Den Hartog D, Weerts B, Verhofstad MHJ, Schepers T. Functional outcome and patient satisfaction after displaced intra-articular calcaneal fractures: a comparison among open, percutaneous, and nonoperative treatment. J Foot Ankle Surg. 2015;54(3):298-305.
14. Buckley R, Tough S, McCormack R, Pate G, Leighton R, Petrie D, et al. Operative compared with nonoperative treatment of displaced intra-articular calcaneal fractures: a prospective, randomized, controlled multicenter trial. J Bone Joint Surg Am. 2002;84(10):1733-44.
15. Hildebrand KA, Buckley RE, Mohtadi NG, Faris P. Functional outcome measures after displaced intra-articular calcaneal fractures. J Bone Joint Surg Br. 1996;78(1):119-23.
16. Howard JL, Buckley R, McCormack R, Pate G, Leighton R, Petrie D, et al. Complications following management of displaced intra-articular calcaneal fractures: a prospective randomized trial comparing open reduction internal fixation with nonoperative management. J Orthop Trauma. 2003;17(4):241-9.
17. O'Brien J, Buckley R, McCormack R, Pate G, Leighton R, Petrie D, et al. Personal gait satisfaction after displaced intraarticular calcaneal fractures: a 2-8 year followup. Foot Ankle Int. 2004;25(9):657-65.
18. Dooley P, Buckley R, Tough S, McCormack B, Pate G, Leighton R, et al. Bilateral calcaneal fractures: operative versus nonoperative treatment. Foot Ankle Int. 2004;25(2):47-52.
19. Csizy M, Buckley R, Tough S, Leighton R, Smith J, McCormack R, et al. Displaced intra-articular calcaneal fractures: variables predicting late subtalar fusion. J Orthop Trauma. 2003;17(2):106-12.
20. Barla J, Buckley R, McCormack R, Pate G, Leighton R, Petrie D, et al. Displaced intraarticular calcaneal fractures: long-term outcome in women. Foot Ankle Int. 2004;25(12):853-6.
21. Griffin D, Parsons N, Shaw E, Kulikov Y, Hutchinson C, Thorogood M, et al. Operative versus non-operative treatment for closed, displaced, intra-articular fractures of the calcaneus: randomised controlled trial. BMJ. 2014;349:g4483.

22. Agren PH, Wretenberg P, Sayed-Noor AS. Operative versus nonoperative treatment of displaced intra-articular calcaneal fractures: a prospective, randomized, controlled multicenter trial. J Bone Joint Surg Am. 2013;95(15):1351-7.

23. Buckley R. Operative care did not benefit closed, displaced, intra-articular calcaneal fractures. J Bone Joint Surg Am. 2015;97(4):341.

24. Brauer CA, Manns BJ, Ko M, Donaldson C, Buckley R. An economic evaluation of operative compared with nonoperative management of displaced intra-articular calcaneal fractures. J Bone Joint Surg Am. 2005;87(12):2741-9.

25. Albin SR, Bellows BK, Van Boerum DH, Hunter S, Koppenhaver SL, Nelson RE, et al. Cost-effectiveness of operative versus nonoperative management of patients with intra-articular calcaneal fractures. J Orthop Trauma. 2020;34:382-8.

26. Ibrahim T, Rowsell M, Rennie W, Brown AR, Taylor GJ, Gregg PJ. Displaced intra-articular calcaneal fractures: 15-year follow-up of a randomised controlled trial of conservative versus operative treatment. Injury. 2007;38(7):848-55.

27. Parmar HV, Triffitt PD, Gregg PJ. Intra-articular fractures of the calcaneum treated operatively or conservatively. A prospective study. J Bone Joint Surg Br. 1993;75(6):932-7.

28. Sharma V, Dogra A. Sanders type II calcaneum fractures—surgical or conservative treatment? A prospective randomized trial. J Clin Orthop Trauma. 2011;2(1):35-8.

29. Thordarson DB, Krieger LE. Operative vs. nonoperative treatment of intra-articular fractures of the calcaneus: a prospective randomized trial. Foot Ankle Int. 1996;17(1):2-9.

30. Dhillon MS, Prabhakar S. Treatment of displaced intra-articular calcaneus fractures: a current concepts review. SICOT J. 2017;3:59.

31. Nouraei MH, Moosa FM. Operative compared to non-operative treatment of displaced intra-articular calcaneal fractures. J Res Med Sci. 2011;16(8):1014-9.

32. Bahari Kashani M, Kachooei AR, Ebrahimi H, Peivandi MT, Amelfarzad S, Bekhradianpoor N, et al. Comparative study of peroneal tenosynovitis as the complication of intraarticular calcaneal fracture in surgically and non-surgically treated patients. Iran Red Crescent Med J. 2013;15(10):e11378.

33. Zhang W, Lin F, Chen E, Xue D, Pan Z. Operative versus nonoperative treatment of displaced intra-articular calcaneal fractures: a meta-analysis of randomized controlled trials. J Orthop Trauma. 2016;30(3):e75-81.

34. Meena S, Gangary SK, Sharma P. Review article: operative versus nonoperative treatment for displaced intraarticular calcaneal fracture: a meta-analysis of randomised controlled trials. J Orthop Surg (Hong Kong). 2016;24(3):411-6.

35. Schepers T. Calcaneal fractures: looking beyond the meta-analyses. J Foot Ankle Surg. 2016;55(4):897-8.

36. Gaskill T, Schweitzer K, Nunley J. Comparison of surgical outcomes of intra-articular calcaneal fractures by age. J Bone Joint Surg Am. 2010;92(18):2884-9.

37. Scranton Jr PE. Commentary on an article by Trevor Gaskill, MD, et al.: "Comparison of surgical outcomes of intra-articular calcaneal fractures by age". J Bone Joint Surg Am. 2010;92(18):e40.

38. Open reduction internal fixation of calcaneus fractures with and without bone graft (calcaneus). [online] Available from https://ClinicalTrials.gov/show/NCT00582686. [Last accessed March, 2023].

39. External fixation versus splinting of acute calcaneus fractures. [online] Available from https://ClinicalTrials.gov/show/NCT04063657. [Last accessed March, 2023].

40. Osteosynthesis of intraarticular calcaneal fractures: arthroscopically assisted percutaneous technique versus sinus tarsi approach. [online] Available from https://ClinicalTrials.gov/show/NCT04372251. [Last accessed March, 2023].

41. Sinus tarsi versus extensile lateral approach for calcaneus fractures. [online] Available from https://ClinicalTrials.gov/show/NCT02446470. [Last accessed March, 2023].

42. Weber M, Lehmann O, Sägesser D, Krause F. Limited open reduction and internal fixation of displaced intra-articular fractures of the calcaneum. J Bone Joint Surg Br. 2008;90(12):1608-16.

43. Grala P, Twardosz W, Tondel W, Olewicz-Gawlik A, Hrycaj P. Large bone distractor for open reconstruction of articular fractures of the calcaneus. Int Orthop. 2009;33(5):1283-8.

44. Besch L, Waldschmidt JS, Daniels-Wredenhagen M, Varoga D, Mueller M, Hilgert RE, et al. The treatment of intra-articular calcaneus fractures with severe soft tissue damage with a hinged external fixator or internal stabilization: long-term results. J Foot Ankle Surg. 2010;49(1):8-15.

45. Sharr PJ, Mangupli MM, Winson IG, Buckley RE. Current management options for displaced intra-articular calcaneal fractures: non-operative, ORIF, minimally invasive reduction and fixation or primary ORIF and subtalar arthrodesis. A contemporary review. Foot Ankle Surg. 2016;22(1):1-8.

46. Cottom JM, Douthett SM, McConnell KK. Intraoperative reduction techniques for surgical management of displaced intra-articular calcaneal fractures. Clin Podiatr Med Surg. 2019;36(2):269-77.

47. Weinraub GM, David MS. Sinus tarsi approach with subcutaneously delivered plate fixation for displaced intra-articular calcaneal fractures. Clin Podiatr Med Surg. 2019;36(2):225-31.

48. Kiewiet NJ, Sangeorzan BJ. Calcaneal fracture management: extensile lateral approach versus small incision technique. Foot Ankle Clin. 2017;22(1):77-91.

49. Giannini S, Cadossi M, Mosca M, Tedesco G, Sambri A, Terrando S, et al. Minimally-invasive treatment of calcaneal fractures: a review of the literature and our experience. Injury. 2016;47(Suppl. 4):S138-46.

50. Sampath Kumar V, Marimuthu K, Subramani S, Sharma V, Bera J, Kotwal P. Prospective randomized trial comparing open reduction and internal fixation with minimally invasive reduction and percutaneous fixation in managing displaced intra-articular calcaneal fractures. Int Orthop. 2014;38(12):2505-12.

51. Khurana A, Dhillon MS, Prabhakar S, John R. Outcome evaluation of minimally invasive surgery versus extensile lateral approach in management of displaced intra-articular calcaneal fractures: a randomised control trial. Foot (Edinb). 2017;31:23-30.

52. Shi Z, Zou J, Wenqi GU, Jiang Y. The clinical outcomes comparison of limited open reduction via a sinus tarsi approach and open reduction internal fixation via a lateral extensile L-shape incision for the treatment of Sanders type II calcaneal fracture. Chinese J Orthop. 2013;(12):298-303.

53. Basile A, Albo F, Via AG. Comparison between sinus tarsi approach and extensile lateral approach for treatment of closed displaced intra-articular calcaneal fractures: a multicenter prospective study. J Foot Ankle Surg. 2016;55(3):513-21.

54. Xia S, Lu Y, Wang H, Wu Z, Wang Z. Open reduction and internal fixation with conventional plate via L-shaped lateral approach versus internal fixation with percutaneous plate via a sinus tarsi approach for calcaneal fractures—a randomized controlled trial. Int J Surg. 2014;12(5):475-80.

55. Li LH, Guo YZ, Wang H, Sang QH, Zhang JZ, Liu Z, et al. Less wound complications of a sinus tarsi approach compared to an extended lateral approach for the treatment of displaced intraarticular calcaneal fracture: a randomized clinical trial in 64 patients. Medicine (Baltimore). 2016;95(36):e4628.

56. Jin C, Weng D, Yang W, He W, Liang W, Qian Y. Minimally invasive percutaneous osteosynthesis versus ORIF for Sanders type II and III calcaneal fractures: a prospective, randomized intervention trial. J Orthop Surg Res. 2017;12(1):10.

57. Chen L, Zhang G, Hong J, Lu X, Yuan W. Comparison of percutaneous screw fixation and calcium sulfate cement grafting versus open treatment of displaced intra-articular calcaneal fractures. Foot Ankle Int. 2011;32(10):979-85.

58. Zhan J, Zhu N, Fang W, Jing J. A comparative study of open reduction with internal fixation and percutaneous poking reduction fixation for the treatment of Sanders type II calcaneal fractures. Int J Clin Exp Med. 2016;9(6):11997-2003.

59. Moon JS, Lee WC. A comparison of extensile lateral approach and sinus tarsi approach for the Sanders type II calcaneal fracture. J Korean Fract Soc. 2009;22(1):13-8.

60. Schepers T, Backes M, Dingemans SA, de Jong VM, Luitse JSK. Similar anatomical reduction and lower complication rates with the sinus tarsi approach compared with the extended lateral approach in displaced intra-articular calcaneal fractures. J Orthop Trauma. 2017;31(6):293-8.

61. Takasaka M, Bittar CK, Mennucci FS, de Mattos CA, Zabeu JLA. Comparative study on three surgical techniques for intra-articular calcaneal fractures: open reduction with internal fixation using a plate, external fixation and minimally invasive surgery. Rev Bras Ortop. 2016;51(3):254-60.

62. Zhou HC, Yu T, Ren HY, Li B, Chen K, Zhao YG, et al. Clinical comparison of extensile lateral approach and sinus tarsi approach combined with medial distraction technique for intra-articular calcaneal fractures. Orthop Surg. 2017;9(1):77-85.

63. Rammelt S, Amlang M, Barthel S, Zwipp H. Minimally-invasive treatment of calcaneal fractures. Injury. 2004;35(Suppl. 2):SB55-63.

64. Wu Z, Su Y, Chen W, Zhang Q, Liu Y, Li M, et al. Functional outcome of displaced intra-articular calcaneal fractures: a comparison between open reduction/internal fixation and a minimally invasive approach featured an anatomical plate and compression bolts. J Trauma Acute Care Surg. 2012;73(3):743-51.

65. Yeap EJ, Rao J, Pan CH, Soelar SA, Younger ASE. Is arthroscopic assisted percutaneous screw fixation as good as open reduction and internal fixation for the treatment of displaced intra-articular calcaneal fractures? Foot Ankle Surg. 2016;22(3)164-9.

66. Yeo JH, Cho HJ, Lee KB. Comparison of two surgical approaches for displaced intra-articular calcaneal fractures: sinus tarsi versus extensile lateral approach. BMC Musculoskelet Disord. 2015;16:63.

67. Kline AJ, Anderson RB, Davis WH, Jones CP, Cohen BE. Minimally invasive technique versus an extensile lateral approach for intra-articular calcaneal fractures. Foot Ankle Int. 2013;34(6):773-80.

68. Seat A, Seat C. Lateral extensile approach versus minimal incision approach for open reduction and internal fixation of displaced intra-articular calcaneal fractures: a meta-analysis. J Foot Ankle Surg. 2020;59(2):356-66.

69. Mehta CR, An VVG, Phan K, Sivakumar B, Kanawati AJ, Suthersan M. Extensile lateral versus sinus tarsi approach for displaced, intra-articular calcaneal fractures: a meta-analysis. J Orthop Surg Res. 2018;13(1):243.

70. Bai L, Hou YL, Lin GH, Zhang X, Liu GQ, Yu B. Sinus tarsi approach (STA) versus extensile lateral approach (ELA) for treatment of closed displaced intra-articular calcaneal fractures (DIACF): a meta-analysis. Orthop Traumatol Surg Res. 2018;104(2):239-44.

71. Majeed H, Barrie J, Munro W, McBride D. Minimally invasive reduction and percutaneous fixation versus open reduction and internal fixation for displaced intra-articular calcaneal fractures: a systematic review of the literature. EFORT Open Rev. 2018;3(7):418-25.

72. Zeng Z, Yuan L, Zheng S, Sun Y, Huang F. Minimally invasive versus extensile lateral approach for Sanders type II and III calcaneal fractures: a meta-analysis of randomized controlled trials. Int J Surg. 2018;50:146-53.

73. Nosewicz TL, Dingemans SA, Backes M, Luitse JSK, Goslings JC, Schepers T. A systematic review and meta-analysis of the sinus tarsi and extended lateral approach in the operative treatment of displaced intra-articular calcaneal fractures. Foot Ankle Surg. 2019;25(5):580-8.

74. Zhang F, Tian H, Li S, Liu B, Dong T, Zhu Y, et al. Meta-analysis of two surgical approaches for calcaneal fractures: sinus tarsi versus extensile lateral approach. ANZ J Surg. 2017;87(3):126-31.

75. Clement RC, Lang PJ, Pettett BJ, Overman RA, Ostrum RF, Tennant JN. Sanders II/III calcaneus fractures in laborers: a cost-effectiveness analysis and call for effectiveness research. J Orthop Trauma. 2017;31(6):299-304.

76. Wu J, Zhou F, Yang L, Tan J. Percutaneous reduction and fixation with Kirschner wires versus open reduction internal fixation for the management of calcaneal fractures: a meta-analysis. Sci Rep. 2016;6:30480.

77. Wang XJ, Su YX, Li L, Zhang ZH, Wei XC, Wei L. Percutaneous poking reduction and fixation versus open reduction and

fixation in the treatment of displaced calcaneal fractures for Chinese patients: a systematic review and meta-analysis. Chin J Traumatol. 2016;19(6):362-7.

78. Fan B, Zhou X, Wei Z, Ren Y, Lin W, Hao Y, et al. Cannulated screw fixation and plate fixation for displaced intra-articular calcaneus fracture: a meta-analysis of randomized controlled trials. Int J Surg. 2016;34:64-72.

79. van Hoeve S, Poeze M. Outcome of minimally invasive open and percutaneous techniques for repair of calcaneal fractures: a systematic review. J Foot Ankle Surg. 2016;55(6):1256-63.

80. Leung KS, Chan WS, Shen WY, Pak PP, So WS, Leung PC. Operative treatment of intraarticular fractures of the os calcis—the role of rigid internal fixation and primary bone grafting: preliminary results. J Orthop Trauma. 1989;3(3): 232-40.

81. Longino D, Buckley RE. Bone graft in the operative treatment of displaced intraarticular calcaneal fractures: is it helpful? J Orthop Trauma. 2001;15(4):280-6.

82. Johal HS, Buckley RE, Le ILD, Leighton RK. A prospective randomized controlled trial of a bioresorbable calcium phosphate paste (alpha-BSM) in treatment of displaced intra-articular calcaneal fractures. J Trauma. 2009;67(4):875-82.

83. Cao H, Li YG, An Q, Gou B, Qian W, Guo XP, et al. Short-term outcomes of open reduction and internal fixation for Sanders type III calcaneal fractures with and without bone grafts. J Foot Ankle Surg. 2018;57(1):7-14.

84. Duymus TM, Mutlu S, Mutlu H, Ozel O, Guler O, Mahirogullari M. Need for bone grafts in the surgical treatment of displaced intra-articular calcaneal fractures. J Foot Ankle Surg. 2017;56(1):54-8.

85. Singh AK, Vinay K. Surgical treatment of displaced intra-articular calcaneal fractures: is bone grafting necessary? J Orthop Traumatol. 2013;14(4):299-305.

86. Gusic N, Fedel I, Darabos N, Lovric Z, Bukvic N, Bakota B, et al. Operative treatment of intraarticular calcaneal fractures: anatomical and functional outcome of three different operative techniques. Injury. 2015;46(Suppl. 6):S130-3.

87. Kennedy JG, Jan WM, McGuinness AJ, Barry K, Curtin J, Cashman WF, et al. An outcomes assessment of intra-articular calcaneal fractures, using patient and physician's assessment profiles. Injury. 2003;34(12):932-6.

88. Feng Y, Shui X, Wang J, Cai L, Yu Y, Ying X, et al. Comparison of percutaneous cannulated screw fixation and calcium sulfate cement grafting versus minimally invasive sinus tarsi approach and plate fixation for displaced intra-articular calcaneal fractures: a prospective randomized controlled trial. BMC Musculoskelet Disord. 2016;17:288.

89. Zheng W, Xie L, Xie H, Chen C, Chen H, Cai L. With versus without bone grafts for operative treatment of displaced intra-articular calcaneal fractures: a meta-analysis. Int J Surg. 2018;59:36-47.

90. Thompson MJ, Roukis TS. Management of calcaneal fracture malunion with bone block distraction arthrodesis: a systematic review and meta-analysis. Clin Podiatr Med Surg. 2019;36(2):307-21.

91. Schepers T. The primary arthrodesis for severely comminuted intra-articular fractures of the calcaneus: a systematic review. Foot Ankle Surg. 2012;18(2):84-8.

92. Schepers T. The subtalar distraction bone block arthrodesis following the late complications of calcaneal fractures: a systematic review. Foot (Edinb). 2013;23(1):39-44.

93. Buckley R, Leighton R, Sanders D, Poon J, Coles CP, Stephen D, et al. Open reduction and internal fixation compared with ORIF and primary subtalar arthrodesis for treatment of Sanders type IV calcaneal fractures: a randomized multicenter trial. J Orthop Trauma. 2014;28(10):577-83.

94. Radnay CS, Clare MP, Sanders RW. Subtalar fusion after displaced intra-articular calcaneal fractures: does initial operative treatment matter? J Bone Joint Surg Am. 2009;91(3):541-6.

95. Liu Y, Li Z, Li H, Zhang Y, Wang P. Protective effect of surgery against early subtalar arthrodesis in displaced intra-articular calcaneal fractures: a meta-analysis. Medicine (Baltimore). 2015;94(45):e1984-0.

96. Poeze M, Verbruggen JPAM, Brink PRG. The relationship between the outcome of operatively treated calcaneal fractures and institutional fracture load. A systematic review of the literature. J Bone Joint Surg Am. 2008;90(5):1013-21.

97. Shervin N, Rubash HE, Katz JN. Orthopaedic procedure volume and patient outcomes: a systematic literature review. Clin Orthop Relat Res. 2007;457:35-41.

98. Ahn J, Kim TY, Kim TW, Jeong BO. Learning curve for open reduction and internal fixation of displaced intra-articular calcaneal fracture by extensile lateral approach using the cumulative summation control chart. Foot Ankle Int. 2019;40(9):1052-9.

99. Sanders FRK, Peters JJ, Schallig W, Mittlmeier T, Schepers T. What is the added value of pedobarography for assessing functional outcome of displaced intra-articular calcaneal fractures? A systematic review of existing literature. Clin Biomech (Bristol, Avon). 2020;72:8-15.

<h1 style="text-align:right">Index</h1>

Page numbers followed by *f* refer to figure, *fc* refer to flowchart and *t* refer to table.